SPORTS MEDICINE FOR THE MATURE ATHLETE

Edited by
John R. Sutton, M.D.
Professor, Department of Medicine
McMaster University
Hamilton, Ontario, Canada

Robert M. Brock, M.D.
Orthopaedic Surgeon
North York Hospital
Toronto, Canada

Benchmark Press, Inc.
Indianapolis

Copyright © 1986, by Benchmark Press, Inc.

ALL RIGHTS RESERVED.

Reproduction or translation of any part of this work beyond that permitted by Sections 107 and 108 of the 1976 United States Copyright Act without the permission of the copyright owner is unlawful. Requests for permission should be addressed to Publisher, Benchmark Press, Inc., 8435 Keystone Crossing, Suite 175, Indianapolis, Indiana 46240.

Library of Congress Cataloging in Publication Data:

1. SUTTON, JOHN R. 1941–
SPORTS MEDICINE FOR THE MATURE ATHLETE

Cover Design: Gary Schmitt
Art: Craig Gosling
Typesetting and Production: Edwards Brothers

Library of Congress Catalog Card number: 86-70747
ISBN: 0-936157-04-6

Printed in the United States
10 9 8 7 6 5 4 3 2

About the Editors

Robert M. Brock, M.D., is a consultant orthopaedic surgeon and director of the Sports Medicine Clinic at North York Hospital in Toronto. He is a Fellow of the Royal College of Physicians and Surgeons of Canada, a Fellow of the American College of Surgeons, a member of the Canadian Academy of Sports Medicine, and an executive member of the Sports Medicine Section of the Ontario Medical Association. In the latter capacity, he has been chairman of the annual "Sport Med" conferences for 1984, 1985, and 1986. Dr. Brock is a consultant to the Canadian Figure Skating Association and has accompanied members on tour to Europe and Japan. He was a physician with the Canadian team at the 1984 Los Angeles Olympics.

John R. Sutton, M.D., is a Professor of Medicine and consultant to the Intensive and Coronary Care Units of McMaster University. He was co-founder of the Sydney Human Performance Laboratory in Australia and the McMaster University Cardiac Rehabilitation Programme and Exercise Laboratory. He is a Fellow of the Royal Australasian College of Physicians, the Royal College of Physicians and Surgeons of Canada, and the Royal Geographic Society; and a member of the Canadian Academy of Sports Medicine, the Canadian Association of Sports Sciences, and the Sports Medicine Section of the Ontario Medical Association. In 1972 he was a member of the International Biological Programme for the Munich Olympics; he is currently president of the American College of Sports Medicine.

Contributors

Per-Olof Astrand
Dept. of Physiology III
Karolinska Institutet
Lidingovagen 1
S-11433 Stockholm, Sweden

James R. Andrews
Hughston Orthopaedic Clinic
6262 Hamilton Road
P.O. Box 9517
Columbus, GA, U.S.A. 31908

Anne C. Balcomb
Tekoona
Toogong, via Cudal, N.S.W.
Australia. 2864

Claude Bouchard
Physical Activity Sciences Laboratory—
 PEPS
Faculte d'education physique
Faculte des Sciences de l'Education
Universite Laval
Quebec, P.Q., Canada. G1K 7P4

Joseph J. Calandra
Hughston Orthopaedic Clinic
6262 Hamilton Road
P.O. Box 9517
Columbus, GA, U.S.A. 31908

Albert V. Carron
Faculty of Physical Education
Thames Hall
University of Western Ontario
London, Ontario, Canada. N6A 3K7

William G. Carson
Division of Orthopaedics
Sports Medicine Section
Tulane University School of Medicine
New Orleans, LA, U.S.A

Geoffrey Coates
Room 1P14
McMaster University Medical Centre
Box 2000, Station A
Hamilton, Ontario, Canada. L8N 3Z5

Stafford W. Dobbin
Suite 504
5400 Portage Road
Niagara Falls, Ontario, Canada.
 L2G 5X7

Deanna L. Dorsey
Nutrition and Metabolism
Dept. of Medicine
Brown University
The Miriam Hospital
164 Summit Ave.
Providence, RI, U.S.A. 02906

Barbara L. Drinkwater
Dept. of Medicine
Pacific Medical Center
1200 12th Ave. S.
Seattle, WA, U.S.A. 98144

Carl V. Gisolfi
Dept. of Physical Education
204 Field House
University of Iowa
Iowa City, IA, U.S.A. 52242

Howard J. Green
Dept. of Kinesiology
University of Waterloo
Waterloo, Ontario, Canada. N2L 3G1

David Hastings
Dept. of Orthopaedic Surgery
Room 418
E. K. Jones Building
The Wellesley Hospital
160 Wellesley St. E.
Toronto, Ontario, Canada. M4Y 1J3

George J. F. Heigenhauser
Room 3U27
McMaster University Medical Centre
Box 2000, Station A
Hamilton, Ontario, Canada. L8N 3Z5

Richard L. Hughson
Dept. of Kinesiology
University of Waterloo
Waterloo, Ontario, Canada. N2L 3G1

Robert W. Jackson
Division of Orthopaedic Surgery
Suite 405
Toronto Western Hospital
25 Leonard Ave.
Toronto, Ontario, Canada. M5T 2R2

Frank W. Jobe
Suite 200
Kerlan-Jobe Orthopedic Clinic
501 East Hardy St.
Englewood, California 90301

Norman L. Jones
Room 3U1,
McMaster University Medical Centre
Box 2000, Station A
Hamilton, Ontario, Canada. L8N 3Z5

M. J. Kenney
Dept. of Physical Education
204 Field House
University of Iowa
Iowa City, IA, U.S.A. 52242

Gilbert Lang
Roosevelt Community Hospital
Boston, MA, U.S.A.

Larry M. Leith
School of Physical Education and
   Outdoor Recreation
Lakehead University
Thunder Bay, Ontario, Canada.
   P7B 5E1

Lydia Makrides
School of Physiotherapy
Forrest Building
5869 University Ave.
Halifax, N.S., Canada. B3J 3J5

Neil McCartney
Dept. of Physical Education
McMaster University
Hamilton, Ontario, Canada. L8S 4K1

Robert S. McKelvie
Room 3U9
McMaster University Medical Centre
Box 2000, Station A
Hamilton, Ontario, Canada. L8N 3Z5

R. S. McLean
British Columbia Sport Medicine Clinic
University of British Columbia
3055 Wesbrook Mall
Vancouver, B.C., Canada. V6T 1W5

Thomas Pashby
Suite 215
1 Medical Place
20 Wynford Dr.
Don Mills, Ontario, Canada. M3C 1J4

Dirk Pette
Fakultat fur Biologie
Universitat Konstanz
Postfach 5560
D-7750 Konstanz 1
West Germany

David A. B. Richards
c/o Suite 310
84 Pacific Highway
North Sydney, N.S.W., Australia. 2060

C. Rowland B. Richards
Suite 310
84 Pacific Highway
North Sydney, N.S.W., Australia. 2060

James H. Roth
Orthopaedic Associates
Suite 312, Victoria Building
111 Waterloo St.
London, Ontario, Canada. N6B 2M6

Rick K. St. Pierre
Hughston Orthopaedic Clinic
6262 Hamilton Road
P.O. Box 9517
Columbus, GA, U.S.A. 31908

Digby G. Sale
Dept. of Physical Education
McMaster University
Hamilton, Ontario, Canada. L8S 4K1

Bengt Saltin
August Krogh Institute
University of Copenhagen
13 Universitetsparken
DK-2100 Copenhagen O, Denmark

Robert B. Schoene
Pulmonary Function and Exercise
   Laboratory
Harborview Medical Center
325 Ninth Ave.
Seattle, WA, U.S.A. 98104

Arthur J. Siegel
Medical Director
Hahnemann Hospital
1515 Commonwealth Ave.
Brighton, MA, U.S.A. 02135

Maria Stokes
Dept. of Medicine
University of Liverpool
Liverpool, England

John R. Sutton
Room 3U26
McMaster University Medical Centre
Box 2000, Station A
Hamilton, Ontario, Canada. L8N 3Z5

Jack E. Taunton
British Columbia Sport Medicine Clinic
University of British Columbia
3055 Wesbrook Mall
Vancouver, B.C., Canada. V6T 1W5

Paul D. Thompson
Nutrition and Metabolism
Dept. of Medicine
Brown University
The Miriam Hospital
164 Summit Ave.
Providence, RI, U.S.A. 02906

Dan S. Tunstall-Pedoe
Cardiac Department
St. Bartholomew's Hospital
West Smithfield, London, England.
 EC1A 7 BE

Michael J. Warhol
Dept. of Pathology
Brigham and Women's Hospital
Boston, MA, U.S.A. 02115

Colin Webber
Room 1P13
McMaster University Medical Centre
Box 2000, Station A
Hamilton, Ontario, Canada. L8N 3Z5

Howard A. Wenger
Dept. of Health Services
University of Victoria
P.O. Box 1700
Victoria, B.C., Canada. V8W 2Y2

Jack H. Wilmore
Dept. of Physical and Health Education
222 Bellmont Hall
The University of Texas at Austin
Austin, TX, U.S.A. 78712

Archie Young
Dept. of Geriatric Medicine
Royal Free Hospital School of Medicine
New End Hospital
Hampstead, London, England.
 NW3 1JB

Foreword

As our population ages, the health and welfare of senior citizens has become of major medical, social and economic concern. The medical problems of the aged have tended to dominate the thinking of politicians and health planners; however, recently a gradual redirection in emphasis has begun toward the maintenance of the health of this group. An important aspect of the health of the mature population is the role played by physical activity. This was placed in international focus when the inaugural World Masters Games were held in Toronto in the summer of 1985, attracting 10,000 participants from around the world.

As part of the Games celebration, an international Masters Sports Medicine Symposium was also held in Toronto at that time. The symposium attracted participants from all continents and was an outstanding scientific and social success. It focused on the unique physiological and sports medicine aspects of the aging population, addressed by authorities with first-hand clinical and research experience in these areas. In bringing these papers to publication, we wish to make the deliberations of the world-renowned speakers on increasingly important but poorly documented topics available to a much wider audience.

Acknowledgements

The inaugural World Masters Games International Sports Medicine Symposium was sponsored by the Ontario Medical Association, the Masters Games organization, and North American Life Assurance Company. The success of the symposium was due to the outstanding caliber of the faculty and the cooperation of many individuals.

We especially wish to thank Dr. Maureen O'Bryan, President of the Masters Games; Mr. Andrew McCaughey, President and Chief Executive Officer of the North American Life Assurance Co.; Mr. Bruce Stock, Public Relations Officer of the North American Life Assurance Co.; Dr. Andrew Pipe; and Mr. Eugene O'Keefe of the Ontario Medical Association.

We also wish to acknowledge the assistance given by the following individuals

Denise Aziz, North American Life
Gord Brock, North American Life
John Cole, M.D., North American Life
Sandi Davis, Burson-Marsteller
Edward Gould, Burson-Marsteller
Linda Hall, Masters Games
Ken Henry, North American Life
Albert Hummel, North American Life
Pat Indart, Masters Games
Paul Leonard, North American Life
Ron Martin, North American Life
Kerri MacDonald, North American Life
Barry Noble, North American Life
Ken O'Bryan, Masters Games
Vicky Park, North American Life
Nan Percival, Masters Games
Doug Philpott, North American Life
Sheila Robb, Burson-Marsteller
Joyce Rutledge, Masters Games
Paul Statler, North American Life
Teresa Zaroda, Masters Games

In addition to the unstinting support of North American Life, financial support was also provided by the Fitness and Amateur Sport Branch of the Government of Canada, the Ministry of Sport and Tourism of Ontario, and Syntex Limited.

Finally, we wish to express our sincere thanks to Cathy Labbett, who coordinated the symposium, and Janet Burke, who has worked tirelessly to bring this book to publication.

                        Robert M. Brock
                        John R. Sutton
                        Co-Chairmen
                        International Sports Medicine Symposium
                            of the Masters Games

Contents

Contributors iv
Foreward vii
Acknowledgements ix

Section I—Keynote Address

1. Exercise Physiology of the Mature Athlete. *Per-Olof Astrand* — 3

Section II—The Mature Muscle

2. Morphological, Ultrastructural, and Functional Characteristics of the Aging Human Skeletal Muscle. *Howard J. Green* 17
3. Adaptability of Skeletal Muscle to Long-term Use. *Dirk Pette* 27
4. Muscle Injury and Repair in Ultra-long Distance Runners. *Arthur J. Siegel, Michael J. Warhol, Gilbert Lang* 35
5. Non-Invasive Measurement of Muscle in the Rehabilitation of Masters Athletes. *Archie Young, Maria Stokes* — 45

Section III—Testing the Mature Athlete

6. Physiological Characteristics of the Masters Athlete. *Bengt Saltin* 59
7. Heredity and Trainability. *Claude Bouchard* 81
8. Testing the Elite Masters Athlete. *Jack H. Wilmore* 91
9. The Canadian Association of Sports Sciences Guidelines: "Physiological Testing of the Elite Athlete." *Howard A. Wenger* — 109
10. Special Cardiovascular Precautions for the Masters Athlete. *Robert S. McKelvie* 113

Section IV—Environmental Stresses

11. Thermal Problems in the Masters Athlete. *John R. Sutton* 125
12. Thermal Regulation: Effects of Exercise and Age. *Carl V. Gisolfi, M. J. Kenney* 133
13. Heat Stroke in Northern Climates. *Richard L. Hughson* 145
14. Prevention of Exercise-induced Heat Stroke. *C. Rowland Richards, David Richards* 151
15. Providing Medical Care in Fun Runs and Marathons in Australasia. *C. Rowland Richards, David Richards* 167
16. Medical Support for Marathons in the United Kingdom: The London Marathon. *Dan S. Tunstall Pedoe* 181

17. Providing Medical Services for Fun Runs and Marathons in North America. *Stafford W. Dobbin* 193
18. Road Racing Medical Management. *Jack E. Taunton, R. S. McLean* 205
19. Advanced Age and Altitude Illness. *Anne C. Balcomb, John R. Sutton* 213
20. Exercise Performance at High Altitude. *Robert B. Schoene* 225

Section V—Mind and Eye

21. Psychology of the Masters Athlete: Motivational Considerations. *Albert Carron, Larry M. Leith* 233
22. Cognitive Psychology: A Viable Alternative to Overtraining in Masters Runners? *Larry M. Leith* 241
23. Eyeball to Eyeball-Acute Eye Injuries. *Thomas Pashby* 247

Section VI—Knee and Shoulder

24. The Masters Knee: Past, Present and Future. *Robert W. Jackson* 257
25. Instability of the Knee in Mature Athletes. *David Hastings* 265
26. Synthetic Materials Used in Intra-articular Anterior Cruciate Ligament Knee Surgery. *James H. Roth* 271
27. Osteoarthritis, Athletes, and Arthroscopic Management. *James R. Andrews, Rick K. St. Pierre* 279
28. Principles of Resistance Exercise in Rehabilitation Following Knee Injuries. *Digby G. Sale* 287
29. Factors Influencing the Throwing Arm of the Masters Athlete. *Frank W. Jobe* 295
30. Arthroscopy of the Shoulder. *James R. Andrews, William G. Carson, Joseph J. Calandra* 299

Section VII—Heart and Lung

31. The Heart of the Masters Athlete. *Paul D. Thompson, Deanna L. Dorsey* 309
32. The Lung of the Masters Athlete. *Norman L. Jones* 319

Section VIII—Bone

33. Nuclear Medicine Techniques to Detect Exercise-induced Changes in the Skeleton. *Geoffrey Coates, Colin Webber* 331
34. Osteoporosis and the Female Masters Athlete. *Barbara L. Drinkwater* 353

North American Life Research Award Paper

35. Physical Training in Young and Older Healthy Subjects. *Lydia Makrides, George J. F. Heigenhauser, Neil McCartney* 363

Section I
Keynote Address

1

Exercise Physiology of the Mature Athlete

PER-OLOF ASTRAND

Karolinska Institute

IS REGULAR PHYSICAL ACTIVITY PROMOTING GOOD HEALTH?

I am a veteran of meetings devoted to papers and discussions dealing with the effects of physical exercise on human performance, organ function, and health. Sooner or later at such meetings a pertinent question arises: what is the role of habitual physical activity in the primary and secondary prevention of diseases, particularly cardiovascular diseases? A quite typical flux of presentations and thoughts is the following: at one stage almost everyone is very enthusiastic about the many positive effects of training on various functions. Then the epidemiologist comes on stage and presents many data in favor of the beneficial effects of regular exercise, but so far there is no conclusive proof that physical training per se can prevent disease. Then we enter the third phase of the meeting when many harmful effects of exercise are discussed.

The result is often confusion and some sort of a despair in those who at the beginning participated in the love songs devoted to regular exercise. The final recommendation is that anyone, particularly those no longer young and the untrained, should undergo a careful medical examination including a so-called stress test to get some sort of certificate that she or he can join an exercise program without risk. My standard comments have been: (1) if a drive to stimulate people to exercise is successful, there are not enough physicians qualified to execute this particular examination; (2) there is, so far, no medical examination that in a foolproof manner can exclude hazardous effects of vigorous exercise on the cardiovascular organs in a particular individual. Even very advanced examinations give too many both false positive and false negative diagnoses to be absolutely reliable in this connection; (3) from a psychological point of view, an emphasis on the importance of a health examination to evaluate whether or not exercise is recommendable gives a definite impression that exercise is more of a threat to health than a sedentary life style.

Therefore, sometime in the 1960s, I presented the following recommendation, and I quote myself: "The question is frequently raised whether a medical examination is advisable before commencing a training program. Certainly anyone who is doubtful about his state of health should consult a physician. In principle, however, there is less risk in activity than in continuous inactivity. In a nutshell, our opinion is that it is more advisable to pass a careful medical examination if one intends to be sedentary in order to establish whether one's state of health is good enough to stand the inactivity." (2, 1st ed., p. 608).

When asking a physician whether or not there are scientific data proving that physical training is beneficial, it is apparently inevitable that she or he concentrates on the question of whether or not such training is useful in the primary and secondary prevention of disease. As mentioned, the epidemiological studies in this field are inconclusive. For this reason most physicians do not actively recommend exercise and I shall add, provocatively, that too many of them know too little about exercise physiology. If you go through the standard basic textbooks in physiology for medical students, you will find one explanation of this lack of knowledge: very few pages of the text are devoted to a discussion of the acute and chronic effects of exercise on different structures and functions. In many ways this almost total exclusion of exercise physiology in the textbooks is remarkable considering that a physiological analysis of an exercise situation gives a unique opportunity to learn how different functions are coordinated and integrated. In the teaching it is natural that one tear the body into small pieces at one stage, but it is definitely as important to put all the pieces together again. Here the teaching of exercise physiology becomes very useful and natural.

As an exercise physiologist I can list dozens of positive effects of regular exercise, positive today and tomorrow—whether positive one month from now if the training is interrupted I do not know. However, my point is that there is a total, unanimous agreement among all exercise physiologists that regular exercise is essential for optimal function of the human body.

I think that this is a quite common situation: There was in West Germany an international symposium devoted to the epidemiology of cardiovascular diseases. Professor Wildor Hollmann reported that there were hardly any discussions on the role of physical inactivity and activity respectively in such diseases. In contrast, in June 1985 there was another symposium in Sweden dedicated to "Physical Activity in Health and Disease" (sponsored by Acta Medica Scandinavica). Positive effects of habitual physical exercise were well documented, but it was concluded that its role in primary and secondary prevention of cardiovascular diseases is not definitely settled. There are, however, many indications and much evidence that regular exercise is also important from a clinical aspect (as summarized by Drs. W. Haskell, J. Morris, R. Paffenbarger, and I. Vuori at that particular symposium).

One reason for this introduction is that at one stage of a discussion on the effects of training it is important to separate physiological and clinical aspects. Thereby some of the confusion mirrored in the mass media can be avoided. Then, of course, it is essential that the physiologists and clinicians join in the discussions. This symposium serves a very important purpose by its integration of different disciplines in human biology, treated as both basic and applied sciences. For instance, by exposing the cardiologist who does not believe that physical inactivity is a risk factor behind coronary heart disease to papers on exercise physiology in general, it is hoped that she or he will prescribe exercise because of its many positive effects on body structures and functions. When prescribing pills, many physicians do not demand so much scientific proof that the medicine is justified for a particular patient as when it is a question of influencing the patient's life style.

I have been asked to present a paper on "Exercise Physiology of the Mature Athlete." Actually, Bengt Saltin has a similar title on his paper. I will not steal his and his co-workers' excellent data from longitudinal studies on athletes (even though it is tempting). He and other speakers will discuss the effects of chronic exercise on lung function, heart morphology, and function of the skeletal muscle, to mention a few topics. It is inevitable that there will be some overlap in the presentations even if I only, for evident reasons, take up some aspects of this particular physiology. For me the mature athlete is someone of middle age or older who is physically active at least three times per week for a minimum of 30 minutes each time. When the purpose is to train the oxygen transport system, the intensity of the exercise should be approximately 75% of the maximal oxygen uptake or higher. For the psychologist yes, but for the physiologist it is not essential whether or not the person has participated in one or many competitions.

AEROBIC POWER

The highest oxygen uptake a person can attain when exercising large muscle groups at sea level is by definition her or his maximal oxygen uptake or aerobic power. There is at present good support for the hypothesis that the central circulation is the limiting factor for this power. In other words, the potential of the skeletal muscles to consume oxygen in their mitochondria exceeds the capacity of the oxygen transport system to deliver oxygen (2, 3rd ed. Chap. 4; Saltin, B.).

In many laboratories maximal aerobic power has been measured in unselected persons of different ages. A common finding is a peak at 15 to 20 years of age, with women at the lower range. It should be pointed out that: (1) oxygen uptake gives quite accurate information about the aerobic energy output (1 liter O_2 consumed in the tissue yields approximately 20 kJ), and (2) the oxygen uptake is highly correlated to the cardiac output. When related to body weight ($\dot{V}O_2$, ml $\times$ kg^{-1} $\times$ min^{-1}), this peak appears at still lower ages (2, Chap. 7). In most studies there is a gradual decline in maximal oxygen uptake (1 $\times$ min^{-1}) from the age of approximately 20 years onward.

It is well documented that training can improve maximal aerobic power by a few percent up to 100% depending on the individual's initial fitness and the intensity and duration of the training (2, Chap. 9). Therefore, it is not surprising that athletes in endurance disciplines at any age have significantly higher maximal aerobic power than is found in the population in general. In addition to a training effect on this power, the athletes are usually, from a genetic point of view, endowed with a relatively high maximal aerobic power even without training.

It is interesting to note that young athletes tested when they have just qualified for a national team in endurance events have a high maximal aerobic power. In the years which follow they train daily and intensively. There are seasonal fluctuations in this power, but usually the highest value recorded in those years is not significantly different from the one first observed. No doubt there is a definite maximum dependent on the individual's natural endowment. Data obtained in the laboratory and statistics of world records and personal best performances reveal that after the age of 30 to 35 years, there is an inevitable decline in maximal aerobic power (in individuals who were well-trained before).

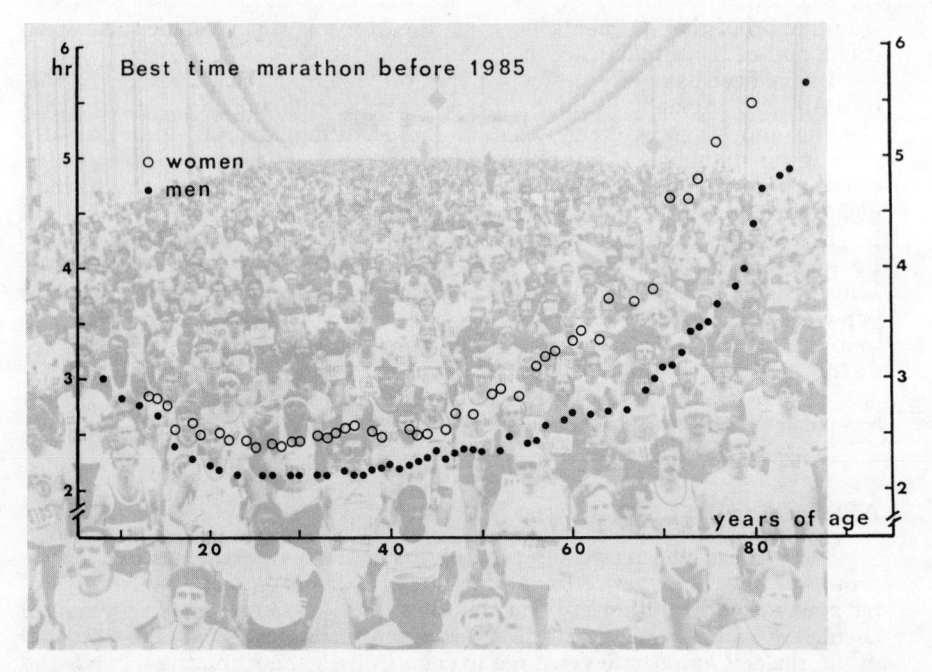

Fig. 1-1. *The best times recorded for marathon runners of different ages. It should be noted that the profile of the courses and weather conditions can be very different in races. One runner, Jack Forster, holds 8 records in the 40-to-50-years-age class and another, Erik Östby, has 4 of the records in the 47-to-60-years-age class. Background: Some of the more than 14,000 entrants pass the Verrazano Bridge at the start of the 10th New York City Marathon race in October, 1983. (United Press International photo.)*

The best times in the marathon distance are noted in the range from 23 up to approximately 35 years of age (Fig. 1-1). A high maximal aerobic power per kilogram (kg) body weight is important, but a somewhat low maximum can be compensated for by good running efficiency, ability to maintain high speed with energy demands close to maximal aerobic power, and smart tactics.

Table 1-1 presents data from Child et al. (4) on master track runners, and they are quite representative. For 70 to 80-year-old male athletes, an average of approximately 40 ml $\times$ kg^{-1} $\times$ min^{-1} has been reported (1, 15). Individuals up to 70 years of age respond positively to endurance training (Fig. 1-2). At

TABLE 1-1. *Age, maximal oxygen uptake (ml $\times$ kg^{-1} $\times$ min^{-1}), and maximal heart rate for master athletes and sedentary individuals respectively*

Age	Endurance N = 9 54 (40–69)	Sprinters N = 13 45 (41–58)	Untrained 55 (40–69)
$\dot{V}_{O2}$	56 (44–71)	47 (39–63)	35
HR$_{MAX}$	162 (146–177)	168 (154–178)	

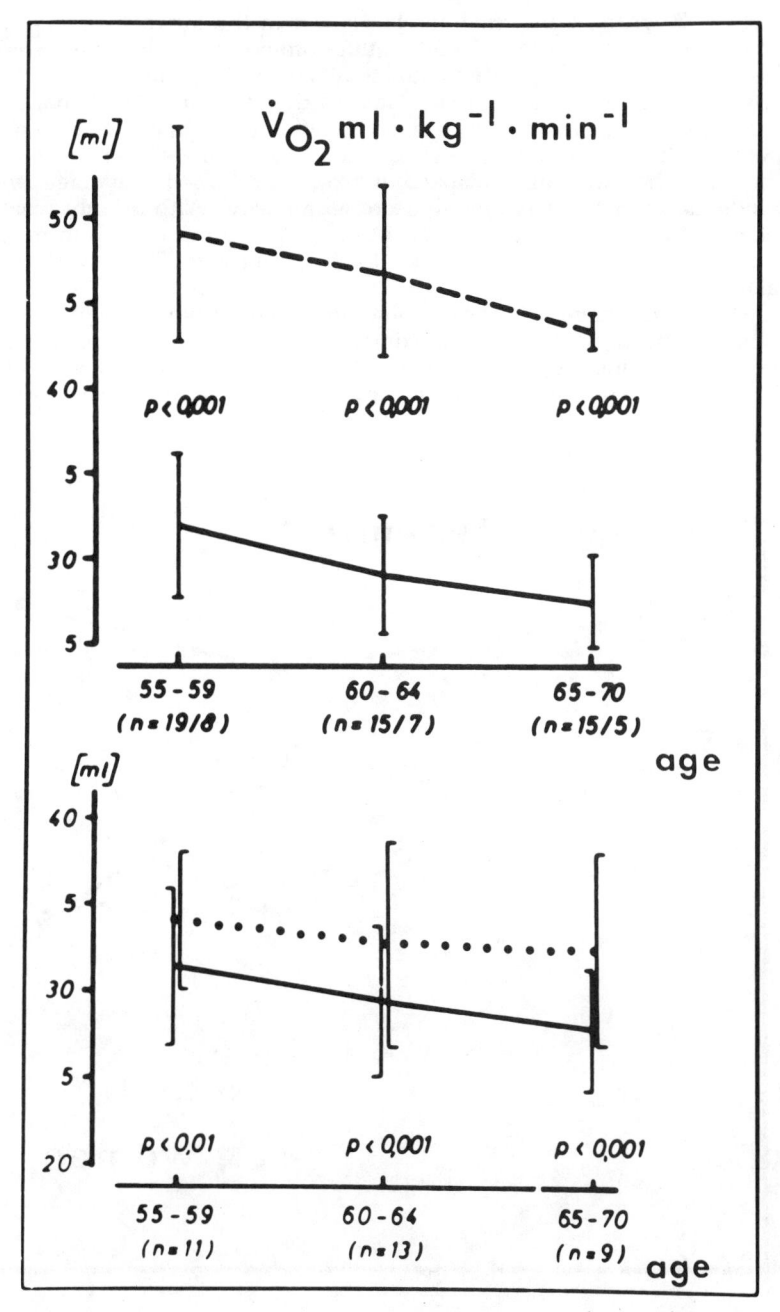

Fig. 1-2. The upper panel shows maximal oxygen uptake in ml $\times$ kg^{-1} $\times$ min^{-1} for well-trained individuals in different age groups (broken line) and sedentary "controls" (full line). The lower panel demonstrates the effect on maximal oxygen uptake of a 10-week training period, 3 times per week, 30 minutes each time (full line before and broken line after training). n = number of subjects (14).

the age of 70 years, a maximal aerobic power in the range 1.3 liters/ min^{-1} (women) to (2.0 liters/min^{-1} (men) is quite common in healthy but sedentary individuals. The stress on various functions when exercising at a submaximal intensity (e.g., when walking) is related to the ratio of submaximal aerobic power/maximal aerobic power. The same holds true for perceived exertion. A person with a body weight of 65 kg needs approximately 1 liter of oxygen per minute when walking at a speed of 5 km $\times$ hr^{-1}. For the average 70-year-old individual, that is a moderate exercise intensity. With a body weight of 100 kg, that walk will tax the aerobic power of many persons up to maximal. It is quite evident that it is important for the aging individual to try to keep fit and slim.

In our department we have a longitudinal study which includes former students of physical education. Maximal oxygen uptake, lung function, and some other parameters were measured first in 1949, then again in 1970 and 1982. (Fig. 1-3). For one male subject a reduction in maximal oxygen uptake

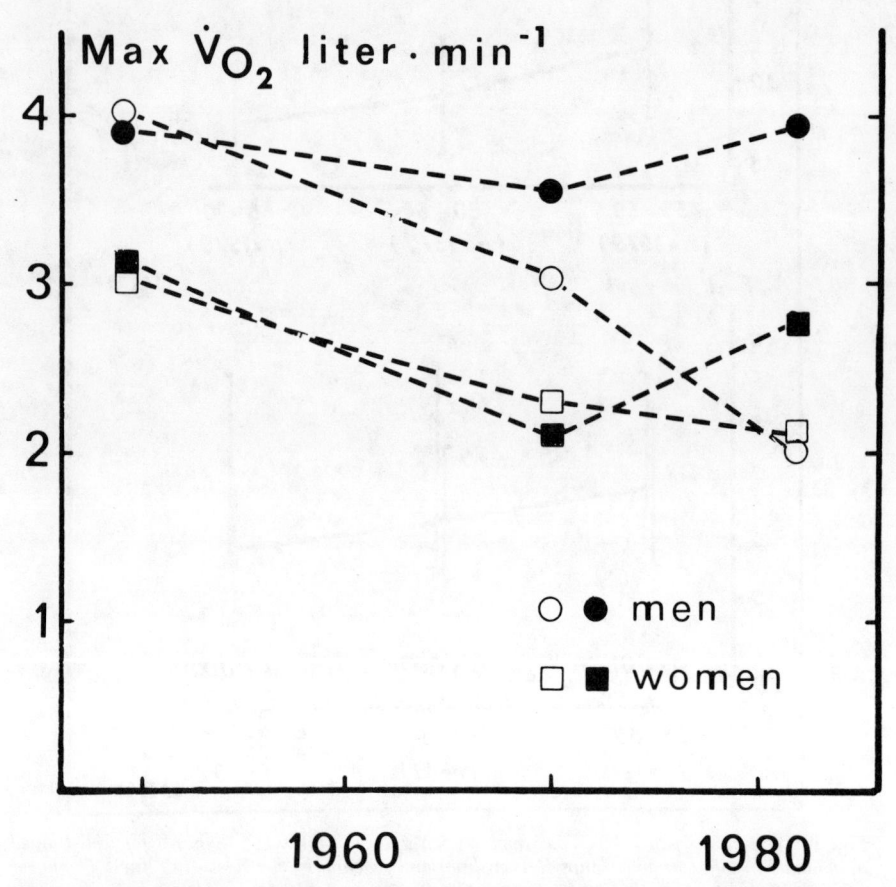

Fig. 1-3. *The maximal oxygen uptake measured on 4 subjects in 1949, 1970, and 1982 respectively. In 1949 they were students in physical education, approximately 25 years old. (See the text.)*

from 3.95 to 3.56 1 × min^{-1} was noted during the first 21-year period. When studied again 12 years later, he was back to the 3.95 1 × min^{-1} level, probably as a result of intensified training (age then 61 years). In contrast, one subject dropped from 4.0 down to 2.0 1 × min^{-1}. He was gradually forced into a relatively sedentary life due to rheumatoid arthritis (age 65 years). These two cases illustrate how critical life style can be for the aging effect on the oxygen transport system.

With age there is a gradual decline in maximal heart rate. With unchanged stroke volume and arterio-venous oxygen difference (a-v̄O$_2$ diff), this reduction will result in a decrease in maximal cardiac output and, therefore, in maximal aerobic power. Heath et al. (9) report that the O$_2$ pulse during maximal exercise was identical in masters endurance athletes (59 plus or minus 6 years) and young athletes. Evidently the stroke volume and a-v̄O$_2$ difference were similar in the two groups. The decline in maximal heart rate could explain the masters lower maximal aerobic power. In a subject with similar maximal oxygen uptake in 1949 and 1982, the maximal heart rate had declined from 200 via 188 to 182 in 1982 (Fig. 1-3). The calculated O$_2$ pulse was 19.7 milliliters (ml) in 1949 and actually 21.7 ml in 1982. On echocardiographic evaluation, endurance athletes of any age have a significantly greater left ventricular volume and mass than untrained people of the same age (4, 9).

(At the symposium a more detailed presentation was given of our longitudinal study, but due to the policy of journals not to accept papers that have partly been published elsewhere, the data have been omitted in this manuscript.)

ANAEROBIC POWER

As mentioned, a measurement of oxygen uptake gives a good estimate of aerobic power. In contrast, there is no method available to measure accurately anaerobic power and capacity. A high concentration of lactate in exercising muscle and in the blood is only a signal indicating that there has been a substantial anaerobic breakdown of glycogen. A high motivation is essential to attain high concentrations of lactate. It is typical that an athlete usually reaches a higher lactate level after an important competition than after an all-out test in the laboratory, exercise time being the same. There is a trend after a maximal effort that: (1) the peak blood lactate concentration is higher after a period of training, and (2) this peak concentration is lower at higher ages.

It is well documented that at a given submaximal relatively high work rate, trained individuals have a lower blood lactate concentration than when untrained. Also when subjects exercise at a given percentage of maximal aerobic power, training can reduce the lactate level. As a consequence the trained individual can run, bicycle, ski, or swim at a relatively high speed without a continuous accumulation of lactate in muscles and blood. At least two factors can explain this finding: an increase in maximal oxygen uptake and, as mentioned, the ability to exercise at a higher percentage of this maximum without lactate production. In addition, an improved technique will reduce the energy cost to maintain a given speed (2).

It has been noticed that training can reduce (normalize) the pulmonary ventilation at a given relatively high oxygen uptake (subject's age was 63 plus or minus 2 years) (19). One factor behind such an effect could be a reduced metabolic hydrogen ion (H+) production after training.

MUSCLE MASS AND STRENGTH

Beyond the age of approximately 50 years there is a significant reduction in muscular strength. A peak is usually reached at the age of 20 for men and a few years earlier for women. The strength of a 65-year-old person is, on the average, 75 to 80% of that attained between the ages of 20 and 30, with a further decline to about 60% in leg and back muscles, and to 70% in arm muscles from 30 to 80 years of age (7). Certainly, there are also large individual variations, and different states of training can highly influence test results. Chronological age is in many ways a poor instrument for a classification of individuals, including athletes. The decline in maximal muscle strength with age seems to parallel the reduction in muscle mass. The individual muscle fibers have a relatively normal cross-sectional area during adult life, up to the age of 80 years, with some diminution in the area of the fast-twitch fibers (type II) (7). The reason for reduced muscle mass, and hence reduced strength in older persons, is a loss of muscle fibers, perhaps down to some 60% of the initial number. It is not surprising that older individuals have a relatively poor power potential for the performance of a vertical jump.

A loss of motoneurons is most likely the cause of this type of degeneration. Muscle fibers which have been deprived of their nervous supply can be reinnervated by the process of fiber sprouting. Nearby, intact nerve terminals can start sprouting and form new synapses. As a consequence, with age there can be an increase in the number of muscle fibers in a motor unit (motoneuron plus the muscle fibers it innervates). It is an open question whether or not activation or training of a muscle group can promote fiber sprouting and thereby minimize the reduction of muscle mass in old age.

There are observations that during the first weeks of strength training, the improvement is not associated with an increase in the cross-sectional area of the muscle groups involved. Then there is often a gradual increase in both strength and the cross-sectional area, particularly of the type II fibers. There is also a specificity in the training so that improved strength is more pronounced in the type of activity that was trained than in other exercises. Both these phenomena can be explained by the fact that the activity in the central nervous system (CNS) is of decisive importance to the number of motor units and the frequency at which they are activated at a given time. As a result of training, the CNS can apparently command more muscle cells to activity by removing inhibitions and the same muscle mass can then produce more strength (2, chap. 10).

TECHNIQUE, COORDINATION

Once one has learned bicycling, a swim stroke, the tennis serve or golf swing, it is remarkable how well the skill is maintained even if not practiced for years. However, without training one tires quickly and the technique may deteriorate, (e.g., in swimming, playing the piano, or the guitar). What about well-maintained agility in old age? Many musicians demonstrate that remarkable performances are possible in later years. Artur Rubenstein played brilliantly technically very demanding Chopin compositions when almost 90 years old. Andrés Segovia still gave concerts on his classic guitar at the age of 91 years. These are just two examples. Musicians usually practice several hours daily. Apparently such training can maintain agility. Most aging individuals do not include agility in their daily activities and their movements become slow and clumsy. We believe that this is an inevitable consequence of aging, but it may not be so. It may be the result of inactivity. Perhaps hours of muscle activity can, as mentioned, promote fiber sprouting and maintain the muscle mass and a high-level CNS-muscle function?

It should be mentioned that efficiency in walking and running at a given speed is similar from the age of approximately 15 up to at least the age of 70 years in individuals without medical problems in the locomotor organs.

NUTRITIONAL ASPECTS

Many masters endurance runners run 50 to 200 kilometers (km) per week (3, 4, 13). They are high energy consumers and of necessity their food intake is high. The substrates for active muscles are carbohydrate and free fatty acids (FFA). One effect of endurance training is an increased utilization of FFA during exercise at a given percentage of maximal aerobic power. This shift in the utilization of substrates is glycogen saving, and it will take longer to consume a given store of glycogen, thereby improving the potential for good performance in endurance events. A reasonable daily energy intake for the 50-km-per-week runner is 12.5 MJ and for the 200-km-runner, 20 MJ (body weight approximately 70 kg). On a well-balanced diet, 10 MJ is supposed to be enough to cover the demand for essential nutrients. Runners are apparently on the safe side. In contrast, sedentary individuals with little physical activity in their job and leisure time must restrict their energy intake to levels below 10 MJ if they want to avoid obesity. They are in the risk zone of malnutrition. With age there is a reduced resting metabolism, but the demand for essential nutrients seems to be the same as at younger ages. If physically inactive, the older individual is therefore particularly exposed to the risk of malnutrition with respect to some essential nutrients.

It should be emphasized that an individual with a high energy output certainly needs more carbohydrate, fat, and water, but the demand for other nutrients is essentially the same as for sedentary individuals. There is a trend for endurance training athletes to have a subnormal hemoglobin concentration (10). The etiology of this anemia is not known. One possible explanation could be an increased mechanical destruction of red cells (hemolytic anemia). Why then is it not compensated for? Hallberg and Magnusson (8) have launched an interesting hypothesis: the trained person has a higher concentration of 2,3-DPG, shifting the oxygen dissociation curve of the hemoglobin to the right. At any level of blood oxygen tension this shift leads to an increased delivery of oxygen to the tissue. The sensor responsible for the erythropoietin level, regulating the rate of red cell production, will receive the same information about the oxygen delivery potential of the arterial blood of the athletes as if, at a normal level of 2,3-DPG, their hemoglobin concentrations were normal. In other words, the regulatory mechanisms are cheated. The increased level of 2,3-DPG would therefore be associated with a decrease in the production of erythropoietin and thus induce a lower hemoglobin concentration. These events would explain the development of a "sports anemia" even if the supply of iron is sufficient. Hallberg concludes that ". . . during the development of the human race—by selection of the fittest—the ability to run very long distances was not decisive for survival. Running short distances fast, to catch or escape wild animals, was probably far more important for our predecessors."

MISCELLANEOUS

Physical training has a positive effect on insulin-carbohydrate metabolism interactions which can be important for patients with diabetes or individuals with the potential to develop diabetes. The training may cause an increased glucose tolerance. As a consequence, the individual may get along with less insulin due to an increased insulin sensitivity (11).

There are data indicating that physical training can increase the blood concentration of high-density lipoprotein and the ratio of high-density lipoproteins/low density lipoproteins. That may reduce the risk of developing atherosclerosis (18).

An interesting new field is the study of endorphins and their effects in the CNS. There are many supporters of the statement that "exercise is the best tranquilizer." It appears well established that the release of beta-endorphins is elevated after prolonged, strenuous exercise (5). These neurohormones (beta-endorphin, encephalin, and dynorphin), which have an effect resembling that of certain opiates, play an important role in general physiological stress reactions. They serve to reduce pain and enhance the feeling of well being. The increased release of endorphins during strenuous exercise may thus, at least in part, explain the feeling of well-being commonly experienced at the end of a training session. As a matter of fact, attachment of endorphins to specific receptors in the brain has been demonstrated in individuals following long distance running. It is also of interest to note that the endorphin antagonist nalaxone has the opposite effect (12, 17).

CONCLUDING REMARKS

The history of Hominids covers millions of years. During more than 99% of our existence we have been hunters and food gatherers. For survival, brisk daily walking of 5 to 10 to 15 km was essential. I believe that running was an exceptional event in the daily activities, not as essential for survival as the more economical walking. Conclusion: habitual brisk walking is a basic activity to promote optimal function. That may be an unpopular statement at a symposium organized in conjunction with Masters Games. However, it is an open question how critical the intensity of habitual physical activity need be to promote optimal function. Presently we can not evaluate the effects of two hours at a moderate work rate compared with one hour at twice that energy demand on vital functions. At any rate, regular physical activity is essential for optimal physical fitness. Therefore, go out and walk or run your dog, even if you don't have one!

REFERENCES

1. Asano, K., S. Ogawa, J. Furuta, T. Yano, and M. Tomihara. Aerobic work capacity and blood composition in middle and old-aged runners. *Bull. Inst. Sport Sci.* (Tokyo Univ. Education) 14:21–34, 1976.
2. Astrand, P. O. and K. Rodahl. *Textbook of Work Physiology.* New York: McGraw-Hill Book Company, 1st ed. 1970, 3rd ed, 1985.
3. Barnard, R. J., G. K. Grimditch, and J. H. Wilmore. Physiological characteristics of sprint and endurance master runners. *Med. Sci. Sports* 11:167–171, 1979.

4. Child, J. S., R. J. Barnard, and R. L. Taw. Cardiac hypertrophy and function in master endurance runners and sprinters. *J. Appl. Physiol.*: REEP 57:176–181, 1984.
5. Dearman, J., and K. T. Francis. Plasma levels of catecholamines, cortisol, and beta-endorphins in male athletes after running 26.2, 6 and 2 miles, *J. Sports Med. Phys. Fitness* 23:30–38, 1983.
6. Drinkwater, B. L., S. M. Horvath, and C. L. Wells. Aerobic power of females, ages 10 to 68. *J. Gerontology* 30:385–394, 1975.
7. Grimby, G. and B. Saltin. The aging muscle. *Clin. Physiol.* 3:209–218, 1983.
8. Hallberg, L., and B. Magnusson: The etiology of "sports anemia." *Acta Med. Scand.* 216:145–148, 1984.
9. Heath, G. W., J. M. Hagberg, A. A. Ehsani, and J. O. Holloszy. A physiological comparison of young and older endurance athletes. *J. Appl. Physiol.*: REEP. 51:634–640, 1981.
10. Hunding, A., R. Jordal, and P. E. Paulev. Runner's anemia and iron deficiency. *Acta Med. Scand.* 209:315–318, 1981.
11. James, D. E., E. W. Kraegen, and D. J. Chisholm. Effect of exercise training on whole-body insulin sensitivity and responsiveness. *J. App. Physiol.*: REEP. 56:1217–1222, 1984.
12. Janal, M. N., E. W. D. Colt, W. C. Clark, and M. Glusman. Pain sensitivity, mood, and plasma endocrine levels in man following long-distance running: effects of naloxone. *Pain* 19:13–25, 1984.
13. Kavanagh, T., and R. J. Shephard. The effects of continued training on the aging process. *Ann. N. Y. Acad. Sci.* 301:656–670, 1977.
14. Liesen, H., and W. Hollmann. Leistungsverbesserung und Muskelstoffwechseladaptationen durch Ausdauertraining im Alter. *Geriatric* 6:150–157, 1976.
15. Pollock, M. L. Physiological characteristics of older champion track athletes. *Am. Assoc. Health Phys. Educ.* 45:363–373, 1974.
16. Robinson, S., D. B. Dill, R. D. Robinson, S. P. Tzankoff, and J. A. Wagner. Physiological aging of champion runners. *J. Appl. Physiol.* 41:46–51, 1976.
17. Surbey, G. D., G. M. Andrew, F. W. Cervenko, and P. P. Hamilton. Effects of naloxone on exercise performance. *J. Appl. Physiol*: REEP. 57:674–679, 1984.
18. Wood, P. D., R. B. Terry, and W. L. Haskell. Metabolism of substrates: diet, lipoprotein metabolism, and exercise. *Fed. Proc.* 44:358–363, 1985.
19. Yerg II, J. E., D. R. Seals, J. M. Hagberg, and J. O. Holloszy. Effect of endurance exercise training on ventilatory function in older individuals. *J. Appl. Physiol.* 58:791–794, 1985.

Section II
The Mature Muscle

2

Characteristics of Aging Human Skeletal Muscles

HOWARD J. GREEN

University of Waterloo

INTRODUCTION

An inevitable consequence of aging is a reduction in physical performance capability. During volitional activity, cross-sectional studies are generally consistent in describing declines in maximal static and dynamic strength, maximal speed, and the peak ability to generate energy through aerobic and anaerobic metabolic pathways (40). For the expression of all of these functional indices, skeletal muscle recruitment and contraction are fundamental. However, there still remains considerable uncertainty about the role played by aging skeletal muscles in contributing to the observed physiological impairment. (12).

The reasons are severalfold. Emphasis on research directed at characterization of human skeletal muscle and aging skeletal muscle at the structural, ultrastructural and biochemical levels is relatively recent. Although impressive advances have been made in describing and characterizing specific fiber types in young adult muscle (35), few studies have been conducted on the aging adult. For those that have been completed, the limitations inherent in ascribing the changes observed to the aging process per se on the basis of cross-sectional sampling are most evident. Problems in obtaining representative samples of sufficient size free from the bias of factors known to affect muscle character and function such as illness, physical activity level, and nutritional status continue to be major obstacles. The problem is further compounded in muscle physiology, since in most research studies an invasive procedure, the needle biopsy, has been used to obtain tissue samples. The limited sampling sites that are safe for the application of this procedure and the very small tissue sample obtained mean that conclusions must be restricted to only a few of the larger muscles, such as the gastrocnemius, vastus lateralis and deltoid. Indeed, if regional differences exist within a muscle as has been observed for the vastus lateralis (22), erroneous conclusions may occur if the sample is considered representative of the whole muscle. The small piece of tissue obtained also limits the range of analyses that can be performed. Consequently, our knowledge is somewhat fragmentary and uncoordinated. At present we do not have the basis on which to describe the pattern of organization of properties within human muscle and in specific fiber types and the manner in which this organization is affected by aging. However, substantial progress has been made, as is illustrated in the accompanying review.

MUSCLE FIBER TYPE CHARACTERISTICS—AN OVERVIEW

Skeletal muscle motor units and muscle fibers may be divided into different types based on physiologic, metabolic, and ultrastructural criteria. In the human, the most popular procedures employed for separation of fiber types are based on the pH sensitivity of the histochemical reaction for myofibrillar (actomyosin) ATPase (7). With this procedure two major classifications of fibers are recognized (Type I vs Type II) as well as several subclassifications of Type II fibers (Type IIA, IIB, IIC).

The histochemical myofibrillar ATPase procedure permits initial recognition of individual fiber types which may then be further characterized using a variety of techniques. Specific histochemical and immunological preparations can be examined by light and electron microscopy for structural, ultrastructural, and biochemical features. In addition, single fiber dissection and analysis of specific types has proved very valuable, most notably for the determination of biochemical properties (9, 24).

In the human, major differences exist in biochemical specialization between Type I and Type II fibers. The capacity for ATP hydrolysis, as measured by maximal myofibrillar ATPase activity, is approximately threefold higher in Type II fibers (9). The large potential for ATP hydrolysis is accompanied by specialized metabolic systems designed for rapid ATP re-synthesis. The enzymes involved in ATP synthesis, creatine phosphokinase (CPK) and adenylate kinase (AK), range from 30 to 80% higher (41), while the glycogenolytic and glycolytic potentials as measured by phosphorylase (PHOSP) and phosphofructokinase (PFK) are approximately twofold higher in the fast contracting (FT) Type II fibers (9, 24).

Metabolic specialization is also accompanied by extensive differentiation in other cellular constituents. The contractile and regulatory proteins including both the myosin light and heavy chain composition (6) and tropomyosin (33) are different between the fiber types. Although data on the characteristics of the human sarcoplasmic reticulum between the different fiber types are generally lacking, the results in other mammals indicate both qualitative and quantitative differences (17). In general, all properties examined support the functional designation of Type II fibers as fast contracting, high force output mechanical generators backed by highly specialized metabolic pathways for instantaneous and large ATP turnover rates.

In slow contracting Type I fibers (ST), ATPase activity and consequently ATP turnover rates are comparatively low (35). Characteristically, these fibers have a metabolic profile more specialized for the aerobic oxidation of fats and carbohydrates. These fibers have a high mitochondrial density with correspondingly high activities of enzymes on the citric acid cycle, the respiratory chain, and free fatty acid oxidation (9, 24). Type II fibers can also be differentiated on the basis of aerobic potential (35). One subgroup of Type II fibers, commonly referred to as fast oxidative-glycolytic (FOG), possesses a similar metabolic pattern to Type I in terms of aerobic metabolic potential. At the other extreme are Type II fibers with a low mitochondrial density and a low respiratory capacity. These fibers have been designated fast-glycolytic (FG). It should be evident that the subclassifications used by Brooke and Kaiser for

Type II fibers (7), which are based on myosin properties, are not compatible with the schema using metabolic criteria (28).

In terms of size, only a small difference is noted between the principal fiber types in the young healthy adult. Type II fibers generally average 15 to 20% larger than Type I (10). In contrast, diffusion potential as represented by capillaries per fiber area is approximately 15 to 20% higher in Type I fibers (10). At present there are no human studies comparing size to aerobic potential of Type II fibers.

Specialized muscle cells with highly ordered subcellular properties provide for optimization and efficiency in the performance of diverse physical tasks. Slow contracting Type I fibers are ideally suited for sustained usage in situations in which ATP turnover is low and oxygen is not limiting. In these fibers ATP production is aerobically based with exogenous free fatty acids and blood glucose serving as key fuels. At the other extreme, the Type II FG fibers are capable of rapid and large bursts of power output. Excitation-contraction-relaxation processes in these fibers are extremely rapid. The high ATP requirements are supplied in large part by anaerobic combustion of endogenous glycogen. Between these extremes exist the FOG fibers which are fast contracting but have a metabolic pattern specialized for the production of ATP by both aerobic and anaerobic processes. These fast fibers appear to have a greater ability to alter the mode of ATP production depending on the availability of oxygen.

In the untrained young adult, most muscles contain a mixture of various types of motor units. Selectivity of motor unit and muscle fiber involvement in specific tasks is provided by a highly stereotyped recruitment pattern (18). Accordingly, Type I fibers are preferentially recruited at low force outputs while Type II fiber populations are progressively involved as the requirements for force increase. This hierarchy in recruitment thresholds of the various motor unit types provides for an appropriate match between task demands and type of fiber recruited. In recent years it has become obvious that the properties of muscle fibers are not stable but rather can be altered by a number of factors. Phenotypic plasticity is most evident in response to persistent alterations in contractile activity (11, 32). This sensitivity of the muscle fiber properties to adapt to altered usage suggests that the specific character and composition of the fiber is a response to the nature of the demand placed upon the muscles collectively and at the level of the individual motor unit. Whether aging acts as an independent influence in altering human muscle structure and function or whether age-associated alterations in selected environmental factors are primarily responsible for defining the character of muscle is presently unknown.

MUSCLE FIBER CHARACTERISTICS—THE AGING ADULT

Fiber Number

Perhaps the least controversial finding in studies of aging human muscle is the loss of muscle fibers that occurs. This finding is supported by direct evidence obtained by counting muscle fibers in autopsied whole vastus lateralis muscle in previously healthy individuals representing two age groups: 30 years and 72 years (23). In these two age groups, the 25% lower fiber number in the older group could account completely for the smaller muscle size. This work is also supported by the findings of Sato et al. (36) in 200 females ranging in age from 26 to 80 years involved in surgical resection of the minor pectoral muscle. In this study, reductions in fiber number become evident only after 60 years of age, with overall reductions approximating 25% during the seventh decade. Other workers (8, 38), using noninvasive physiological techniques to estimate motor unit counts in the extensor digitorum brevis, the thenar, and hypothenar muscles of the hand, have observed an initial decline at a similar age. In these studies, the decrease in the number of motor units amounted to at least 50% in individuals in their seventh decade. The associated decrease in both motor unit number and fiber number has promoted the proposition that at least part of the reduction in fiber number is due to loss of functioning motoneurons. Whether or not the loss of more motoneurons than muscle fibers is indicative of a greater age-associated innervation ratio, possibly mediated by collateral sprouting of surviving motoneurons, is speculative. Data obtained from non-humans, particularly rats and mice, suggest that this is the case (15).

Fiber Type Distribution

Alterations in fiber type distribution in specific muscles are possible either as a consequence of a transformation of one fiber type to another, as has been observed with the conversion of Type II (FT) to Type I (ST) fibers in chronic electrical stimulation experiments (32), or by a preferential loss of a specific motor unit type. There has been a general consensus that aging in the human results in progressive increases in ST fiber population. However, this conclusion, based largely on the studies of Larsson et al. (21), is not supported by several recent studies (12, 13, 23, 36). In the study by Sato et al. (36), Type I fiber distribution remained remarkably stable both during the period prior to 60 years of age when the estimated total fiber number remained constant and during the sixth and seventh decades when total fiber number decreased. The subjects studied by Grimby et al. (13, 14) ranged from 66 to 100 years, an age range in which a pronounced loss of muscle fibers would have been expected (23). However, no alteration in the distribution of major fiber types was evident. Similarly, Lexell et al. (23), using the same muscle, the vastus lateralis, were not able to conclude that the loss was preferential to Type II fibers. These results support the conclusion that in aged human muscles where a loss of muscle fiber occurs, the loss is not fiber type-specific, at least to specific types as classified by the histochemical myofibrillar ATPase reaction (7).

Perhaps the most influential study supporting the notion that aging is associated with a loss of Type II fibers has been published by Larsson et al. (21), who found a 60 to 45% reduction in the Type II fiber population between the third and seventh decades. Since these changes were initiated and became pronounced during an age period when no significant loss of fiber number would have been expected, it would appear that either an FT or ST transformation has occurred or FT fibers have been lost and replaced by ST. Currently, there is very little evidence to support either of these hypotheses. The fact that physical activity levels generally show dramatic reductions in the middle-to-older age groups renders an explanation based on altered usage patterns somewhat remote.

Muscle Fiber Size

Several studies (4, 21) agree that Type I fibers are relatively insensitive to an age-associated change in size up until the age of 60 to 70 years in both males and females. For Type II fibers, however, the results are not as conclusive. Larsson et al. (21) have found a progressive decline with age in Type II fiber area such that at 60 to 65 years of age, mean areas were only 58% of those measured at 20 to 29 years. This general finding has also been supported by Sato et al. (36). Other studies have revealed only minor changes in Type II fiber area up until at least the seventh decade (4, 14). Beyond 70 years of age, dramatic reduction in fiber size appears evident in all fiber types and most particularly in the Type II fibers, both Type IIA and Type IIB. The results of Grimby et al. (13) suggest that major fiber size reductions occur at some critical age and then remain relatively stable with further aging. The suggestion that Type I fiber hypertrophy occurs with aging is not supported in studies on the human vastus lateralis muscle (4, 14), but may occur in other muscles, as Sato et al. (36) have found size increases in this fiber type in the minor pectoral muscles of females.

Capillarization

Capillarization of skeletal muscle most often has been expressed in terms of the number of capillaries in a defined cross-sectional area of the muscle, the number of capillaries per fiber, and the number of capillaries per cross-section area of the fiber. This latter index provides an indication of the specific cross-sectional area in a fiber served by a capillary. No definite conclusions appear possible at this time regarding alterations in capillarization with aging for any of the criteria cited. In one of the earliest studies in this area, Parizková et al. (31) concluded that although the number of capillaries per square millimeter (mm) was the same in young and old subjects, the reduction in fiber size and greater number of fibers per square mm promoted a significantly higher capillary-to-fiber ratio. Aniansson et al. (4) found decreases in the number of capillaries per fiber in males but not in females.

When comparisons are made between old age groups (78 to 81 years), both male and female (14), and between young adult males (2) and females (29), comparative values are found for the number of capillaries per fiber and the capillaries per fiber area. This result is somewhat surprising in view of the large differences in fiber area. However, it must be realized that age comparisons have been based on a single study of relatively small size. It seems premature at this time to draw any conclusions based on the limited experimental data.

Energy Metabolic Potential

The most comprehensive studies of age-associated changes in energy metabolic potential of human skeletal muscle have been published by Larsson et al. (21) and Örlander et al. (30). These authors, utilizing the same sample group, have found that maximal activities of several enzymes involved in the citric acid cycle (citrate synthase, CS) and the electron transport chain (cytochrome oxidase, CO), anaerobic glycolysis (phosphofructokinase, PFK; lactate dehydrogenase, LDH), ATP synthesis (adenylate kinase, AK), and ATP hydrolysis (Mg^{2+}-stimulated myofibrillar ATPase) did not change over the age range of 25 to 65 years. Only an enzyme involved in β-oxidation (3-hydroxy CoA dehydrogenase, HAD) and an isozyme of LDH (M-LDH) showed a significant trend with age. Although the age trend for enzymes involved in aerobic end oxidation was in a similar positive direction to HAD, the change was not of sufficient magnitude to be significant. The conclusion that age does not provoke a decline in energy metabolic potential also appears to apply even to older groups. Aniansson et al. (3) have reported no change in either males (66 to 76 years) or females (61 to 71 years) in the maximal activities of Mg^{2+} ATPase, AK and LDH, while Grimby et al. (14) reported similar findings for hexokinase (HK), LDH, HAD, and CS in a similar muscle (vastus lateralis) in men and women aged 78 to 81 years. These conclusions were based on comparisons with a group of young subjects of comparable sex (39) using identical procedures for measurement of enzymatic activities. Further evidence of general biochemical stability with age is provided by the findings of Möller et al. (26), who found that in the resting vastus lateralis muscle of 52 to 79 year-olds, resting ATP, AMP, and energy charge potential were all comparable to a group of 18 to 36 year-olds (16). A small but significant reduction was noted for the total adenine nucleotides (TAN) and for phosphocreatine (PC).

It seems reasonable to conclude, at least, based on the relatively limited data base, that energy metabolic potential and in particular the capacity for aerobic substrate end oxidation and anaerobic glycolysis do not deteriorate with age. This seems to occur regardless of whether fiber type distribution is altered (14, 30). It is possible that the trend towards higher β-oxidative and aerobic oxidative capacities noted by Örlander et al. (30) may have been biased by the increase in Type I fiber distribution noted with advancing age. Since little change in the maximal enzyme activities has been found over a wide age range, it seems apparent that any loss of muscle fibers noted with age (14) must consist of fibers of representative metabolic potentials. The collective effect of the loss of muscle fibers will be a lowering of the absolute maximal ATP turnover rate generated by both aerobic and anaerobic metabolism without a loss of metabolic potential in each fiber type. Since muscle fiber atrophy has also been found in the older ages (13), probably resulting from the loss of contractile protein, it would appear that maximal enzyme activities are adjusted to maintain a constant metabolic potential in relation to the amount of contractile protein.

It must be emphasized that these conclusions, although appealing, are speculative at best. A much more comprehensive analysis of maximal enzyme activities is needed, with representation given to all metabolic segments in conjunction with appropriate studies of metabolic control, mitochondrial respiration, and the coupling between electron transport and phosphorylation.

Muscle Fiber Composition and Structure

Örlander et al. (30) have examined a number of ultrastructural features in adult aging vastus lateralis muscle, including selected mitochondrial characteristics in the interfibrillar and sarcolemma space. In the interfibrillar space, reductions in the volume fraction of mitochondria (Vv) and the mean mitochondrial volume ($\tilde{V}_{mit}$) are apparent over the age range of 16 to 76 years. No change is evident in either the apparent number (Nv) of mitochondria or in the number per sarcomere (Ns). A similar age-dependent decline was also noted for the mitochondrial volume fraction in the subsarcolemma region. In the intermyofibrillar space, reductions appear to occur as a result of a loss of mitochondrial volume per se, as the number of mitochondria was uninfluenced by age. Since there was a trend toward an increased potential for β-oxidation and aerobic oxidation as measured by the maximal activities of representative enzymes, this would imply an increased capacity per unit of mitochondrial volume (30), possibly indicating an increase in the density of respiratory assemblies on the inner mitochondrial membranes. In the case of the subsarcolemma, the decline in the mitochondrial volume fraction is not as clear. A decreasing trend is evident for both the apparent number of mitochondria and the apparent mean volume of mitochondria. Subcellular compartmentalization of energy metabolic pathways in muscle cells is well established (19). Whether the decline in the subcellular mitochondria fraction is associated with a reduced oxidative potential is unclear, as is the potential effect of this reduction on sarcolemma excitation and impulse. Several additional alterations in ultrastructure have been observed in senile human muscle (42, 43). Fiber type grouping, characterized by the appearance of compact fields of distinct fiber types, has been observed in aging muscle. The incidence of this grouping phenomenon appears to be related to the age of the muscles, as Grimby et al. (14) have observed a substantially higher incidence of grouping in subjects 78 to 81 years of age as compared to Aniansson et al. (3) and Lexell (23), who examined the muscles of subjects approximately 10 to 15 years younger. This phenomenon has been interpreted as a neurogenic disturbance resulting from denervation and atrophy of FT fibers and re-innervation by motor axons supplying ST fibers (14). Atrophy of single fibers is commonly observed in senile human muscle (33).

Shafiq et al. (37), using biopsy samples obtained from subjects aged 70 to 83 years, have found the general architecture of the muscle to be generally well preserved with fiber constituents and differentiation of fiber types similar to young subjects. However, a number of atypical features were noted in senile muscles. These included focal myofibrillar degeneration with streaming of Z lines or its accumulation into irregular dense structure, and increases in lipid and lipofuscin granules. Increases in lipofuscin granules are well established in aging muscle (30) and are thought to result from peroxidation of unsaturated lipids (37). Although the lipofuscin granules appear to possess lysosomal activity, their specific function in skeletal muscle is questionable.

Muscle Function

Few would disagree with the statement that age has a deleterious effect on a wide range of physiological attributes of muscle. Not well established, however, is the time course with which different functional characteristics are affected and the relationship between specific age-induced alterations in muscle structure and composition and muscle function.

In humans, muscle function studies have been focused primarily on determining the mechanical characteristics of the aging muscle in terms of both maximal force capabilities (MVC) and fatigue resistance or endurance.

Descriptions of aging pattern in maximal force capabilities in selected muscles and muscle groups have appeared in the literature since the turn of the century, and it has generally been accepted that declines in maximal voluntary static contraction (MVC) begin as early as the third decade (5). More recent studies employing more controlled sampling techniques and more sophisticated measurement devices are consistent in observing that strength declines with age are considerably more delayed (44). The magnitude of the decline still remains speculative. Larsson et al. (20) have reported losses in both static and dynamic strength of 26 to 38% in the quadriceps over the age range of 20 to 65 years, with most of the loss occurring after the fourth decade. In contrast, Vandervoort (44) reported that 80 to 90% of maximal voluntary static strength of both the dorsi flexors and plantar flexors is retained in both males and females to the seventh decade. Rapids dropoffs in strength are observed only in the older age groups, 80 to 100 years. Vandervoort (44) has also found that the reduction in maximal strength is not due to an inability to recruit the full motor neuron pool, as most subjects did not demonstrate an increase in force output in response to a superimposed electrical stimulus during the effort. It thus appears that a major reason for the pronounced loss of strength observed in the older age group is due to a loss of muscle fibers and a reduction in muscle cross-sectional area (12). This is supported by the finding that there is also a reduction in muscle compound action potentials (M waves) suggestive of a decrease in the number of functioning units (44). It is of interest that a prolongation in both contraction time (CT) and one-half relaxation time (1/2 RT) were found for both the dorsi flexors and plantar flexors with advancing age (44). The prolongation of CT with age has also been confirmed by McDonagh and Davies (25) in the leg triceps surae group. Prolongation of either CT or 1/2 RT may have important consequences for the discharge frequency needed to maintain submaximal tension levels. It is possible that specific tension can be maintained at lower discharge frequencies, a possibility suggested by the work of Nelson et al. (27).

In gross motor activities, the ability to produce energy aerobically (aerobic power) shows a progressive decline with age. This decline becomes manifest as early as the third decade, well before there is any apparent change in the muscle fiber cross-sectional area, the total fiber number, and the size or the aerobic metabolic potential of the cell (12, 40). Dissociation between alterations in aerobic power and apparent changes in muscle morphology and biochemistry support the notion that aerobic power is limited by central factors, most notably reduction in maximal cardiac output and maximal heart rate (34). Although skeletal muscle does not appear to be the limiting factor in aerobic production of ATP in maximal exercise involving large muscle groups over a wide age range, there may be differences in muscle energy metabolism during submaximal exercise. Recent (1) evidence suggests that elite endurance athletes are able to perform at a higher percentage of their maximal aerobic power than younger athletes at comparable blood lactate concentrations. Whether or not this observation is due to a larger percentage of energy being derived from aerobic oxidation has not been established.

In summary, there is little evidence to suggest major changes in muscle structure and composition in healthy humans up until approximately 70 years of age. Any changes that do occur prior to this age appear to represent a simple atrophy of existing fiber types. The magnitude of age-associated loss in performance functions appears to be dependent on the type of activity and the degree of muscle involvement. Future studies must isolate the specific role of central versus peripheral factors in contributing to performance deterioration in different physical tasks. A greater emphasis in longitudinal experiments offers the exciting possibility of both specifically delineating the role of the skeletal muscle in maintaining functional capabilities and of determining the specific influence of altered usage patterns on muscle structure, composition, and function.

REFERENCES

1. Allen, W., D. Seals, B. Hurley, A. Ehsani, and J. Hagberg. Lactate threshold and distance-running performance in younger and older endurance athletes. *J. Appl. Physiol.* 58:1281–1284, 1985.
2. Anderson, P., and J. Henriksson. Capillary supply of the quadriceps femoris muscle of man: adaptive response to exercise. *J. Physiol.* 270:677–680, 1977.
3. Aniansson, A., G. Grimby, M. Hedberg, and M. Krotkiewski. Muscle morphology, enzyme

activity, and muscle strength in elderly men and women. *Clin. Physiol.* 1:73–86, 1981.
4. Aniansson, A., G. Grimby, E. Nygaard, and B. Saltin. Muscle fiber composition and fiber area in various age groups. *Muscle and Nerve* 2:271–272, 1980.
5. Asmussen, E., and K. Heebøll-Nielsen. Isometric muscle strength of adult men and women. in: *Communications from the Testing and Observations Institute of the Danish National Association for Infantile Paralysis*, E. Asmussen, A. Fredsted, and E. Ryge (eds.) No. 11, Copenhagen, 1961.
6. Billeter, R., C. W. Heizmann, H. Howald, and E. Jenny. Analysis of myosin light chain types in single human skeletal muscle fibers. *Europ. J. Biochem.* 116:389–395, 1981.
7. Brooke, M. H., and K. K. Kaiser. Three "myosin ATPase" systems: the nature of their pH lability and sulphdryl dependence. *J. Histochem. Cytochem.* 18:670–672, 1970.
8. Campbell, M. J., A. J. McComas, and F. Petito. Physiological changes in aging muscles. *J. Neurol. Neurosurg. Psych.* 36:174–182, 1973.
9. Essen, B., E. Jansson, J. Henriksson, A. W. Taylor, and B. Saltin. Metabolic characteristics of fiber types in human skeletal muscle. *Acta Physiol. Scand.* 95:153–165, 1975.
10. Green, H. J., B. Daub, M. E. Houston, J. A. Thomson, I. Fraser, and D. Ranney. Human vastus lateralis and gastrocnemius muscles. A comparative histochemical and biochemical analysis. *J. Neurol. Sci.* 52:201–210, 1981.
11. Green, H. J., H. Reichmann, and D. Pette. Fiber type specific transformation in the enzyme activity pattern of rat vastus lateralis muscle by prolonged endurance training. *Pflügers Arch.* 399:216–222, 1983.
12. Grimby, G., and B. Saltin. Mini-review. The ageing muscle. *Clin. Physiol.* 3:209–218, 1983.
13. Grimby, G., A. Aniansson, C. Zetterberg, and B. Saltin. Is there a change in relative muscle fibre composition with age? *Clin. Physiol.* 4:189–194, 1984.
14. Grimby, G., B. Danneskold-Samsøe, K. Huid, and B. Saltin. Morphology and enzymatic capacity in arm and leg muscles in 78–81 year old men and women. *Acta Physiol. Scand.* 115:125–134, 1982.
15. Gutman, E., and E. Hanzliková. Fast and slow motor units in ageing. *Gerontology* 22:280–300, 1976.
16. Harris, R., E. Hultman, and L. -O. Nordesjö. Glycogen, glycolytic intermediates and high energy phosphates in biopsy samples of m. quadriceps femoris of man at rest. Methods and variance of values. *Scand. J. Clin. Lab. Invest.* 33:109–120, 1974.
17. Heilmann, C., W. Müller, and D. Pette. Correlation between ultrastructural and functional changes in sarcoplasmic reticulum during chronic stimulation of fast muscle. *J. Membr. Biol.* 59:143–149, 1981.
18. Henneman, E. The size principle. A deterministic output emerges from a set of probabilistic connections. *J. Exp. Biol.* 115:105–112, 1985.
19. Landau, B. R., and E. A. Sims. On the existence of two separate pools of glucose-6-phosphate in rat diaphragm. *J. Biol. Chem.* 242:163–172, 1967.
20. Larsson, L. Morphological and functional characteristics of the ageing skeletal muscle in man. *Acta Physiol. Scand.* Suppl. 457:1–36, 1978.
21. Larsson, L., B. Sjödin, and J. Karlsson. Histochemical and biochemical changes in human skeletal muscle with age in sedentary males, age 22–65 years. *Acta Physiol. Scand.* 103:31–39, 1978.
22. Lexell, J., D. Downham, and M. Sjöström. Distribution of different fibre types in human skeletal muscles. *J. Neurol. Sci.* 65:353–365, 1984.
23. Lexell, J., K. Henriksson-Larsén, B. Winblad, and M. Sjöström. Distribution of different fiber types in human skeletal muscles. Effects of aging studied in whole muscle cross sections. *Muscle and Nerve* 6:588–595, 1983.
24. Lowry, C. V., J. S. Kimmey, S. Felder, M. M-Y. Chi, K. K. Kaiser, P. N. Passoneau, K. A. Kirk, and O. H. Lowry. Enzyme patterns in single human muscle fibers. *J. Biol. Chem.* 253:8269–8277, 1978.
25. McDonagh, M. J. N., M. J. White and C. T. M. Davies. Different effects of aging on the mechanical properties of arm and leg muscles. *Gerontol.* 30:49–54, 1984.
26. Möller, P., J. Bergström, P. Fürst and K. Hellström. Effect of aging on energy-rich phosphagens in human skeletal muscles. *Clin. Sci.* 58:553–555, 1980.
27. Nelson, R., G. Soderberg, and N. Urbscheit. Alteration in motor unit discharge characteristics in aged humans. *Physical Therapy* 64:29–34, 1984.
28. Nemeth, P. M., H. W. Hofer, and D. Pette. Metabolic heterogeneity of muscle fibers classified by myosin ATPase. *Histochem.* 63:191–201, 1979.
29. Nygaard, E. Skeletal muscle fiber characteristics in young women. *Acta Physiol. Scand.* 112:299–304, 1981.
30. Örlander, J., K.-H. Kiessling, L. Larsson, J. Karlsson, and A. Aniansson. Skeletal muscle metabolism and ultrastructure in relation to age in sedentary men. *Acta Physiol. Scand.* 104:249–261, 1978.
31. Parizková, J., E. Eiselt, S. Šprynarová, and M. Wachtlová. Body composition, aerobic capacity, and density of muscle capillaries in young and old men. *J. Appl. Physiol.* 31:323–325, 1971.
32. Pette, D. Activity-induced fast to slow transitions in mammalian muscle. *Med. Sci. Sports Exerc.* 16:517–528, 1984.

33. Romera-Herrera, A. E., S. Nasser, and N. Lieska. Heterogeneity of adult human muscle tropomyosin. *Muscle and Nerve* 5:713–718, 1982.
34. Saltin, B. Hemodynamic adaptations to exercise. *Am. J. Cardiol.* 55:420–470, 1985.
35. Saltin, B., and P. D. Gollnick. Skeletal muscle adaptability. Significance for metabolism and performance. in: *Handbook of Physiology*, L. D. Peacher, R. H. Adrian and S. R. Geiger (eds.). Section 10: Skeletal Muscle. Washington: *Am. Physiol. Society*, Williams and Wilkins, 555–633, 1983.
36. Sato, T. H. Akatsuka, K. Kito, Y. Tokoro, H. Tauchi, and K. Kato. Age changes in size and number of muscle fibers in human minor pectoral muscle. *Mech. Ageing Develop.* 28: 99–109, 1984.
37. Shafiq, S. A., S. G. Lewis, L. C. Dimino, and H. S. Schutta. Electron microscopy study of skeletal muscle in elderly subjects. in: *Aging*, G. Kalder and J. Di Battista (eds). New York: Raven Press, pp. 65–85, 1978.
38. Sica, R. E. P., A. J. McComas, A. R. M. Upton, and D. Longmire. Estimations of motor units in small muscles of the hand. *J. Neurol. Neurosurg. Psych.* 37:55–67, 1974.
39. Sjøgaard, G. Muscle enzyme activity in relation to maximal oxygen uptake. *Acta Physiol. Scand.* 112:12A, 1981.
40. Skinner, J. S., C. M. Tipton, and A. C. Vailas. Exercise, physical training, and the aging process. In: *Lectures on Gerontology*, A. Viiduk (ed.). Vol. 1B. New York: Academic Press, 407–439, 1982.
41. Thorstensson, A., B. Sjödin, P. Tesch, and J. Karlsson. Actomysoin ATPase, myokinase, CPK and LDH in human fast and slow twitch muscle fibres. *Acta Physiol. Scand.* 99:225–229, 1977.
42. Tomlinson, B. E., J. N. Walton, and J. J. Rebeiz. The effect of ageing and of cachexia upon skeletal muscle. A histopathological study. *J. Neurol. Sci.* 9:321–326, 1969.
43. Tomonaga, M. Histochemical and ultrastructural changes in senile human skeletal muscle. *J. Am. Geriat. Soc.* 25:125–131, 1976.
44. Vandervoort, A. Aging and human neuromuscular function. Ph.D. thesis, McMaster University, 1984.

3

Adaptability of Skeletal Muscle To Long-Term Use

DIRK PETTE

University of Konstanz

INTRODUCTION

Endurance training increases the capacity of skeletal muscle for long-term use through adaptational processes which, in addition to skeletal muscle, affect the whole organism. Therefore, an appropriate model is needed to isolate the direct effects of activity upon muscle.

The chronic nerve stimulation experiment described by Salmons and Vrbová (38) is regarded as the most suitable model to investigate the effects of increased contractile activity on skeletal muscle under defined conditions. This approach uses indirect, chronic stimulation of selected muscles or muscle groups via implanted electrodes. Hence, responses to increased contractile activity are limited to the target and are independent of reactions other than in the stimulated muscle. In addition, chronic stimulation allows the application of defined work loads and, thus, the study of dose-response relationships. Unlike endurance training, where the work load must be increased in a stepwise manner for acclimatization, contractile activity can be at maximum from stimulation onset and the work loads can be higher and last longer. Therefore, chronic stimulation is also appropriate for studying the time course of induced changes.

It should be pointed out, however, that chronic nerve stimulation results in a nonphysiological mode of fiber recruitment, especially in those fibers unable to cope with sustained activity (e.g., fast-twitch glycolytic fibers). Electrical stimulation recruits 100% of the fiber population, whereas fibers are recruited asynchronously according to their motor unit thresholds during physiological locomotion. Nevertheless, the stimulation model has proven to

---

Acknowledgements

These studies were supported by Deutsche Forschungsgemeinschaft, Sonderforschungsbereiche 138 and 156. I express my gratitude to all my collaborators for their contributions and I especially thank Dr. Robert S. Staron for his help in preparing this manuscript.

be a useful approach and has been chosen as the topic for the following discussion on adaptational processes in response to increased contractile activity.

ALTERATIONS INDUCED BY CHRONIC STIMULATION

The chronic stimulation model was originally designed to study the influence of specific frequency patterns upon contractile properties. It was shown that chronic low frequency (10 Hz) stimulation had a pronounced slowing effect upon fast-twitch muscles (38). Many studies have since demonstrated that chronic nerve stimulation of fast-twitch muscles elicits a set of remodeling processes which ultimately result in the conversion of a white, fatiguable, fast-twitch muscle into a red, fatigue-resistant, slow-twitch muscle (27). These white-to-red and fast-to-slow conversions affect the major functional systems of the muscle fiber (i.e., the Ca^{2+} handling system, energy metabolism, and the myofibrillar apparatus). The major changes of these systems in response to chronic low frequency stimulation of fast-twitch muscles in the rabbit are summarized in Tables 3-1, 3-2, and 3-3.

Time Course of Fast-to-Slow Transitions

Although stimulation-induced changes result in a fast-to-slow transition, muscle fibers are not transformed as entities (27). Conversions of the different functional elements of the muscle fiber occur asynchronously and in a time-ordered sequence. The earliest changes are those affecting the Ca^{2+} dynamics of the muscle fiber and consist, 1 to 2 days after stimulation onset, of a 50% decrease in both total capacity and rate of Ca^{2+} uptake by the sarcoplasmic reticulum (15). The decrease in Ca^{2+} uptake is accompanied by a fall in the specific activity of Ca^{2+}-pumping ATPase (23) and is succeeded by a drastic reduction in parvalbumin, the major sarcoplasmic Ca^{2+}-binding protein (22). These changes accompany an increase in both half-relaxation time and time to peak of isometric twitch contraction (15). Prolonged stimulation subsequently leads to thorough rearrangements of both the peptide pattern and the phospholipid matrix of the sarcoplasmic reticulum membranes (15, 39).

The changes in enzyme activity levels and isozymes, which signify the metabolic white-to-red conversion and the concomitant increase in resistance to fatigue (17, 31), occur shortly after the onset of alterations in Ca^{2+} dynamics. The earliest detectable metabolic change is a pronounced increase in hexokinase activity (11, 32, 35). This is followed by severalfold increases in mitochondrial creatine kinase (42) and in enzymes representing various metabolic pathways of aerobic substrate oxidation (11, 30, 32, 35). Moderate decreases in enzyme activities of anaerobic carbohydrate catabolism (11, 30, 32, 35) and in extramitochondrial MM-creatine kinase (32, 42) are accompanied by an increase in H-type LDH isozymes at the cost of M-type LDH isozymes (11, 22, 32).

The rearrangement of the isomorph patterns of contractile and regulatory myofibrillar proteins occurs after prolonged stimulation. These changes, which are concomitant with decreases in the rate of tension development, relate to myosin light (2, 26, 30, 36, 37, 44, 45) and heavy chains (2, 26), as well as to the subunits of the regulatory proteins of the thin filament (28, 36). However, the fast-to-slow conversions of the myofibrillar proteins (myosin light chains

TABLE 3-1. *Summary of fast-to-slow transitions of the Ca^{2+}-sequestering system in chronically nerve-stimulated (10 Hz) fast-twitch muscle of the rabbit.*

Sarcoplasmic Reticulum		
T-Tubules, terminal cisternae, longitudinal SR	↓	(5, 6)
7-9 nm particles in freeze-fractured membranes	↓	(14)
Ca^{2+} uptake	↓	(14, 15, 23, 37)
Ca^{2+}-ATPase	↓	(14, 15, 22, 23, 37)
115 000-M_r Ca^{2+}-ATPase monomer	↓	(15, 22, 29, 39)
55 000-M_r peptide	↑	(15, 22, 39)
30 000-M_r peptide	↑	(22, 29)
Sarcoplasm		
Parvalbumin	↓	(22, 24, 29)

TABLE 3-2. *Summary of "white-to-red" transitions in the enzyme activity and isozyme pattern of energy metabolism in chronically nerve-stimulated (10 Hz) fast-twitch muscle of the rabbit (3, 11, 22, 27–33, 35, 42).*

Enzyme Activities:	
Glucose phosphorylation	↑
Fatty acid activation	↑
Fatty acid oxidation	↑
Ketone body utilization	↑
Citric acid cycle	↑
Respiratory chain	↑
mt-Creatine kinase	↑
MM-Creatine kinase	↓
Adenylate kinase	↓
Glycogenolysis	↓
Glycolysis	↓
Glycerol-P oxidation	↓
M-type LDH isozymes	↓
H-type LDH isozymes	↑

TABLE 3-3. *Summary of fast-to-slow transitions of myofibrillar proteins of thick and thin filaments in chronically nerve-stimulated (10 Hz) fast-twitch muscle of the rabbit.*

Myosin ATPase	↓	(37, 45)
Myosin light chains		(2, 26, 29, 36, 37, 44, 45)
fast type	↓	
slow type	↑	
Myosin heavy chains		(2)
fast type	↓	
slow type	↑	
Myosin light chain kinase	↓	(21)
Tropomyosin		
α/β	↓	(36)
slow type α	↑	(28)
Type I protein	↑	(13, 28)

ADAPTABILITY OF SKELETAL MUSCLE TO LONG-TERM USE

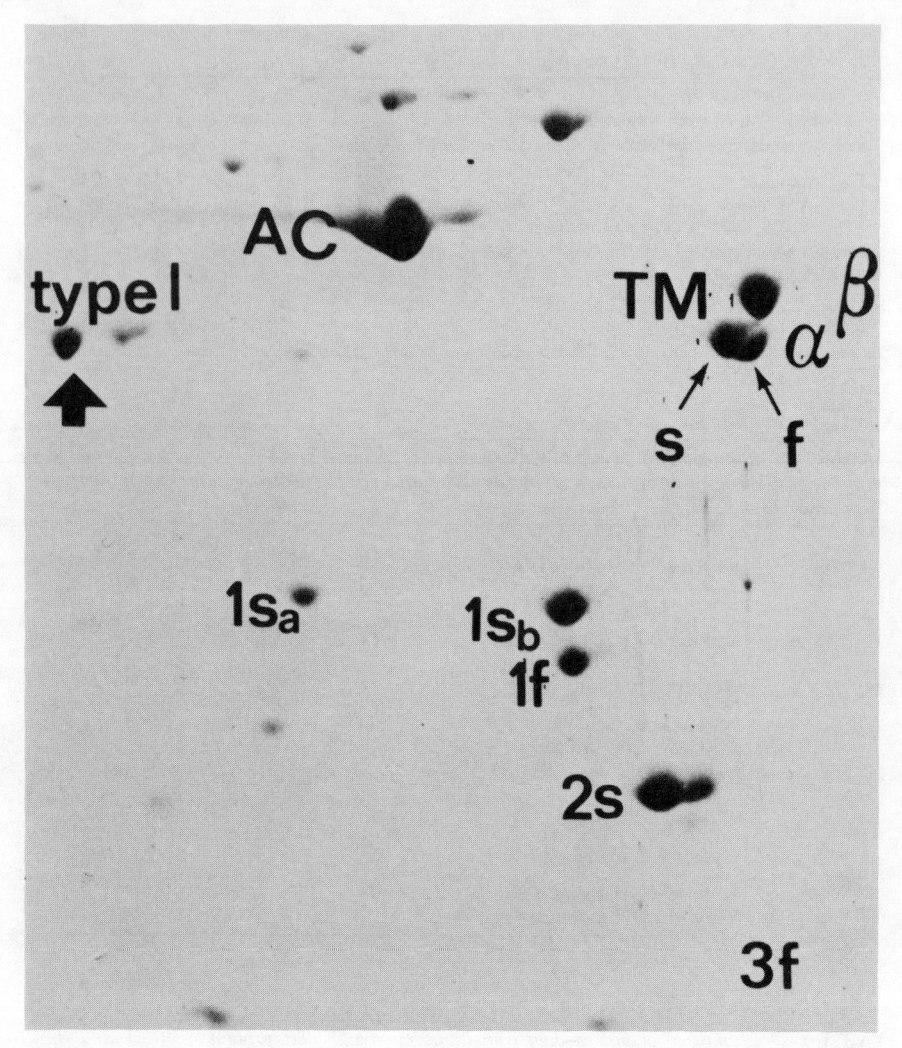

Fig. 3-1. *Two-dimensional electrophoresis of a myofibrillar extract from a 90-day continuously (24 hour day) stimulated rabbit tibialis anterior muscle. Abbreviations: AC: actin; TM: tropomyosin (α- and β-subunits), fast (f) and slow (s) isomorphs; type I: type I protein; 1f, 3f: fast type (alkali) myosin light chains; 1sa, 1sb, 2s: slow type myosin light chains.*

and tropomyosin) are not yet complete after 90 days of continuous (24 hour-a-day) stimulation (Fig. 3-1).

Molecular Mechanisms of Fast-to-Slow Transitions

The changes in expression of phenotype-specific proteins result from alterations in transcription and translation. Chronic stimulation induces pronounced elevations in total poly(A)$^+$RNA with significant increases 6 to 8 days after stimulation onset (12, 13, 24, 29, 34, 43). *In vitro* translations of poly(A)⁺RNA prepared from chronically stimulated fast-twitch muscles show that both decreases and increases in fiber type-specific myofibrillar proteins correlate with changes in the amounts of specific mRNAs. Likewise, changes in tissue levels of several other proteins (e.g., parvalbumin, type I protein, H- and M-subunits of lactate dehydrogenase, citrate synthase) are preceded by changes in the amounts of their *in vitro* translatable mRNAs (13, 24, 29, 43).

A recent study has shown drastic effects of chronic stimulation on ribosome concentration and ribosome profiles (20). Thus, increases in translational efficiency and capacity appear to precede changes in transcriptional activity. Stimulation for 1 to 2 days greatly enhances the assembly of monosomes from existing precursors. Pronounced increases in total RNA and ribosome concentration occur after 4 days' stimulation, with maximal increases between 14 and 21 days (fourfold increase in monosomes, sixfold increase in polysomes).

Fast-to-Slow Fiber Type Conversion

It appears that the changes induced by chronic stimulation of fast-twitch muscle point to the transformation of fast-twitch, fatiguable into slow-twitch, fatigue-resistant fibers. Indeed, qualitative histochemical findings support this notion of fiber type transformation. Thus, the fiber population in chronically stimulated muscle appears homogeneous with regard to high activities of succinate dehydrogenase (31-33) or low myofibrillar actomyosin ATPase typical of type I fibers (3, 27, 30, 36). However, the resolution of these qualitative histochemical methods is insufficient to establish whether a complete and homogeneous transformation of fiber types has occurred.

Quantitative single fiber analyses have confirmed the marked increases in enzymes of aerobic-oxidative metabolism but, additionally, have demonstrated the persistence of a pronounced heterogeneity (3). Moreover, the absolute activity levels of these enzymes in long-term stimulated muscles exceed those in normal slow-twitch muscles (3, 29, 35). Likewise, the fractional volume of total mitochondria in 28-day-stimulated fast-twitch muscle (20%) attains values more characteristic of cardiac than of red, slow-twitch muscle (35). Therefore, chronic stimulation appears to creat a metabolically super-red muscle.

Analyses of myofibrillar peptide patterns (Fig. 3-1) indicate that long-term chronic stimulation does not accomplish a complete fast-to-slow transformation of the myofibrillar apparatus. Although proteins typical of type I fibers are induced after long-term stimulation (e.g., type I protein, slow type myosin light chains, slow type α-subunit of tropomyosin), some proteins characteristic of type II fibers persist (e.g., fast type myosin light chains LC1f and LC3f, fast type α-subunit of tropomyosin). This incomplete transformation may result from an insufficient duration of stimulation. However, it is more likely that altered enzyme activity and isozyme patterns and atypical combinations of fast and slow type myofibrillar proteins represent a specific response to the applied work load in the fast-twitch muscle stimulated at low frequency. The appearance of these atypical fibers indicates that muscle fibers are capable of a large variety of adaptations by multiple altered gene expressions. This suggests a spectrum of fiber types in chronically stimulated muscle, representing various transitional states between the two major fiber populations (type I and type II). Consequently, classification of fiber types in chronically stimulated muscle may not be feasible using categories derived by qualitative histochemistry from normal muscles.

Fiber Transformation versus Fiber Replacement

There is strong evidence that most changes induced by chronic stimulation are due to conversions of existing fibers. However, recent analyses indicate that chronic stimulation can cause fiber degeneration and regeneration (7), predominantly affecting the fast-twitch glycolytic fibers. These fibers, perhaps unable to withstand sustained contractile activity, deteriorate soon after the onset of stimulation and are replaced by new fibers originating from proliferating satellite cells. The occurence of regeneration is supported by the appearance of the MB-heterodimer of creatine kinase in short-term (8-day) stimulated fast-twitch muscle (unpublished observations).

Chronic Stimulation versus Endurance Training

Prolonged endurance training in humans and experimental animals may lead to changes similar to, although quantitatively less pronounced than, those observed in chronically stimulated fast-twitch muscle. An increase in slow-twitch (type I) fibers has been observed by several authors in human (1, 10, 16, 18, 19, 40, 41) and rat (8, 9, 25) muscles in response to prolonged endurance training. In addition, Green et al. have recently demonstrated that long-term, high-intensity running is capable of inducing a whole set of fast-to-slow transitions in rat muscle. These changes occurred to a lesser degree than in chronically stimulated rabbit muscles, but were similar in sequentially affecting the sarcoplasmic reticulum, parvalbumin content, enzymes of energy metabolism, and the myosin light chain pattern (8, 9). It is likely, therefore, that increased contractile activity, whether induced by chronic nerve stimulation or by increased physiological locomotion, represents a common trigger for white-to-red and fast-to-slow conversions. Because fast-twitch fibers have a higher energy cost for contractile work than slow-twitch fibers (4), this type of adaptation seems to represent the ultimate response of fast-twitch muscle to sustained activity. Therefore, the stepwise fast-to-slow conversions may represent adaptive responses providing conditions which are energetically more suitable for sustained contractile activity.

CONCLUSIONS

Although increased work loads may cause isolated fiber damage, most muscle fibers are able to adapt. Thus, contractile activity appears to be a major factor in controlling the expression of phenotype-specific properties of the muscle fiber. In view of this, the changes in phenotypic expression represent a set of specific responses to increased use. These changes are brought about by altered transcriptional and translational activities and affect the major functional systems of the muscle fiber in a time-ordered sequence. This sequence points to the existence of different thresholds and indicates that muscle fibers may respond in a graded manner to best meet their functional demands. The changes induced by low frequency chronic stimulation include the appearance of atypical patterns of metabolic enzyme activities and atypical combinations of myofibrillar proteins. These may be regarded as special adaptations to this type of increased activity and probably reflect only a portion of possible responses. Above all, these adaptations emphasize the pronounced plasticity of skeletal muscle fibers.

REFERENCES

1. Andersen, P., and J. Henriksson. Training induced changes in the subgroups of human type II skeletal muscle fibres. *Acta Physiol. Scand.* 99:123–125, 1977.
2. Brown, W. E., S. Salmons, and R. G. Whalen. The sequential replacement of myosin subunit isoforms during muscle type transformation induced by long term electrical stimulation. *J. Biol. Chem.* 258:14686–14692, 1983.
3. Buchegger, A., P. M. Nemeth, D. Pette, and H. Reichmann. Effects of chronic stimulation on the metabolic heterogeneity of the fibre population in rabbit tibialis anterior muscle. *J. Physiol.* (Lond.) 350:109–119, 1984.
4. Crow, M., and M. J. Kushmerick. Chemical energetics of slow- and fast-twitch muscles of the mouse. *J. Gen. Physiol.* 79:147–166, 1982.
5. Eisenberg, B. R., J. M. C. Brown, and S. Salmons. Restoration of fast muscle characteristics following cessation of chronic stimulation. *Cell Tissue Res.* 238:221–230, 1984.
6. Eisenberg, B. R., and S. Salmons. The reorganization of subcellular structure in muscle undergoing fast-to-slow type transformation. *Cell Tissue Res.* 220:449–471, 1981.
7. Gambke, B., A. Maier, and D. Pette. Transformation and/or replacement of fibres in chronically stimulated fast-twitch rabbit muscle. *J. Physiol.* (Lond.) 361:33P, 1985.
8. Green, H. J., G. A. Klug, H. Reichmann, U. Seedorf, W. Wiehrer and D. Pette. Exercise-induced fibre type transitions with regard to myosin, parvalbumin, and sarcoplasmic reticulum in muscles of the rat. *Pflügers Arch.* 400:432–438, 1984.
9. Green, H. J., H. Reichmann, and D. Pette. Fiber type specific transformations in the enzyme activity pattern of rat vastus lateralis muscle by prolonged endurance training. *Pflügers Arch.* 399:216–222, 1983.
10. Green, H. J., J. A. Thompson, W. D. Daub, M. E. Houston, and D. A. Ranney. Fiber composition, fiber size, and enzyme activities in vastus lateralis of elite athletes involved in high intensity exercise. *Eur. J. Appl. Physiol.* 41:109–117, 1979.
11. Heilig, A., and D. Pette. Changes induced in the enzyme activity pattern by electrical stimulation of fast-twitch muscle. In: *Plasticity of Muscle*, D. Pette. (ed.) 409–420. Berlin, New York: de Gruyter, 1980.
12. Heilig, A., and D. Pette. Changes in transcriptional activity of chronically stimulated fast twitch muscle. *FEBS Lett.* 151:211–214, 1983.
13. Heilig, A., U. Seedorf, and D. Pette. Appearance of type-I-protein and its mRNA in rabbit fast-twitch muscle as induced by chronic stimulation. *J. Muscle Res.* Cell Motil., (in press).
14. Heilmann, C., W. Müller, and D. Pette. Correlation between ultrastructural and functional changes in sarcoplasmic reticulum during chronic stimulation of fast muscle. *J. Membr. Biol.* 59:143–149, 1981.
15. Heilmann, C., and D. Pette. Molecular transformations in sarcoplasmic reticulum of fast-twitch muscle by electro-stimulation. *Eur. J. Biochem.* 93:437–446, 1979.
16. Howald, H. Training-induced morphological and functional changes in skeletal muscle. *Int. J. Sports Med.* 3:1–12, 1982.
17. Hudlická, O., M. Brown, M. Cotter, M. Smith, and G. Vrbová. The effect of long-term stimulation of fast muscles on their blood flow, metabolism and ability to withstand fatigue. *Pflügers Arch.* 369:141–149, 1977.
18. Ingjer, F. Effects of endurance training on muscle fibre ATPase activity, capillary supply and mitochondrial content in man. *J. Physiol.* (Lond.) 294:419–432, 1979.
19. Jansson, E., B. Sjödin, and P. Tesch. Changes in muscle fibre type distribution in man after physical training. *Acta Physiol. Scand.* 104:235–237, 1978.
20. Kirschbaum, B., U. Seedorf, and D. Pette. Effects of chronic stimulation upon the translational apparatus in rabbit fast twitch muscle. *Biochem. J.* (in press).
21. Klug, G. A., M. Houston, J. T. Stull, and D. Pette. Effect of chronic stimulation upon the characteristics of myosin phosphorylation. *Med. Sci. Sports Exerc.* 17:234, (Abst.) 1985.
22. Klug, G., W. Wiehrer, H. Reichmann, E. Leberer, and D. Pette. Relationships between early alterations in parvalbumins, sarcoplasmic reticulum and metabolic enzymes in chronically stimulated fast twitch muscle. *Pflügers Arch.* 399:280–284, 1983.
23. Leberer, E., K. T. Härtner, and D. Pette. Reduced specific activity of sarcoplasmic reticulum Ca^{2+}-ATPase in stimulated rabbit muscle. *J. Muscle Res.* Cell Motil. (in press).
24. Leberer, E., U. Seedorf, G. Klug, and D. Pette. Parvalbumin levels and *in vitro* translation of its mRNA in chronically stimulated rabbit muscle. *J. Muscle Res.* Cell Motil. 6:84, 1985.
25. Luginbuhl, A. J., G. A. Dudley, and R. S. Staron. Fiber type changes in rat skeletal muscle after intense interval training. *Histochemistry* 81:55–58, 1984.
26. Mabuchi, K., D. Szvetko, K. Pinter, and F. A. Sréter. Type IIB to IIA fiber transformation in intermittently stimulated rabbit muscles. *Am. J. Physiol.* 242:C373–C381, 1982.
27. Pette, D. Activity-induced fast to slow transitions in mammalian muscle. *Med. Sci. Sports Exerc.* 16:517–528, 1984.
28. Pette, D. Regulation of phenotype expression in skeletal muscle fibers by increased contractile

activity. In: *Biochemistry of Exercise*, Vol. 14, B. Saltin (ed.) Champaign: Human Kinetics Publishers, (in press).
29. Pette, D., A. Heilig, G. Klug, H. Reichmann, U. Seedorf, and W. Wiehrer. Alterations in phenotype expression of muscle by chronic nerve stimulation. In: *Gene Expression in Muscle*, R. C. Strohman and S. Wolf (eds.) 169–178. New York: Plenum Press, 1985.
30. Pette, D., W. Müller, E. Leisner, and G. Vrbová. Time dependent effects on contractile properties, fibre population, myosin light chains and enzymes of energy metabolism in intermittently and continuously stimulated fast twitch muscles of the rabbit. *Pflügers Arch.* 364:103–112, 1976.
31. Pette, D., B. U. Ramirez, W. Müller, R. Simon, G. U. Exner, and R. Hildebrand. Influence of intermittent long-term stimulation on contractile, histochemical and metabolic properties of fibre populations in fast and slow rabbit muscles. *Pflügers Arch.* 361:1–7, 1975.
32. Pette, D., M. E. Smith, H. W. Staudte, and G. Vrbová. Effects of long-term electrical stimulation on some contractile and metabolic characteristics of fast rabbit muscles. *Pflügers Arch.* 338:257–272, 1973.
33. Pette, D., H. W. Staudte, and G. Vrbová. Physiological and biochemical changes induced by long-term stimulation of fast muscle. *Naturwissenschaften* 59:469–470, 1972.
34. Pluskal, M. G., and F. A. Sréter. Correlation between protein phenotype and gene expression in adult rabbit fast twitch muscles undergoing a fast to slow fiber transformation in response to electrical stimulation *in vivo*. *Biochem. Biophys. Res. Comm.* 113:325–331, 1983.
35. Reichmann, H., H. Hoppeler, O. Mathieu-Costello, F. von Bergen, and D. Pette. Biochemical and ultrastructural changes of skeletal muscle mitochondria after chronic electrical stimulation in rabbits. *Pflügers Arch.* 404:1–9, 1985.
36. Roy, R. K., K. Mabuchi, S. Sarkar, C. Mis, and F. A. Sréter. Changes in tropomyosin subunit pattern in chronic electrically stimulated rabbit fast muscles. *Biochem. Biophys. Res. Comm.* 89:181–187, 1979.
37. Salmons, S., and F. A. Sréter. Significance of impulse activity in the transformation of skeletal muscle type. *Nature* (Lond.) 263:30–34, 1976.
38. Salmons, S., and G. Vrbová. The influence of activity on some contractile characteristics of mammalian fast and slow muscles. *J. Physiol.* (Lond.) 210:535–549, 1969.
39. Sarzala, M. G., G. Szymanska, W. Wiehrer, and D. Pette. Effects of chronic stimulation at low frequency on the lipid phase of sarcoplasmic reticulum in rabbit fast-twitch muscle. *Eur. J. Biochem.* 123:241-245, 1982.
40. Schantz, P., R. Billeter, J. Henriksson, and E. Jansson. Training-induced increase in myofibrillar ATPase intermediate fibers in human skeletal muscle. *Muscle Nerve* 5:628–636, 1982.
41. Schantz, P., and J. Henriksson. Increases in myofibrillar ATPase intermediate human skeletal muscle fibers in response to endurance training. *Muscle Nerve* 6:553–556, 1983.
42. Schmitt, T., and D. Pette. Increased mitochondrial creatine kinase in chronically stimulated fast-twitch rabbit muscle. *FEBS Lett.* 188:341-344, 1985.
43. Seedorf, U., E. Leberer, and D. Pette. *In vitro* translation of mRNAs coding for citrate synthetase and lactate dehydrogenase isozymes in chronically stimulated rabbit muscle. *J. Muscle Res. Cell. Motil.* 6:85, 1985.
44. Seedorf, K., and D. Pette. Coordinate expression of alkali and DTNB myosin light chains during transformation of rabbit fast muscle by chronic stimulation. *FEBS Lett.* 158:321–324, 1983.
45. Sréter, F. A., J. Gergely, S. Salmons, and F. C. A. Romanul. Synthesis by fast muscle of myosin characteristic of slow muscle in response to long term stimulation. *Nature New Biol.* (Lond.) 241:17–19, 1973.

4

Muscle Injury and Repair in Ultra-Long Distance Runners

ARTHUR J. SIEGEL, M.D.

Brigham & Women's Hospital

MICHAEL J. WARHOL, M.D.

Brigham & Women's Hospital

GILBERT LANG, M.D.

Roosevelt Community Hospital

INTRODUCTION

A body of scientific knowledge in exercise physiology documents the sequence of adaptive or positive changes in skeletal muscle with endurance training. The basic metabolic response is enhanced utilization of alternate fuels as sources of ATP to conserve limited but essential stores of intracellular glycogen on which work capacity is dependent. Recent investigations of muscular over-use syndromes in athletes document release of intracellular enzymes as markers of exertional rhabdomyolysis. High resolution electron microscopy of skeletal muscle of long-distance runners shows focal or segmental myofibrillar damage in glycogen-depleted fibers. The mechanism for focal injury is metabolic and leads to a regenerative response through activation of satellite cells.

Repetitive injury, as occurs with the intense endurance training of ultra-long distance runners, leads to micro-fibrosis, the functional significance of which is yet to be determined. Elevated levels of the MB isoenzyme of creatine kinase in trained skeletal muscle may be based upon the persistent presence of regenerating muscle fibers.

Manuscript correspondence should be addressed to Dr. Siegel at Hahnemann Hospital, 1515 Commonwealth Avenue, Brighton, MA 02135.
Janice Murphy provided technical assistance in the preparation of this manuscript.

MUSCLE METABOLISM DURING EXERCISE: POSITIVE ADAPTATIONS

Several decades of research in muscle physiology have informed us about the adaptations which enhance exercise capacity (10). An increase in capillary fiber ratio with augmented muscle myoglobin content enhances delivery and capture of oxygen from the circulation at the cellular level. A sequence of specific biochemical alterations within the cell enhances the oxidation of circulating fuels (glucose, ketones, free fatty acids) to conserve essential intracellular carbohydrate stores (5, 11). The fundamental metabolic training response is enhancement of oxidative phosphorylation to augment the regeneration rate of ATP. Perhaps the most recent and elegant manifestation of the response of muscle fibers to training is the work by Pette and collaborators showing the alteration of muscle fiber types with exercise as a stimulus to the high oxidative histochemical profile (14). The pattern of fuel utilization during prolonged strenuous exercise is shown in Fig. 4-1 (5). This highlights the importance of alternate fuels late in exercise while stressing the obligatory high rate of glycogen utilization at the onset of exercise and its contribution throughout continuous muscular work. The rate of glycogen utilization is dependent upon training, as discussed above, and increases with exercise intensity at any given level of training. Glycogen depletion marks the onset of muscle fatigue, which is dependent on intensity and duration of work performed. The quantitative analysis of fuel utilization suggests that any muscle

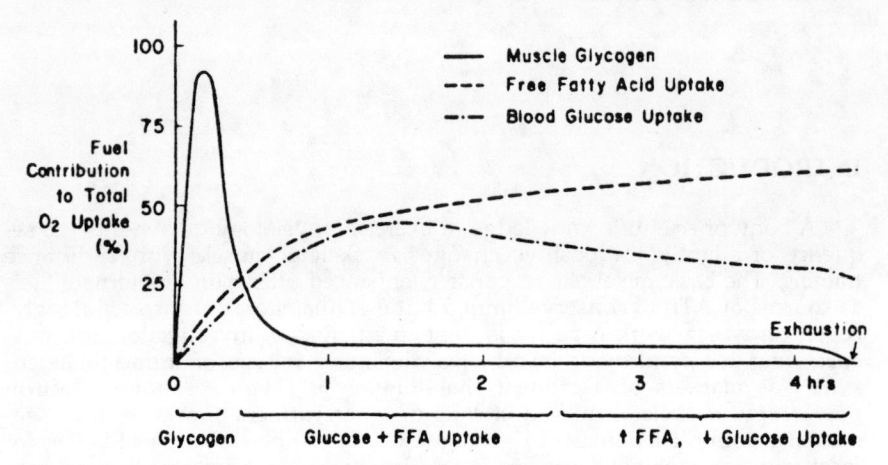

Fig. 4-1. Triphasic response of body fuels to acute exercise. During the first few minutes of exercise, breakdown of muscle glycogen is the major source of ATP for contracting muscle. As exercise extends beyond 10 min, blood-borne fuels in the form of glucose and free fatty acids become increasingly important. As exercise extends beyond 90–120 min (e.g., in marathon runners), there is an increasing dependence on fat and lesser uptake of glucose. Muscle glycogen contributes a small proportion of the fuel requirements even in prolonged exercise, and its depletion is associated with exhaustion. Not shown is the small contribution of body protein breakdown to total fuel utilization in prolonged exercise (generally <5–10% of total caloric utilization).

From: Felig, P. Metabolic and endocrine disorders and exercise. *Exercise Medicine: Physiological Principles and Clinical Application*, 305–320. New York: Academic Press, 1983. With permission.

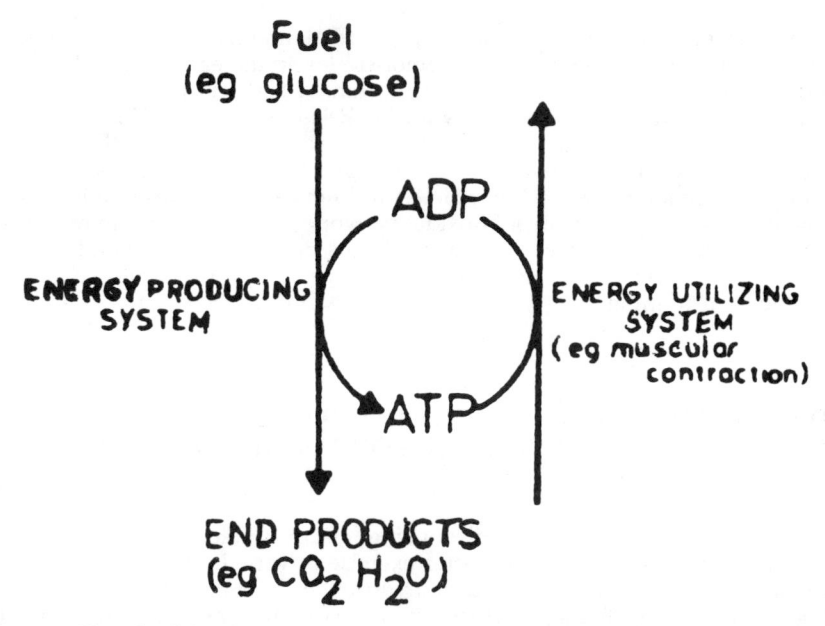

Fig. 4-2. *The role of the ATP/ADP couple in energy transfer to the muscle. The ATP/ADP concentration ratio remains remarkably constant under very different conditions of steady-state flux. There is no store of energy in this system, so that a change in rate of utilization of ATP must cause the same change in rate of production.*

(Reprinted from *Ann. N.Y. Acad. Sci.* 301:82, 1977 with permission of the author and editor.)

or fiber exercised at a sufficient time-intensity level will experience glycogen depletion, after which levels of ATP are insufficient to maintain work efficiency. The delicate balance of oxidative phosphorylation linking energy use to production (Fig. 4-2) is overthrown.

INJURY THRESHOLD ENERGY IMBALANCE AND ENZYME RELEASE

Observations of delayed onset of muscle soreness with modest exercise (especially eccentric) in untrained subjects (13) and muscular overuse syndromes in trained athletes suggest muscle injury related to physical activity (4, 8). Measurements of total serum creatine kinase after a variety of exercise stimuli confirm release of intracellular enzymes into serum, indicating at least transient muscle fiber damage (8, 17). This suggests a susceptibility to transient injury on a continuum from untrained to elite muscle tissue at the threshold of unaccustomed work stress. The eccentric training models suggest a component of biomechanical stress as a contributor to the fiber damage. Muscular overuse syndromes in endurance-trained athletes such as long distance runners are accompanied by marked elevations in serum levels of the MB isoenzyme of creatine kinase (CK) (1, 16). Serum levels of CK-MB in asymptomatic marathon runners after competition are quantitatively similar to peak levels in patients with acute myocardial infarction (3, 15). Biochemical analysis of trained skeletal muscle demonstrates an increase in CK-MB content with training (8 to 10% of total creatine kinase activity) in contrast to trace amounts in untrained or sedentary adult skeletal muscle (2, 15).

The basis for the increase in skeletal muscle content of CK-MB with training might reflect its selective concentration in high oxidative fibers, which are known to predominate in elite athletes and hence to be a positive isoenzyme change reflecting a high level of oxidative work (18). The alternate hypothesis is that CK-MB is a marker for the persistent presence of regenerating fibers due to ongoing exercise-related injury and repair (15). This would validate the well known training adage, "NO STRAIN, NO GAIN!"

HIGH RESOLUTION ELECTRON MICROSCOPY: MORPHOLOGICAL EVIDENCE FOR FOCAL MYOFIBRILLAR INJURY AND REPAIR

Recent morphological studies using electron microscopy document a spectrum of muscle fiber injury after exercise of varied intensity. Modest levels of eccentric exercise may lead to myofibrillar disarray with Z band streaming in untrained subjects (6). Muscle biopsy studies in marathon runners after competition show greater degrees of focal muscle fiber damage including segmental myofibrillar lysis, dilatation and disruption of the T-tubule system, and focal mitochondrial degeneration (9, 20). Such injury is selective for fibers showing evidence of glycogen depletion and occurs segmentally rather than uniformly within the cell. A correlation of injury with glycogen depletion and the minor component of capillary damage suggests a metabolic rather than hypoxic basis for muscular damage. Continued demand for physical work after glycogen depletion places the muscle fiber under a metabolic stress similar to the exercise-related injury in muscle phosphorylase deficiency (12).

Studies in marathon runners using sequential biopsies over several weeks following a race document repair of myofibrillar damage associated with an increase in satellite cells (20). This sequence of injury and repair reflects the peak in release of CK-MB and a return to basal but persistently elevated levels during continued training. The focal nature of injury and repair with a documented regenerative response accounts for the transient release of intracellular enzymes from reversibly injured cells without cell death and scarring as occurs in vascular occlusion injury. The capacity of genetically normal skeletal muscle tissue to repair does not imply cellular dropout with advancing age as has been postulated for the decline in peak muscle function as part of the aging process (7).

ULTRA-MARATHON RUNNERS' STUDY

Participants in this study included 4 men and 1 woman who qualified for the 1984 Western States 100-Mile Run by completing a 50-mile certified race in less than 10 hours. These runners averaged 70 miles per week in training for the year preceding this race and completed an average of 3 standard marathons (26.2 miles) in the year prior to this event. The ages of subjects ranged from 34 to 61 years (mean = 49 years), as shown in Table 4-1.

TABLE 4-1. *Western States' 100-mile Ultra-marathon runners' biopsy study.*

SUBJECT # AGE	1 46	2 61 (F)	3 34	4 34	5 46	NORMAL VALUES	AVERAGE 49
Finishing Time	27:38	29:19	27:46	21:07	22:58		22:45
Total CK	1806	2457	2604	9702	12558	28–100 CNU	5830
CK MB	90	147	130	485	819	5 CNU	335
% MB	5	6	5	5	7	3%	5.6
CK MB (IMMUNO-ASSAY)	36.0	86.0	38.0	336.0	652.0	0–9.0 ng/ml	230

The 1984 Western States 100 Race was run on July 7 and 8, from Squaw Valley to Auburn, California, including an ascent of 5,179 meters (m) to the highest elevation of 2,918 m with a subsequent descent of 6,618 m to the finish. This trans-Sierra ultra-run tranverses a mountain path with intermittent snow at the highest elevations followed by desert with temperatures approaching 41° C on the day of the race.

All runners completed the 160-kilometer (Km) race within the 30-hour cut-off limit and were free of acute cardiorespiratory symptoms. Runners participated in the serum and biopsy studies after appropriate informed consent.

Methods

Serum samples for creatine kinase isoenzyme analysis were obtained within 24 hours of completing the race, which approximates the peak in serum CK activity in marathon runners after competition. Samples were frozen and stored at −20° C until the time of enzyme analysis. Total CK activity was determined on a kinetic enzyme analyzer using optimized CK substrate reagent. Isoenzyme fractionation was done by agarose electrophoresis after appropriate dilution of total enzyme activity to the optimal range for the assay. Normal ranges for total CK and CK-MB in this laboratory are 28 to 100 and less than 3 Iu/ml, respectively. In addition, CK-MB was measured by radioimmunoassay to determine absolute concentration and a relative index.

Percutaneous needle biopsies of the lateral gastrocnemius muscle were performed by the Bergstrom technique. The biopsy specimen was immediately fixed in half-strength Karnovsky's fixative. The tissue was then postfixed in osmium tetroxide, dehydrated in alcohol, and embedded in Epon. Thick sections (1 micron) were stained with toluidine blue for selection of areas for thin sectioning. Thin sections were stained with uranyl acetate and lead citrate, and examined on a JOEL EM-100 microscope. A minimum of 20 fibers were examined from each sample.

Results

Serum values for total creatine kinase and the MB isoenzyme for the runners are shown in Table 4-1. The mean total creatine kinase activity was 5,830 Iu/dl, or roughly 58 times the upper limits of normal. The mean CK-MB by agarose electrophoresis was 335 Iu/dl, accounting for 5.6% of total creatine kinase activity. CK-MB measured by radioimmunoassay was 239 ng/ml, comparable in magnitude to the elevation as measured by conventional electrophoresis.

The ultra-structural appearance of skeletal muscle obtained from the 5 runners on the day following the race was assessed for morphologic markers of injury and repair. Selected fibers showed evidence of light staining due to depletion of intercellular glycogen together with intracellular edema (Fig. 4-3). These substrate-depleted fibers showed evidence of myofibrillar lysis with focal injury to the sarcoplasmic reticulum (Fig. 4-3b). Mitochondrial damage was also manifested by dissolution of cristae and loss of mitochondrial matrix (Fig. 4-3a). Also noted was focal damage to capillary endothelial cells with loss of cytoplasmic substance and the formation of intracellular myelin fibers (Fig. 4-3c).

Qualitative comparison of these markers of acute injury to marathon runners after competition showed a lesser degree of myofibrillar damage. Less than 5% of fibers showed definite focal injury in comparison to roughly 20% of fibers in marathon runners as estimated semi-quantitatively.

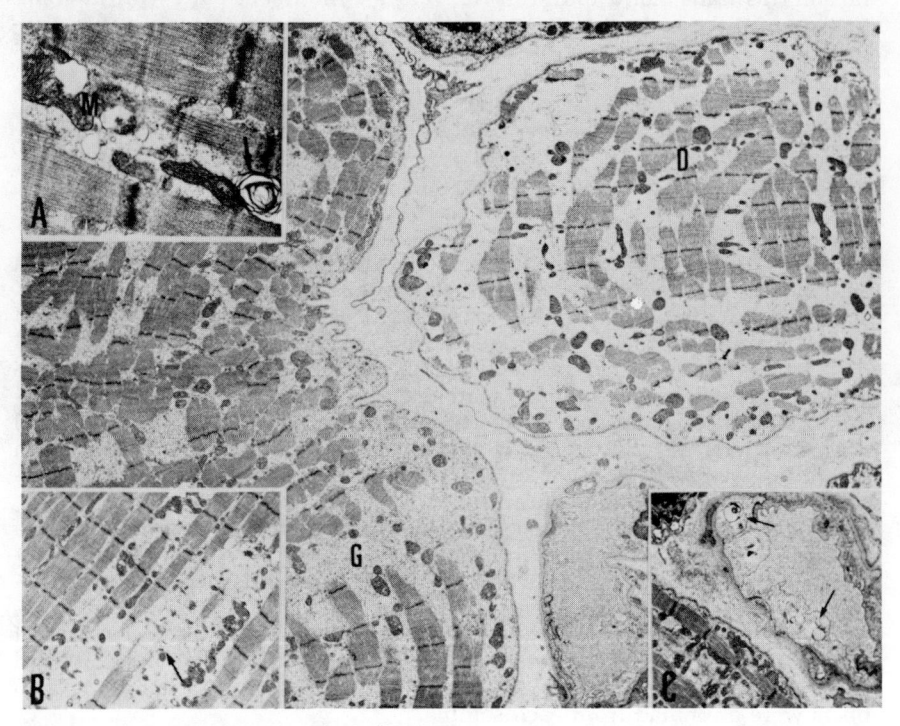

Fig. 4-3. *A low power electron micrograph of two muscle fibers. One fiber (G) has a normal content of glycogen and has largely intact myofibrils. The other "pale" fiber (D) is depleted of glycogen and exhibits intra-cellular edema. (×2,000)*
A. Mitochondrial injury with both lysis of mitochondrial matrix (M), and the formation of intra-mitochondrial myelin figures. (×10,000)
B. A glycogen-depleted fiber with myofibrillar lysis and dilatation of sarcoplasmic reticulum. (arrow) (×2,000)
C. A capillary with injury to one endothelial cell characterized by loss of cytoplasmic density and the formation of intracellular myelin figures. (arrow) (×2,000)

In addition to focal injury, all 5 biopsies from these ultra-long distance runners showed simultaneous evidence for fiber regeneration and repair. Satellite cells, the presumed precursor of skeletal muscle cells, were prominent in these biopsies as a marker for the reparative response to prior injury (Fig. 4-4, inset). These cells can be recognized because of their characteristic location immediately outside the basal lamina of the muscle cells. These satellite cells showed many polysomes and the development of endoplasmic reticulum (Fig. 4-4), the morphologic markers of "metabolically active" cells with high rates of protein synthesis. This evidence of regenerative activity was similar to findings in marathon runners observed 10 to 12 weeks after competition. Findings in these ultramarathon runners showed concurrent injury and repair, reflecting the higher level of training intensity engaged in by these athletes. The post-race regenerative changes reflect a reparative response to injury occurring during long distance training weeks prior to the time of the 100-mile run.

These electron microscopic findings in ultra-long distance runners show a balanced process of injury and repair. In addition, there was evidence of ongoing cell injury in variable amounts of interstitial collagen deposition (Fig. 4-4). Capillaries also displayed the markers of previous injury, such as lipofuchsin deposition in endothelial cells and thickening of basal lamina. Collagen deposition was particularly prominent in a perivascular distribution. Similar findings of micro-fibrosis were evident only in selected marathon run-

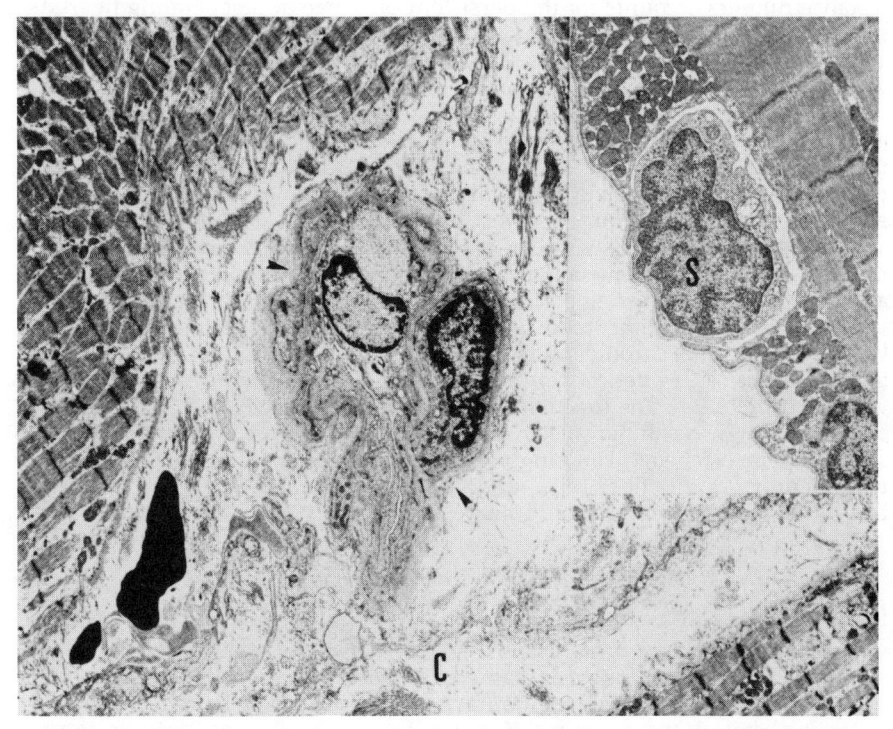

Fig. 4-4. *The changes of chronic injury. There are numerous collagen fibers (C) in the interstitial space. The capillary basal lamina is thickened and irregular. (arrowheads) (×4,000). Inset— Satellite cells (S), located inside the basal lamina were a prominent feature of these biopsies. (×8,000)*

ners who had been competing at high intensity over long periods of time. None of the biopsy specimens revealed evidence of cellular inflammation, as has been variably noted in other studies (9).

Discussion

While the sample size reported in this study is limited, the serologic and morphologic findings suggest a balanced process of injury and repair in endurance-trained skeletal muscle. Peak levels in serum CK-MB measured 24 hours after the race by agarose and immunoelectrophoresis confirm isoenzyme levels quantitatively similar to those in patients undergoing acute myocardial infarction (3, 15). Previous studies confirm negative myocardial infarction avid scintigraphy using technitium pyrophosphate and evidence for quadriceps muscle damage by this same radionucleide technique (16).

The morphologic evidence of glycogen depletion in selected fibers associated with focal myofibrillar injuries is consistent with substrate depletion as the basis for metabolic injury to fibers on a focal basis. Earlier studies of marathon runners showed normal morphology prior to the race, acute injury in the days and weeks following a marathon, and regenerative changes in the 10-to-12-week time frame. Biopsies performed one day after a 160 km run showed the sequence of changes reported in marathon runners telescoped into a single time frame. The intensity and duration of training in ultra-long distance runners accounts for the persistent presence of regenerating fibers as the basis for elevations in serum CK-MB. Direct biochemical measurement of CK-MB in skeletal muscle tissue, as reported in marathon runners, was not attempted in these subjects, however.

Developing or fetal skeletal muscle tissue is known to be rich in the MB isoenzyme of creatine kinase (19), perhaps on the basis of a metabolic advantage. An increase in tissue skeletal muscle CK-MB occurs in various myopathic states, (12) consistent with this isoenzyme as a marker of the regenerating fiber. Ongoing injury and repair in skeletal muscle might then lead to an increase in CK-MB, as has been reported in dystrophies, myopathies, and myositis. The combined metabolic and biochemical stress placed upon normal adult skeletal muscle during prolonged strenuous training can lead to a similar balanced process of injury and repair, as seen in these specimens. Morphological evidence for chronic injury was also identified in these ultra-long distance runners, as evidenced by inter-cellular collagen deposition in a perivascular distribution. The functional or clinical significance of such microfibrosis as seen by high resolution electron microscopy is as yet unknown. Further studies on the biochemical and morphological changes in trained skeletal muscle may identify specific fiber types at risk and lead to strategies for protecting this tissue from exercise-related injury.

SUMMARY

Much information has been gathered in recent years about the muscular overuse syndrome in endurance-trained athletes, especially long-distance runners. Biochemical and morphological evidence supports focal muscle injury on the basis of metabolic substrate depletion during prolonged strenuous training and competition. Studies in long-distance runners show a balanced process of injury and repair resulting in micro-fibrosis seen on a high resolution electron microscopic level. Similar biochemical and morphological evidence for muscle fiber injury has been reported in untrained subjects after unaccustomed exercise, suggesting a continuum of muscle fiber injury and repair as an adaptation to muscular work at each stage of endurance participation and training. The findings in long-distance runners suggest that injury and repair is a background dynamic essential to improved exercise performance.

On a simpler level, these findings merely provide a morphological and biochemical correlate to the athletes' appreciation of the training adage, "NO STRAIN, NO GAIN!" This translates into the need for adequate rest and recovery as key components of any intense training program. The more intense the training, the greater the need for a phase of rest and recovery. Future investigations in single fiber type susceptibilities to fatigue may provide breakthroughs in enhancement of endurance performance.

REFERENCES

1. Apple, G. S., and M. K. McGue. Serum enzyme changes during marathon training. *Am. J. Clin. Pathol.* 79:716–719, 1983.
2. Apple, F. S., M. A. Rogers, W. M. Sherman, D. L. Costill, F. C. Hagerman, and J. L. Ivy. Profile of creatine kinase isoenzymes in skeletal muscles of marathon runners. *Clin. Chem.* 30:413–416, 1984.
3. Apple, F. S., M. A. Rogers, W. M. Sherman, and J. L. Ivy. Comparison of serum creatine kinase and creatine kinase MB activities post marathon race versus post myocardial infarction. *Clin. Chem. Acta* 138:111–118, 1984.
4. Dressendorfer, R. H., and C. E. Wade. The muscular overuse syndrome in long-distance runners. *Phys. Sportsmed.* 11:116–130, 1983.
5. Felig, P. Metabolic and endocrine disorders and exercise. In: *Exercise Medicine: Physiological Principles and Clinical Application*, 305–320. New York: Academic Press, 1983.
6. Friden, J., M. Sjostrom, and B. Ekblom. A morphologic study of delayed muscle soreness. *Experientia* 37:506–507, 1981.
7. Grimby, G., and B. Saltin. Mini Review: The ageing muscle. *Clin. Physiol.* 3:209–218, 1983.
8. Hansen, K. N., J. Bjerre-Knudsen, U. Brodthagen, R. Jordal, and P. E. Paulev. Muscle cell leakage due to long-distance training. *Eur. J. Appl. Physiol.* 48:177–188, 1982.
9. Hikida, R. S., R. S. Staron, F. C. Hagerman, W. M. Sherman, and D. L. Costill. Muscle fiber necrosis associated with human marathon runners. *J. Neurol. Sci.* 59:185–203, 1983.
10. Holloszy, J. O. Muscle metabolism during exercise. *Arch. Phys. Med. Rehab.* 63:231–234, 1982.
11. Holloszy, J. O. Adaptation of skeletal muscle to endurance exercise. *Med. Sci. Sports Exerc.* 7:155–164, 1975.
12. Layzer, R. B., and S. F. Lewis. Clinical disorders of muscle energy metabolism. *Med. Sci. Sports Exerc.* 16:451–455, 1984.
13. Newman, D. J., D. A. Jones, and R. H. T. Edwards. Large delayed plasma creatine kinase changes after stepping exercise. *Muscle Nerve* 6:380–385, 1983.
14. Pette, D. Activity-induced fast to slow transitions in mammalian muscle. *Med. Sci. Sports Exerc.* 16:517–528, 1984.
15. Siegel, A. J., L. M. Silverman, and W. J. Evans. Elevated skeletal muscle creatine kinase MB isoenzyme levels in marathon runners. *J.A.M.A.* 250:2835–2837, 1983.
16. Siegel, A. J., L. M. Silverman, and B. L. Holman. Elevated creatine kinase MB isoenzyme levels in marathon runners. *J.A.M.A.* 246:2049–2051, 1981.
17. Siegel, A. J., L. M. Silverman, and R. E. Lopez. Creatine kinase elevations in marathon runners: Relationship to training and competition. *Yale J. Biol. Med.* 53:275–279, 1980.
18. Sylven, C., E. Jansson, and C. Olin. Human myocardial and skeletal muscle enzyme activities: Creatine kinase and its isoenzyme MB as related to citrate synthesis and muscle fiber types. *Clin. Physiol.* 3:461–468, 1983.
19. Tzvetanova, E. Creatine kinase isoenzymes in muscle tissue of patients with neuromuscular diseases and human fetuses. *Enzyme* 12:279–284, 1971.
20. Warhol, M. J., A. J. Siegel, W. J. Evans, and L. M. Silverman. Skeletal muscle injury and repair in marathon runners after competition. *Am. J. Pathol.* 118:331–339, 1985.

5

Non-Invasive Measurement of Muscle in the Rehabilitation of Masters Athletes

ARCHIE YOUNG

Royal Free Hospital School of Medicine

MARIA STOKES

University of Liverpool

ABSTRACT

Objective measurements of the size, strength, and activation of individual muscles allow a rational approach to the rehabilitation of the athlete with muscle weakness after joint injury and/or immobilization. This may be of particular importance for the older athlete, whose safety margin for strength has already been eroded by an obligatory age-related atrophy.

Changes in the cross-sectional area of an individual muscle cannot be measured with a tape measure but can be measured with transverse imaging techniques, such as computerized axial x-ray tomography or compound ultrasound B-scanning. The importance of the latter is its acceptability for repeated measurements. The degree of activation achieved by a maximal voluntary effort can be quantified by integrated surface electromyography.

The repeatability of measurements made with these techniques, and with isometric dynamometry, is sufficiently good for them to be valuable clinical

---

Based on work conducted while the authors were associated with the Nuffield Departments of Orthopedic Surgery and Clinical Medicine, University of Oxford. (Dr. Stokes is now in the Department of medicine, University of Liverpool.)

Acknowledgment

We are pleased to acknowledge the collaboration of numerous co-authors in the work on which this paper is based. We also thank the Office of the Chief Scientist, Department of Health and Social Security, for financial support.

tools. Conventional age-related normal values, however, may be inappropriate for highly trained older subjects. This chapter describes how sequential and bilateral measurements may be used instead.

INTRODUCTION

Joint injury and/or immobilization results in weakness and wasting of muscles acting across the joint. Conversely, the integrity of a joint depends on the strength and function of its muscles. Any deficiency in the size, strength, or activation of a muscle may render its joints more susceptible to further injury (Fig. 5-1). There is a loss of muscle mass and, therefore, of strength with advancing age. Therefore, the masters athlete may be considered to be at increased risk of joint injury and, when injured, it is especially important that the restoration of his muscle size, strength, and activation is complete. Those responsible for the masters athlete's rehabilitation require accurate, noninvasive techniques by which to assess the severity of the problem and to follow its response, or lack of response, to treatment.

This chapter reviews the measurement of quadriceps size and strength in healthy elderly people and considers how this information may be applied to monitoring the rehabilitation of the injured masters athlete. Afferent stimuli from in and around the damaged knee inhibit both reflex and voluntary activation of the quadriceps' anterior horn cells. The chapter also describes how inhibition may be measured and suggests ways such measurements may be used to guide rehabilitative efforts.

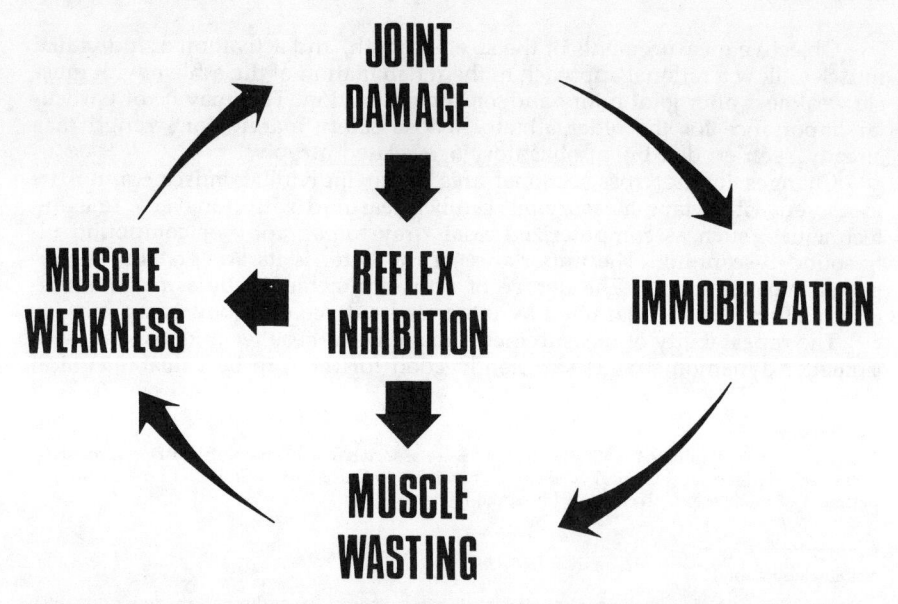

Fig. 5-1. *Vicious circles of muscle weakness following joint injury. (By permission of the Editor, Clinical Science) (25).*

QUADRICEPS STRENGTH

Cross-sectional studies suggest that over a 30-to-50-year period after their mid-20s, men and women lose isometric quadriceps strength at a rate of 0.6 to 0.9% per year (2, 11, 12, 16, 33, 34). The rate of loss of strength probably accelerates after the age of 40 and seems to be similar whether measured as isometric or isokinetic strength (12).

It is not known how much of the age-related decline in muscle strength is obligatory and how much may be ascribed to inactivity. Age-related norms are of limited value, therefore, when dealing with highly trained older adults. It is probably more useful to make repeated or bilateral measurements in the same individual. Information on the symmetry of quadriceps strength in normal subjects of different ages is, therefore, included in slightly greater detail than in our original communications (33, 34).

Symmetry

None of the healthy men and women in their 70s whom we have studied (33, 34), had had a lower limb joint immobilized for more than 1 week in the preceding 20 years. In three-quarters of the women, the left and right quadriceps differed in isometric strength by 12% or less (Table 5-1). In three-quarters of the men the difference was 16% or less. (Nevertheless, a few healthy elderly subjects had differences in strength as great as 25%).

Repeatability

The simplest way to measure quadriceps strength is to record the force exerted at the ankle during isometric contractions made with the knee flexed to 90° and the subject seated in an adjustable, straight-backed chair (6, 27). The day-to-day variability of quadriceps strength, defined as the best of at least 3 contractions on each occasion, seems to be rather similar for women in their 20s, women in their 70s, and men in their 70s (Table 5-2). Aniansson and her colleagues (1) reported a slightly greater variability for isometric contractions by 70-year-old men and women: the coefficients of variation (CV) were 12% and 14% respectively. In isokinetic contractions at different angular velocities, she reported CV = 6 to 7% and 9 to 14% respectively.

Although this degree of variability is not unacceptable, it does mean that

TABLE 5-1. *Symmetry of quadriceps strength in healthy men and women in their 20s and 70s (33, 34).*

	n	*Between-limbs difference (%)			
		Least	1st Quartile	Median	3rd Quartile	Greatest
Elderly men	12	0.3	4	7	16	25
women	25	0	2	5	12	24
Young men	12	0.7	2	7	12	15
women	25	0.3	3	5	8	13

*Between-limbs difference calculated as (greater value-lesser value) × 100/greater value.

TABLE 5-2. *Day-to-day variability of repeated measurements of isometric quadriceps strength in healthy men and women in their 70s and healthy women in their 20s (33, 34).*

	No. of Subjects	No. of Days	Coefficient of variation (%) Right	Left
Elderly men	10	3	8	8
Elderly women	12	3	8	8
	12	2	4	12
Young women	12	3	8	9
	12	2	4	3

it is not sufficient simply to make "before" and "after" measurements. A series of measurements, repeated over a period of time, is required in order to follow changes in strength with any degree of accuracy. On the other hand, it would be wise to avoid testing elderly subjects on successive days lest they show an apparent loss of strength as a result of tenderness of the semitendinosus tendon where it presses on the edge of the seat (34).

QUADRICEPS CROSS-SECTIONAL AREA

The loss of muscle cross-sectional area (CSA) with advancing age can be measured by compound ultrasound B-scanning (29, 31). Computed x-ray tomography could also be used (7). Cross-sectional studies show an average quadriceps CSA loss of 0.5 to 0.7% per year over the 50 years from the mid-20s (33, 34). This is in keeping with figures of 0.4% (from a cadaver study of vastus lateralis) (13) and 0.6% (calculated from changes in creatinine excretion) (28). In elderly women, quadriceps CSA at mid-thigh correlates significantly with body weight ($r = 0.79$) (33), but the scatter around this relationship is such that, once again, it is better to make bilateral measurements to identify asymmetry or repeated measurements to identify changes in muscle size over a period of time. (Of course, for repeated measurements, ultrasonic imaging is safer than x-ray tomography.)

Symmetry

In all 37 young adults studied (33, 34), the between-sides difference in quadriceps CSA was less than 13% of the larger muscle. This was also true of three-quarters of the elderly subjects (Table 5-3). In 37 healthy men and women in their 70s, the greatest difference in quadriceps CSA was 20% (33, 34).

To the best of my knowledge, no one has measured the disparity in quadriceps cross-sectional area between the two limbs of elderly subjects with unilateral knee injury and/or immobilization. In young subjects, differences of 30 to 50% are not uncommon (31). Because this loss of muscle bulk is virtually confined to the quadriceps, its severity is seriously underestimated by measurements of thigh circumference (31).

Circumference measurements are not even valid predictors of the severity of quadriceps wasting in the individual patient. Accurate measurement of

TABLE 5-3. *Symmetry of quadriceps CSA in healthy men and women in their 20s and in their 70s (33, 34).*

	n	Least	1st Quartile	Median	3rd Quartile	Greatest
Elderly men	12	0.4	4	9	13	18
women	25	0.8	5	9	12	20
Young men	12	0.2	1	5	7	12
women	25	0	1	4	6	12

*Between-limbs difference calculated as (greater value − lesser value) × 100/greater value.

quadriceps wasting requires a transverse imaging technique, such as compound ultrasound B-scanning or computerized x-ray tomography (9, 14).

Repeatability

The repeatability of measurements of quadriceps CSA made by compound ultrasound B-scanning at mid-thigh is good: CV = 4% (31) or less (21). The latter value was obtained by improving the accuracy with which the scanning level was relocated (by marking it on a transparent sheet on which were also mapped the positions of naevi, scars, and other skin blemishes) (5). These estimates of variability, however, were both determined with young subjects. Older subjects have smaller muscles and, since some of the technical sources of measurement error will remain unchanged, the percentage variability of repeated measurements in elderly subjects may be slightly greater.

STRENGTH/SIZE RELATIONSHIP

It seems that the relationship between the quadriceps' isometric strength and its CSA at mid-thigh is the same for healthy, untrained women in their 70s as it is for women in their 20s (33). Indeed, it is possible to use the data from these two groups of women to assess whether quadriceps weakness in a female patient aged between 20 and 80 years is commensurate with the size of her muscle (Fig. 5-2). The precise relationship may be influenced slightly by the effects of training (34) or by the choice of specialist event (15), but not sufficiently to preclude its practical clinical application.

Unfortunately, the situation is not quite as easy with male subjects. Some young men have quadriceps strength which is greater than one would have predicted from the size of the muscle had the relationship been the same as in women (Fig. 5-3) (34). In elderly men, however, the relationship appears to be the same as that which holds in women of either age (34). We do not know at what age the male relationship changes. Nor do we know the explanation for the apparent additional strength of some young men. The topic is discussed more fully elsewhere (34). Briefly, it could be an artifact of the CSA measurement technique if young male muscles have an intrinsically different shape, or it may reflect differences in fiber-type composition (30).

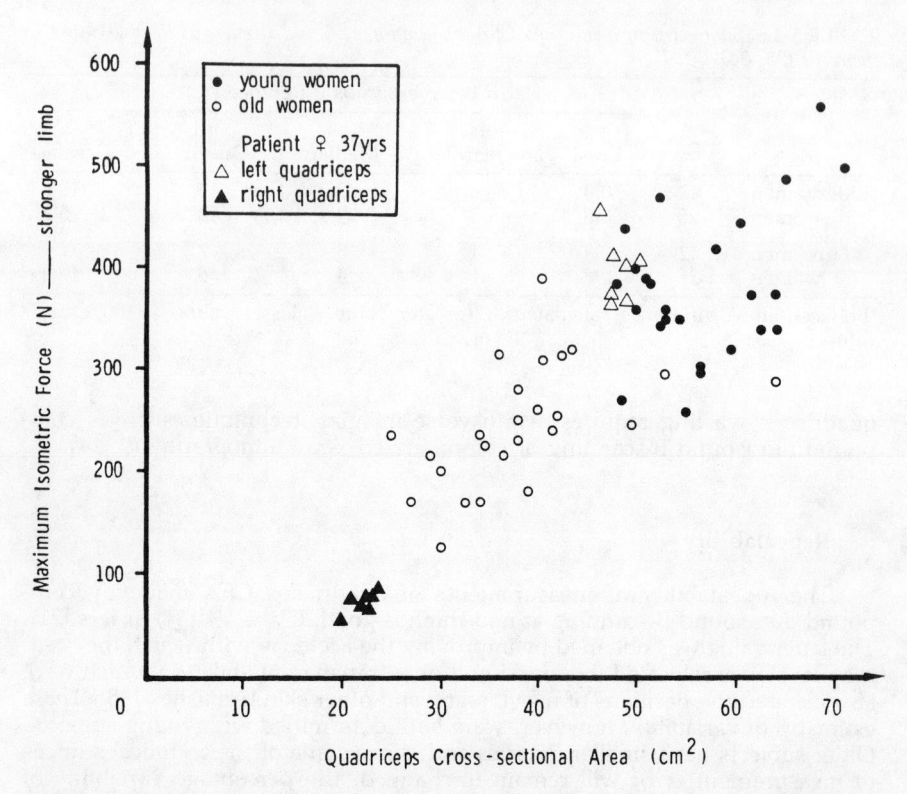

Fig. 5-2. *The relationship between quadriceps strength and CSA in normal women of different ages (33) may be used to evaluate measurements made in an individual patient. In contractions made with the knee at 90°, the unilateral weakness of this 37-year-old woman was commensurate with her atrophy.*
The measurements also confirmed her failure to respond to the treatments tried over a 16-month period, despite occasional subjective impressions of benefit.

QUADRICEPS ACTIVATION

Patients often experience great difficulty activating the extensor of an injured joint. This does not mean that the patient lacks self-discipline or motivation; it is the reflex effect of activity in afferents arising in or around the damaged joint, inhibiting the muscle's anterior horn cells. The inhibitory afferents are probably of larger diameter than nociceptive afferents and the inhibitory effect does not depend upon the perception of pain. Recent studies of the underlying pathophysiology and their historical antecedents have been reviewed elsewhere (22, 25, 32, 35) and their treatment here will be brief. First, however, the measurement technique and its repeatability will be considered.

Method

Surface electromyography (EMG) can be used to measure changes in the ability to activate a muscle voluntarily. Surface electrodes are placed at a re-

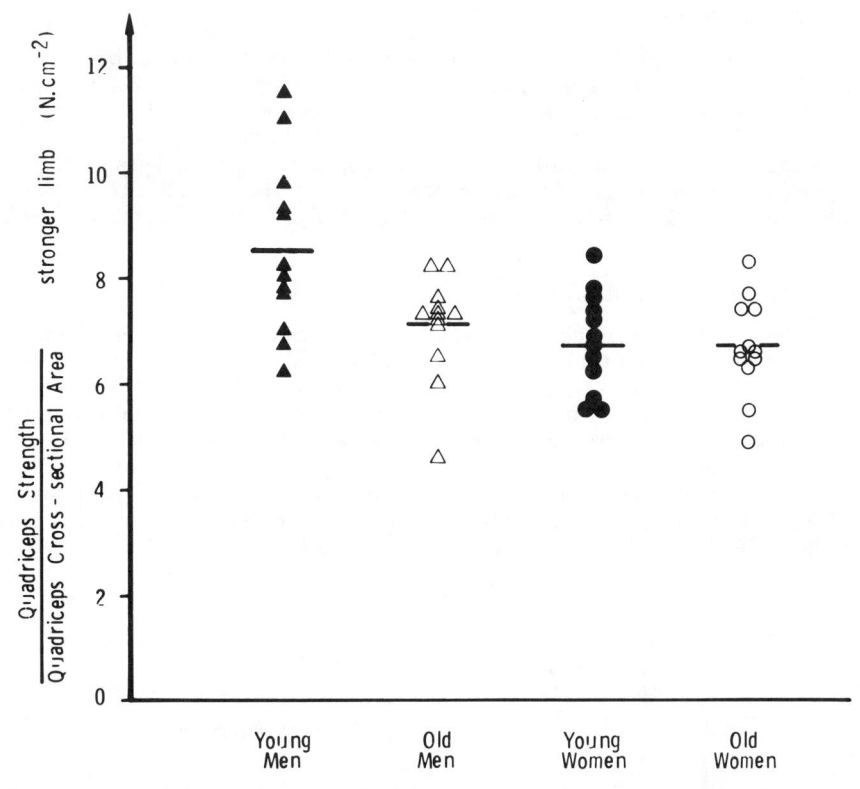

Fig. 5-3. *Ratio of the isometric strength of the stronger quadriceps to its mid-thigh cross-sectional area. Data for healthy men (34) and women (33) in their 20s and 70s. (For the women, only the data from the first 12 in each age group have been illustrated.) The horizontal lines indicate group means.*

produceable site over the muscle, and the patient is instructed to make a maximal, voluntary, isometric contraction. That is, in the case of the quadriceps, he does a maximal quadriceps setting maneuver. The EMG signal is rectified and integrated, producing a measure of the "maximal voluntary activation" (MVA) of the muscle. This is a function of both the number of motor units being activated and their firing frequency; it is relatively independent of the degree of atrophy. Recordings are made from both quadriceps, allowing comparison of one limb with the other. Of greater value, however, are repeated measurements of the MVA of the quadriceps of the injured limb. The validity of such longitudinal comparisons depends upon accurate relocation of the same electrode site. This can be done by marking the electrode position on the skin and by marking it on a transparent skin map (5), as described above for the scans.

Each maximal contraction lasts 4 to 5 seconds. We usually have our patients perform two such contractions with each muscle on each measurement occasion and record the MVA as the greatest integrated EMG signal recorded over any 0.9-seconds period during either of the contractions.

Repeatability

For normal limbs, the CV for measurements of MVA made on different days is 6%, even if measurements are made as early as 1 to 2 hours post-operatively (32). Measurements of MVA on 8 occasions over a 15-month-period in a 37-year-old woman with severe unilateral quadriceps weakness and wasting due to inhibitory afferent stimuli arising in a prepatellar scar showed a high degree of consistency (25). Mean MVA in the inhibited muscle was 10 EMG units (SD 2.4) and in the contralateral muscle was 39 units (SD 1.3).

Severity of Inhibition

Many of the recent clinical studies were conducted on young or middle-aged adults who had undergone meniscectomy by open arthrotomy. This experimental model for quadriceps inhibition had the advantage that post-operative measurements of quadriceps MVA could be compared with those made on the same muscle pre-operatively, as well as with those made on the contralateral muscle. Such studies have shown that inhibition of voluntary activation of the quadriceps is severe for at least 3 days (a 70-to-80% reduction of MVA is typical), and persists for at least 2 weeks, when it may still be reduced by 35 to 40% (25) or even more (Fig. 5-4).

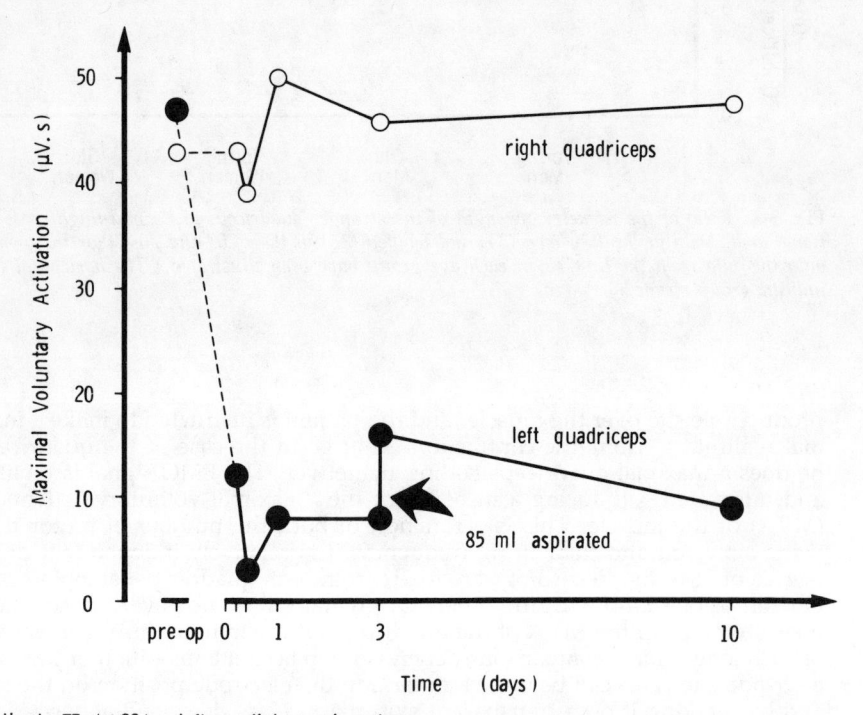

Patient: TF (♂ 33) left medial meniscectomy

Fig. 5-4. Bilateral measurements of quadriceps MVA before and after left arthrotomy and medial meniscectomy in a 33-year-old man. On the third post-operative day, MVA of the left quadriceps was recorded before and after aspiration of an effusion. None of the other measurements was associated with a clinically apparent effusion. (Reproduced with permission) (32).

Pain and Local Anesthesia

During the first 24 hours after meniscectomy, pain during a maximal quadriceps contraction may be quite severe but, unlike inhibition, it is usually only mild by 3 to 4 days. By two weeks post-operatively, pain is usually absent although inhibition may still be obvious (18, 25).

If sufficient local anesthetic is used, both inhibition and pain may be largely prevented by infiltration of the meniscal bed and the tissues around the incision (18). A smaller dose demonstrates a dose-related dissociation of the effects of local anesthetic on inhibition and on pain; pain is more readily prevented than is inhibition (18). The location of a peri-articular source of inhibitory afferent stimuli may be identified by selective infiltration of local anesthetic into the areas under suspicion (25).

Joint Position

Inhibition of voluntary quadriceps activation after meniscectomy is much less severe when isometric contractions are attempted with the knee in flexion than with it rather fully extended (25). Similarly, in the patient with unilateral quadriceps inhibition due to stimuli arising in a prepatellar scar, inhibition was virtually absent when the isometric quadriceps contractions were performed with the knee flexed (25). This explains why her quadriceps weakness with the knee at 90° was commensurate with the severity of atrophy (Fig. 5-2) although MVA in extension was severely inhibited (see Repeatability, above).

Surgical Procedures

Quadriceps inhibition after meniscectomy seems unrelated to the use of intra-operative tourniquet ischemia (23) despite some claims to the contrary (4, 17). The severity of inhibition may be approximately halved by performing meniscectomy by arthroscopy rather than by arthrotomy (19).

Effusions

The severity of post-meniscectomy quadriceps inhibition in the presence of a clinically apparent knee joint effusion is reduced (but only occasionally abolished) by aspirating the effusion (Fig. 5-4) (25). As expected from the earlier work of de Andrade, Grant, and Dixon (3) and of Jayson and Dixon (10), infusion of sterile saline into the knees of normal volunteers produces increasing inhibition of voluntary activation of the quadriceps as the volume of the infusion increases, even in the absence of pain (35). The quadriceps can be inhibited by knee infusions so small that they are still not clinically apparent (35).

It is not only voluntary activation of the quadriceps that is inhibited. Reflex activation of the quadriceps (as demonstrated by its H-reflex) is increasingly inhibited as fluid is infused (8, 20, 22). There is no indication of a threshold intra-articular pressure, and undetectably small infusions (as small as 10 milliliters) can inhibit reflex activation of the quadriceps (22). Inhibition of the H-reflex is greater during submaximal voluntary contractions than at rest (8, 22).

Clinical Applications

It is important to realize that it requires only a very small knee effusion, and that it does not require any perception of pain, for the quadriceps to be profoundly inhibited. This implies that we should be much more aggressive in dealing with effusions if we wish our rehabilitation exercises to be effectively performed. Moreover, it would seem most unwise to allow a return to active sport if significant inhibition is still present. Pain, therefore, cannot be an adequate guide to the appropriate time for resumption of sporting activity. This would be particularly true if techniques were being used to relieve pain which might have little (24) or no effect on inhibition.

The effect of joint angle on inhibition has yet to be convincingly exploited in rehabilitation practice. It seems likely that it has considerable potential relevance to the positions in which injured joints are immobilized.

Future neurophysiological studies of spinal connections of the inhibitory afferent pathways from the infused joint may well indicate potential applications for ice, vibration, and other sources of sensory stimulation in rehabilitation practice (8, 22, 35). Meantime, in the absence of generally applicable guidelines, the techniques used in our studies of voluntary quadriceps activation after meniscectomy can be applied readily to assessing the efficacy of specific measures in the individual patient. Similarly, they can be used to assist the clinician in deciding when inhibition is sufficiently mild that a return to sporting activity may be entertained.

REFERENCES

1. Aniansson, A., G. Grimby, and Å. Rundgren. Isometric and isokinetic quadriceps muscle strength in 70-year-old men and women. *Scand. J. Rehab. Med.* 12:161–168, 1980.
2. Asmussen, E., and K. Heebøll-Nielsen. Isometric muscle strength of adult men and women. In: *Communications from the Testing and Observation Institute of the Danish National Association for Infantile Paralysis*, E. Asmussen, A. Fredsted, and E. Ryge (eds.). No. 11:40. Copenhagen, 1961.
3. de Andrade, J. R., C. Grant, and A. St. J. Dixon. Joint distension and reflex muscle inhibition in the knee. *J. Bone Jt. Surg.* 47-A:313–322, 1965.
4. Dobner, J. J., and A. J. Nitz. Postmeniscectomy tourniquet palsy and functional sequelae. *Am. J. Sports Med.* 10:211–214, 1982.
5. Dons, B., K. Bollerup, F. Bonde-Petersen, and S. Hancke. The effect of weight-lifting exercise related to muscle fibre cross-sectional area in humans. *Eur. J. Appl. Physiol.* 40:95–106, 1979.
6. Edwards, R. H. T., A. Young, G. P. Hosking, and D. A. Jones. Human skeletal muscle function: description of tests and normal values. *Clin. Sci. Mol. Med.* 52:283–290, 1977.
7. Häggmark, T., E. Jansson, and B. Svane. Cross-sectional area of the thigh muscle in man measured by computed tomography. *Scand. J. Clin. Lab. Invest.* 38:355–360, 1978.
8. Iles, J. F., M. Stokes, and A. Young. Reflex actions of knee-joint receptors on quadriceps in man. *J. Physiol. (Lond.)* 360:48P, (Abs.) 1985.
9. Ingemann-Hansen, T., and J. Halkjaer-Kristensen. Computerized tomographic determination of human thigh components. The effects of immobilization in plaster and subsequent physical training. *Scand. J. Rehab. Med.* 12:27–31, 1980.
10. Jayson, M. I. V., and A. St. J. Dixon. Intra-articular pressure in rheumatoid arthritis of the knee. III. Pressure changes during joint use. *Ann. Rheum. Dis.* 29:401–408, 1970.
11. Johnson, T. Age-related differences in isometric and dynamic strength and endurance. *Phys. Ther.* 62:985–989, 1982.
12. Larsson, L., G. Grimby, and J. Karlsson. Muscle strength and speed of movement in relation to age and muscle morphology. *J. Appl. Physiol.* 46:451–456, 1979.
13. Lexell, J., K. Henriksson-Larsén, B. Winblad, and M. Sjöström. Distribution of different fiber types in human skeletal muscles: Effects of ageing studied in whole muscle cross sections. *Muscle & Nerve* 6:588–595, 1983.
14. LoPresti, C., D. Kirkendall, G. Street, J. Lombardo, G. Weiker, J. Bergfeld, and J. Andrish. Degree of quadriceps atrophy at 1 year post anterior cruciate repair. *Med. Sci. Sports Exerc.* 16:204, (Abs.) 1984.
15. Maughan, R. J., J. S. Watson, and J. Weir. Relationships between muscle strength and muscle

cross-sectional area in male sprinters and endurance runners. *Eur. J. Appl. Physiol.* 50:309–318, 1983.
16. Murray, M. P., G. M. Gardner, L. A. Mollinger, and S. B. Sepic. Strength of isometric and isokinetic contractions. Knee muscles of men aged 20 to 86. *Phys. Ther.* 60:412–419, 1980.
17. Saunders, K. C., D. L. Louis, S. I. Weingarden, and G. W. Waylonis. Effect of tourniquet time on post-operative quadriceps function. *Clin. Orthop. Rel. Res.* 143:194–199, 1979.
18. Shakespeare, D. T., M. Stokes, K. P. Sherman, and A. Young. Reflex inhibition of the quadriceps after meniscectomy: Lack of association with pain. *Clin. Physiol.* 5:137–144, 1985.
19. Sherman, K. P., A. Young, M. Stokes, and D. T. Shakespeare. Joint injury and muscle weakness. *Lancet ii:* 646, (Letter) 1984.
20. Spencer, J. D., K. C. Hayes, and I. J. Alexander. Knee joint effusion and quadriceps reflex inhibition in man. *Arch. Phys. Med. Rehab.* 65:171–177, 1984.
21. Stokes, M. *Reflex Inhibition of the Human Quadriceps in the Presence of Knee Joint Damage.* Ph.D. thesis. The Polytechnic of North London, 1984.
22. Stokes, M., J. F. Iles, and A. Young. Actions of knee joint afferents during contraction of the human quadriceps. *Brain* (in press).
23. Stokes, M., K. Mills, D. Shakespeare, K. Sherman, M. Whittle, and A. Young. 'Post-meniscectomy inhibition': Voluntary ischemia does not alter quadriceps function in normal subjects. In: *Biomechanical Measurement in Orthopaedic Practice,* 188–193. M. Whittle and D. Harris (eds.). Oxford: Clarendon Press, 1985.
24. Stokes, M., D. T. Shakespeare, K. P. Sherman, and A. Young. Transcutaneous nerve stimulation (TNS) and post-meniscectomy quadriceps inhibition. *Int. J. Rehab. Res.* 8:248, (Abs.) 1985.
25. Stokes, M., and A. Young. The contribution of reflex inhibition to arthrogenous muscle weakness. *Clin. Sci.* 67:7–14, 1984.
26. Stratford, P. Electromyography of the quadriceps femoris muscles in subjects with normal knees and acutely effused knees. *Phys. Ther.* 62:279–283, 1981.
27. Tornvall, G. Assessment of physical capabilities with special reference to the evaluation of maximal voluntary isometric muscle strength and maximal working capacity. *Acta Physiol. Scand.* 58:Suppl. 201, 1963.
28. Tzankoff, S. P., and A. H. Norris. Effect of muscle mass decrease on age-related BMR changes. *J. Appl. Physiol.* 43:1001–1006, 1977.
29. Vandervoort, A. A., A. J. McComas, A. Toi, and K. Viviani. Measurement of triceps surae muscle cross-sectional area in young and very old adults using ultrasonic imaging. *Can. J. Appl. Sport Sci.* 8:211, (Abs.) 1983.
30. Young, A. The relative isometric strength of type I and type II muscle fibres in the human quadriceps. *Clin. Physiol.* 4:23–32, 1984.
31. Young, A., I. Hughes, P. Russell, M. J. Parker, and P. J. R. Nichols. Measurement of quadriceps muscle wasting by ultrasonography. *Rheumatol. Rehabil.* 19:141–148, 1980.
32. Young, A., and M. Stokes. Reflex inhibition of muscle activity and the morphological consequences of inactivity. In: *Proceedings of 'Biochemistry of Exercise' 6th International Symposium (Copenhagen, 1985).* Champaign, IL: Human Kinetics Publishers, (in press).
33. Young, A., M. Stokes, and M. Crowe. Size and strength of the quadriceps muscles of old and young women. *Eur. J. Clin. Invest.* 14:282–287, 1984.
34. Young, A., M. Stokes, and M. Crowe. The size and strength of the quadriceps muscles of old and young men. *Clin. Physiol.* 5:145–154, 1985.
35. Young, A., M. Stokes, and J. F. Iles. Effects of joint pathology on muscle. *Clin. Orthop. Rel. Research,* (in press) 1986.

Section III
Testing the Mature Athlete

6

The Aging Endurance Athlete

BENGT SALTIN

University of Copenhagen

Performances of older people can be outstanding, indeed beyond comprehension. However, such performances cannot curtail the fact that even the most well-trained aging athletes experience a decline in function capabilities and results. The mechanisms responsible for decreased performance with age will be examined in this article, with the discussion limited to endurance performance in men.

It would have been ideal to present data from longitudinal studies; however, such investigations have not been done. Instead, the account has to be based primarily on cross-sectional studies of top-performing endurance athletes of various ages. Some of these have been followed for almost 20 years, which makes it possible—at least in part—to "validate" the cross-sectional data. The group of endurance athletes who form the focus of this examination consists of still-active orienteers studied first in the early 1960s, when they were 45 to 65 years old (21), and then again in the early 1980s (24, 52).

Orienteering is an endurance sport in which the competitor runs through the forest, finding certain features in the terrain with the aid of a detailed map and a compass. Top orienteers can navigate essentially without stopping, and the distance covered demands a running time of 1 to 2 hours. Typical for the sport is that many athletes continue for a lifetime. From 35 years of age and above, five-year interval age classes are available for competitors in orienteering, up to the age of 70 years. Another group of subjects to which reference will be made is that of the master runners studied by Heath, Hagberg, Holloszy, and associates in St. Louis (26, 29).

MAXIMAL OXYGEN UPTAKE

Figure 6-1 depicts the results from measurements of maximal oxygen uptake ($\dot{V}O_2$ max) in the very best male orienteers as well as from healthy

---

Acknowledgments

My thanks go to all the Swedish orienteers who through almost three decades have willingly participated in various studies. The follow-up studies performed recently were supported by grants from the research councils of the Danish and the Swedish Sports Federations.

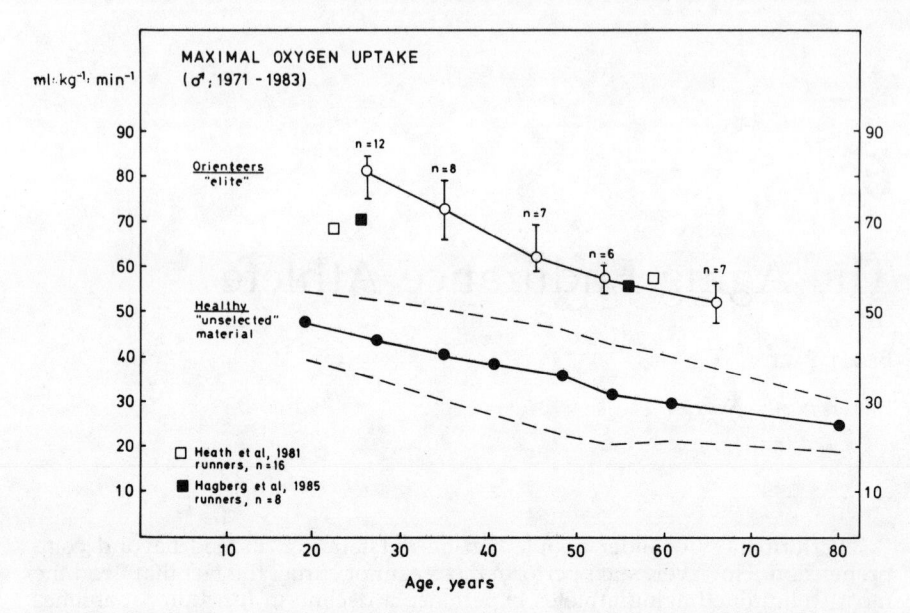

Fig. 6-1. Mean values (with range) for maximal oxygen uptake in elite orienteers in Sweden. The data are taken from various cross-sectional studies of the very best in each age category (1, 13, 16, 21, 24, 45). The youngest orienteers all belonged to the national team and the measurements were performed when they were in optimal condition. Included in the graph are mean values for the runners studied in St. Louis by Heath et al. (29) and Hagberg et al. (26). For comparison, data are included from cross-sectional studies of men randomly selected from ongoing population studies in Sweden and Denmark (unpublished data from the laboratory; 25, 36). Mean values ±1SD are given.

men of various ages. The young orienteers average 81 ml kg^{-1} min^{-1} in maximal oxygen uptake. A gradual decline with age can be noted, resulting in 29 ml kg^{-1} min^{-1} lower values for the oldest orienteer, who was 66 years old. The average decline with age is 0.73 ml kg^{-1} min^{-1} per year or about 0.9% per year. The close to 70-year old male orienteer is still above sedentary healthy young men in maximal aerobic power. Further, although the young orienteers have extremely high maximal oxygen uptakes, they are not—in relative terms—as much above their age-matched, more sedentary counterparts as are the older orienteers. The difference is about 70% in the young whereas the oldest have a $\dot{V}O_2$ max twice that of the sedentary "controls."

The data on the healthy men have been collected over a little more than a decade, and special precautions have been made to obtain a representative material. Thus, all subjects were recruited from ongoing population studies in Scandinavia, a fact which made it possible to evaluate exactly that the studied group in fact reflected the whole population of healthy men. Of note is that the mean values do not represent sedentary men but a mixture of men with markedly different physical activity pattern and fitness. The orienteers, on the other hand, are the very best in their age class. Their values for maximal oxygen uptake are as high as ever reported for any endurance athletes (8, 48). Included in the graph are mean values for some of the groups studied in St. Louis (26, 29). Their older runners have maximal oxygen uptake values similar to the orienteers, but their younger runners have lower values than those found in the orienteers.

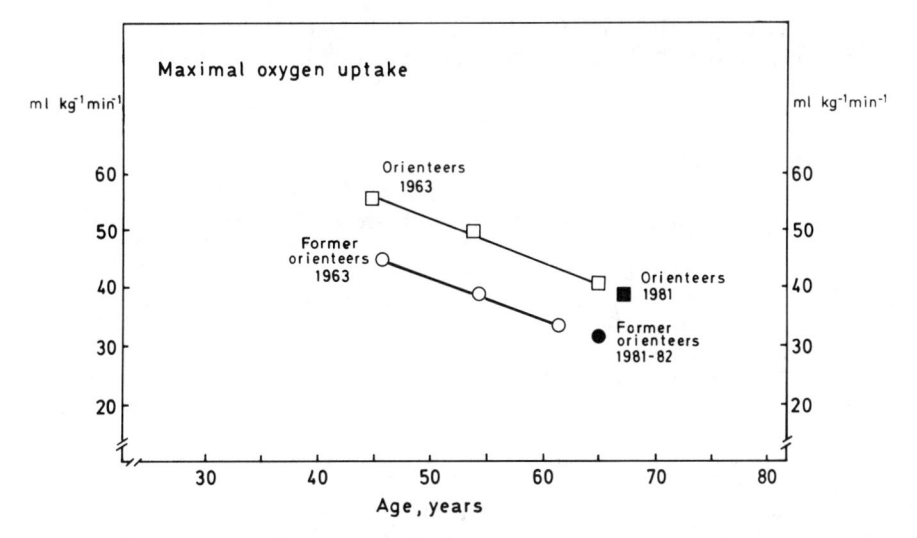

Fig. 6-2. *Mean values are depicted for maximal oxygen uptake in still-active orienteers studied in 1963, and 19 of them again 1981 (21, 24, 52). Included also are data for former orienteers studied in 1963, and 9 of them again 1981 (24, 50, 52).*

It is well documented that today's champion endurance athletes, such as cyclists, runners, and cross-country skiers, have maximal oxygen uptakes close to 80 ml kg^{-1} min^{-1} (8), but what values were obtained 30 to 50 years ago when the present master orienteers and runners were young? Robinson et al. reported in 1937 (42) that champion runners of that time were above 80 ml kg min^{-1}; and in 1954 Astrand (6) observed similar high values. In the late 1950s the first measurements on orienteers revealed that the very best competitors all were above 73 ml, with 83 ml kg^{-1} min^{-1} as the highest reported individual value in maximal oxygen uptake (1, 13, 45). It seems likely that the middle-aged and older orienteers discussed here were in this range when they were young as they also were among the very best in their young age groups then.

The data in Fig. 6-1 are all from cross-sectional studies. The question is then, how well they describe true changes with age. Fig. 6-2 shows the results for 19 still-active orienteers who were studied in 1963, remained active thereafter, and were restudied in 1981. It is quite apparent that the average decline with age was essentially the same when evaluated from the cross-sectional data obtained in 1963 and the results observed in 1981. A similar conclusion is reached when viewing the data from the follow-up of former top orienteers which was made at the same time. Those who remained "inactive" and were restudied in 1981 fell on the extrapolated line based on the results from 1963.

The maximal oxygen uptake of the former orienteers is higher than that found in the healthy controls despite the fact that nearly all have stopped regular training and competition. This could be explained either by maintained endurance fitness level from a training period earlier in life or by the fact that the former orienteers are more physically active than the healthy controls. The latter explanation appears to be true. The former orienteers were found to have quite active lifestyles with long walks, bicycle rides, and hiking in the mountains as regular leisure time activities. If endurance athletes take up sedentary lifestyles, following successful sports careers, their maximal oxygen uptakes would also soon reflect their new, lower activity levels (4, 10, 14, 41, 55). This particular topic has been discussed by others (38, 39, 59).

MAXIMAL OXYGEN PULSE

The oxygen pulse is a measure of both stroke volume and a-v oxygen difference. In 1981 it was claimed by Heath et al. (29) that older, very well-trained runners could maintain a maximal oxygen pulse as high (0.35 ml kg^{-1} min^{-1} beat^{-1}) as the very best young runners. Later, the same researchers partly changed this conclusion as they found slightly lower maximal oxygen pulse values in the 56-year old runners compared to the 26-year old runners (Fig. 6-3). These studies demonstrate the difficulty in drawing conclusions about alterations with age based on cross-sectional data. Although Heath et al. (29) had been extremely careful in matching their two groups of subjects, it must be questioned whether their young runners really represent the very top among endurance athletes. In the present data of orienteers, the oxygen pulse fell from 0.42 to 0.32 ml kg^{-1} min^{-1} beat^{-1} from the age of 26 to 66 years. Healthy men are in the range of 0.25 at the age of 20 years and decline to around 0.15 at the age of 70 to 80 years.

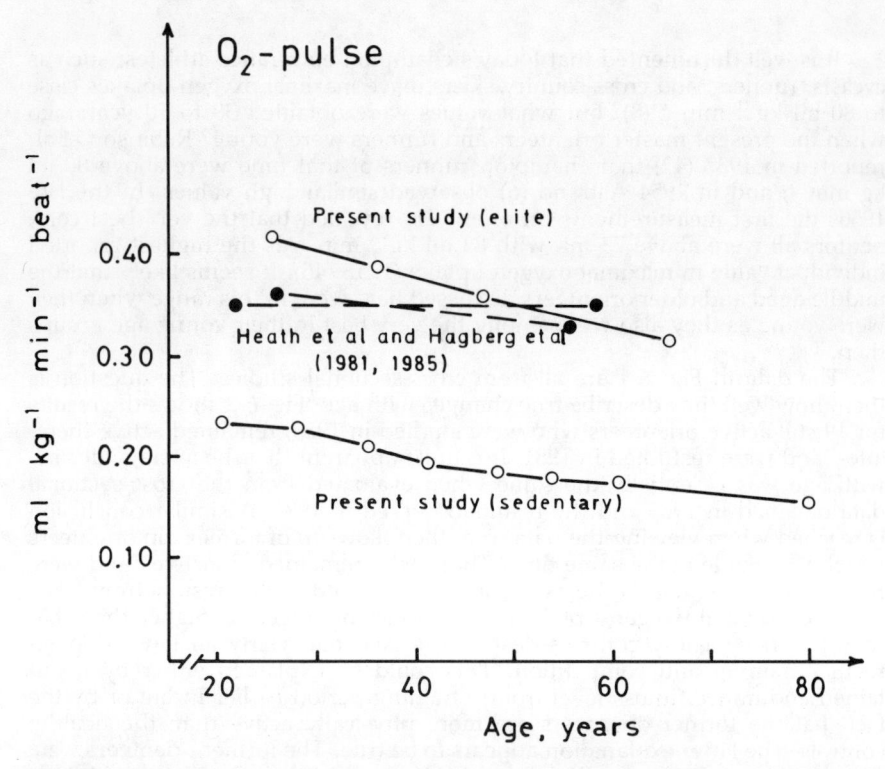

Fig. 6-3. *Mean values for the oxygen pulse in the present study of orienteers and healthy sedentary men, as well as mean values published on master runners by Heath et al. (29) and Hagberg et al. (26).*

TABLE 6-1. *Mean values for some hemodynamic variables from trained middle-aged orienteers (22) young orienteers (11, 31, 45) and middle-aged sedentary men (28).*

VARIABLE	TRAINED ≈25 yrs	TRAINED ≈50 yrs	YOUNG VS MIDDLE-AGED Δ %	SEDENTARY ≈50 yrs	SEDENTARY VS TRAINED MIDDLE-AGED Δ %
maximal oxygen uptake 1/min	5.05	3.56	30	2.68	−25
ml kg^{-1} min^{-1}	73	52	30	35	−33
cardiac output 1 min^{-1}	31.8	26.6	16	18.7	−30
heart rate, bpm	193	171	11	180	+5
stroke volume ml	165	156	5	103	−35
a-v$_{o_2}$ diff. ml · l^{-1}	159	134	14	142	+5

So far little has been said about the reduction in maximal heart rate with age. The question that is pertinent in this regard is whether trained individuals behave differently than sedentary people. The answer appears to be no. Some small variations may be observed between various studies (compare also data in Table 1), but the overall picture is that, regardless of training status, there is a gradual decline in maximal heart rate with age (5, 40). This can be substantiated by the findings in the longitudinal studies of the still-active and former athletes (Fig. 6-4). At the age of 50 years, healthy, but not especially trained, men have the same mean maximal heart rates as former and still-active orienteers, and all exhibit lower mean values at the age of 70. The in-

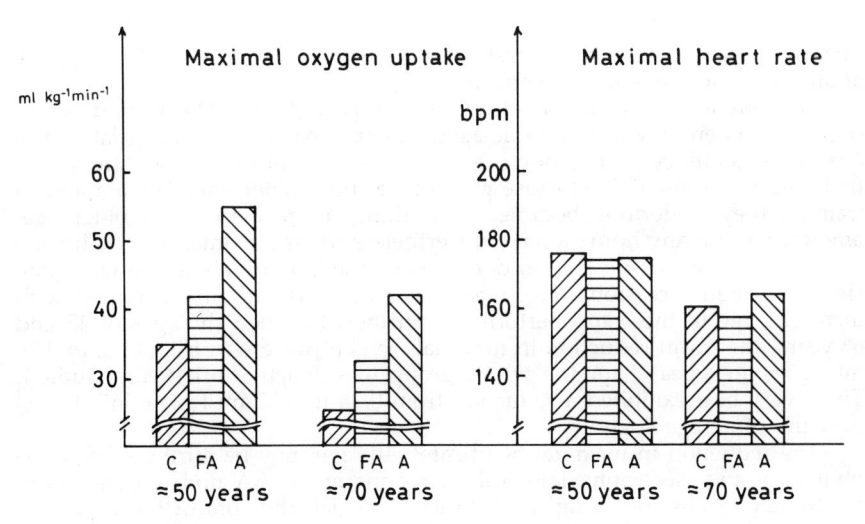

Fig. 6-4. *Comparison of maximal oxygen uptake and heart rate in 50- and 70-year-olds who were either sedentary (C), former orienteeers (FA), or still-active orienteers (A). Note that the data on the orienteers are from a longitudinal study (as in Fig. 6-2), whereas the data on the sedentary men are cross-sectional (as in Fig. 6-1).*

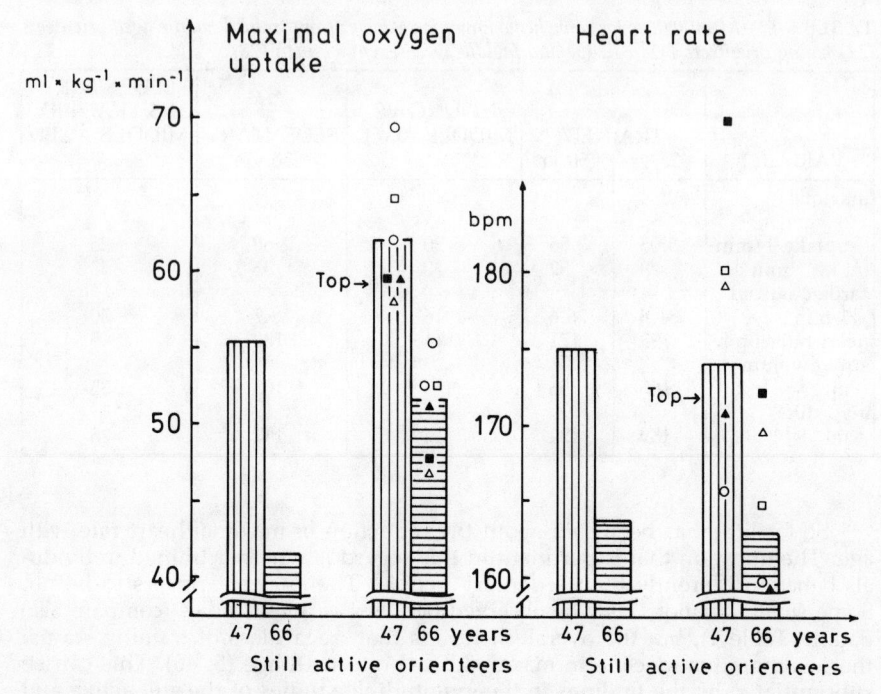

Fig. 6-5. *The reduction in maximal oxygen uptake and heart rate from the age of 47 to 66 years in still active orienteers is depicted. Comparisons are made for the whole material (n = 19) and the six best top orienteers at the age of 47 and 66 years (21, 25, 53). For this last group, mean and individual data are presented. The subject denoted by a filled circle had a maximal heart rate of 151 bpm in 1961. Twenty years later (1981) it was 146 bpm.*

dividual variation is large, and training intensity—very hard, moderate or not at all—does not appear to be crucial.

Of some interest in this context is to compare the very best middle-aged orienteers when they were middle-aged and approximately 20 years later. The 6 runners examined were among the 10 best in the country at the time of the first study and maintained those positions at their older age. The amount of training they undertook became, if anything, more extreme in older age, amounting to many hours a day. Nevertheless, their maximal oxygen uptake fell, and of note was the rank order between the individuals which was quite similar on both occasions (Fig. 6-5). Maximal heart rate also dropped with increased age in these top performers. Further, between the ages of 47 and 66 years, the mean reduction in maximal oxygen pulse was from 0.32 to 0.26 ml kg^{-1} min^{-1} $beat^{-1}$ for the whole group of still-active orienteers studied. The 6 very best exhibited a reduction from 0.36 to 0.32 ml kg^{-1} min^{-1} $beat^{-1}$ over the same age span.

The reduction in maximal heart rate with age may be attributed to morphological and electrophysiological alterations in the SA node as well as in the bundle of His, reducing the velocity by which the conduction of an impulse can be propagated (35). Further, it has been proposed that the sensitivity of the SA node for sympathetic stimulation is reduced with age (43).

From the above account it is clear that maximal heart rate and, more importantly, maximal oxygen uptake also decline with age in master endurance athletes who train extremely hard. Nevertheless, this does not alter the fact that regular physical training can improve aerobic fitness in middle-aged and older men (27, 46, 53, 56), as well as maintain aerobic fitness in active elderly men (9, 34, 38, 39). Of note, however, is that this occurs only if the men are below the upper range of maximal oxygen uptake for their age group. This is nicely demonstrated in several studies, for example by Kasch et al. (34) and Pollock et al. (38). In the former study 45-year-old men maintained their maximal oxygen uptakes of 44 ml kg^{-1} min^{-1} until the age of 55 years. Pollock et al. (38) followed middle-aged runners over 5 years (43 to 48 years and 55 to 61 years) and "controlled" their training. Although these runners were approximately 10% below the mean values presented for endurance runners in Fig. 6-1, they averaged a 2.5 ml kg^{-1} min^{-1} reduction in maximal oxygen uptake over the 5 years; the maximal oxygen pulse was 0.34 ml kg^{-1} min^{-1} $beat^{-1}$ in the 43-year-olds as compared to 0.31 ml kg^{-1} min^{-1} $beat^{-1}$ in 61-year-old runners.

HEMODYNAMIC RESPONSE

The reduction in oxygen pulse during maximal work in aging athletes is due to a decline in maximal stroke volume as well as to a reduction in systemic oxygen extraction, the latter contributing the most (Table 6-1). This conclusion is based on the only available invasive study of the hemodynamic response to exercise in middle-aged athletes (23). These orienteers were 51 years old and had a maximal oxygen uptake of 52 ml kg^{-1} min^{-1} as compared to young elite orienteers studied in a similar fashion who had a VO_2 max of 73 ml kg^{-1} min^{-1}. Thus, both groups were approximately 10% lower in maximal oxygen uptake than the orienteers presented in Fig. 6-1. Part of the difference (<5%) relates to the fact that peak values for maximal oxygen uptake were not achieved in the study when invasive measurements were performed. With these limitations the following may be stated. Maximal cardiac output was about 5 liters per min^{-1} lower in the middle-aged athletes, compared to the young orienteers. This was due mainly to a lowering of the maximal heart rate, but also to a reduced stroke volume. The 30% reduction in maximal oxygen uptake was almost equally related to a lowered maximal cardiac output and systemic arterio-venous oxygen difference. Compared with sedentary middle-aged men, active orienteers of the same age had markedly higher maximal oxygen uptakes, due almost exclusively to a larger stroke volume and thus maximal cardiac output.

In Fig. 6-6, data are collected from some studies in which hemodynamic responses were studied at various exercise levels in sedentary subjects and orienteers of different ages. What is apparent is that the relationship between cardiac output and oxygen uptake is very similar regardless of age and training status, and the pattern for a change in stroke volume with exercise is also much the same. Equally apparent is that both maximal cardiac output and stroke volume are reduced with age which, in part, can be counteracted by training.

It is well demonstrated that blood pressure at rest and during exercise is elevated in aging men (27, 28), an observation made also in the older athlete (Fig. 6-7). It is true that mean arterial pressure increases are slightly less in middle-aged orienteers than in age-matched, sedentary subjects during exercise, but compared to young, well trained or sedentary men, the difference

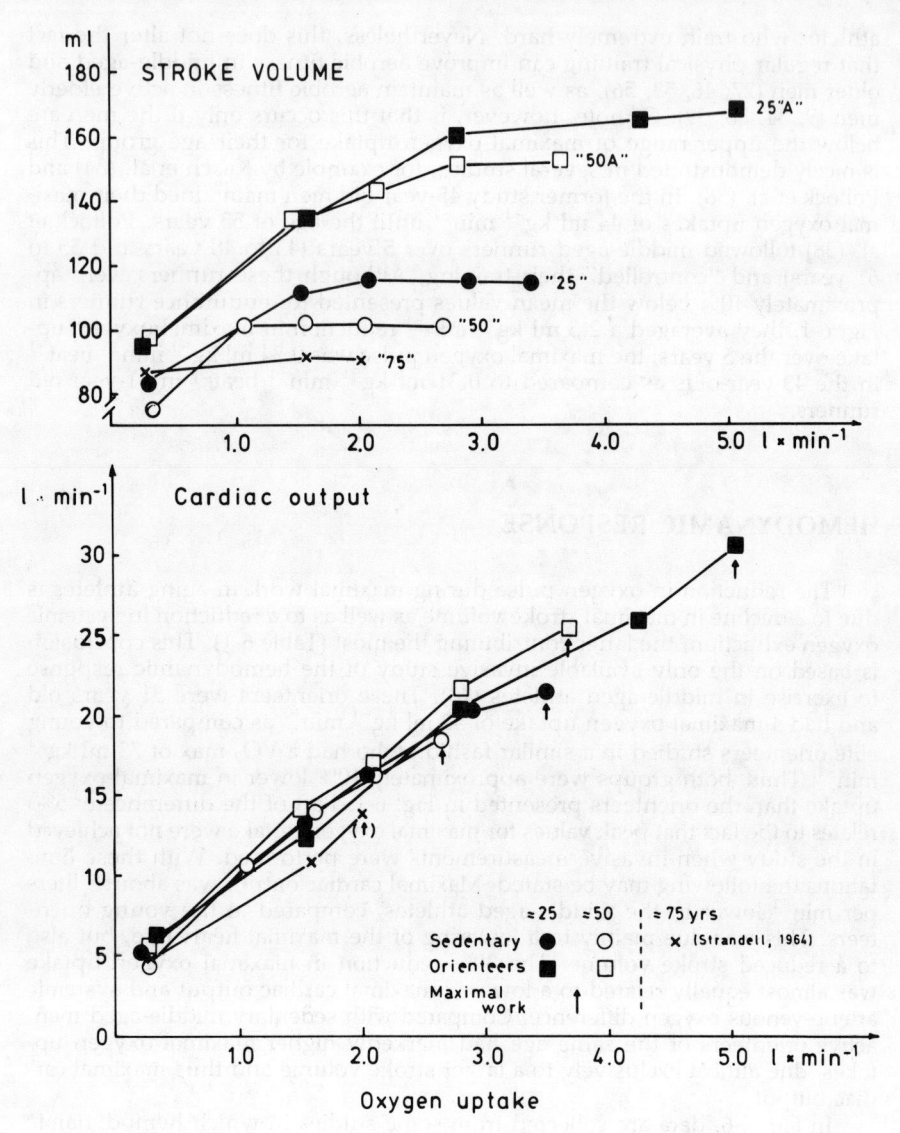

Fig. 6-6. Cardiac output and stroke volume at rest and during submaximal and maximal exercise in some subjects of different ages and training status. (7, 11, 12, 19, 23, 28, 31, 44, 60).

is quite apparent. When total peripheral resistance is calculated, the picture changes as follows. The middle-aged orienteers have equally low total peripheral resistance during submaximal and maximal exercise as the young men. This is due to the fact that they can maintain a large stroke volume and cardiac output. Thus, the low peripheral resistance is more a sign of maintenance of pump capacity of the heart than of unaltered stiffness of the arterial tree.

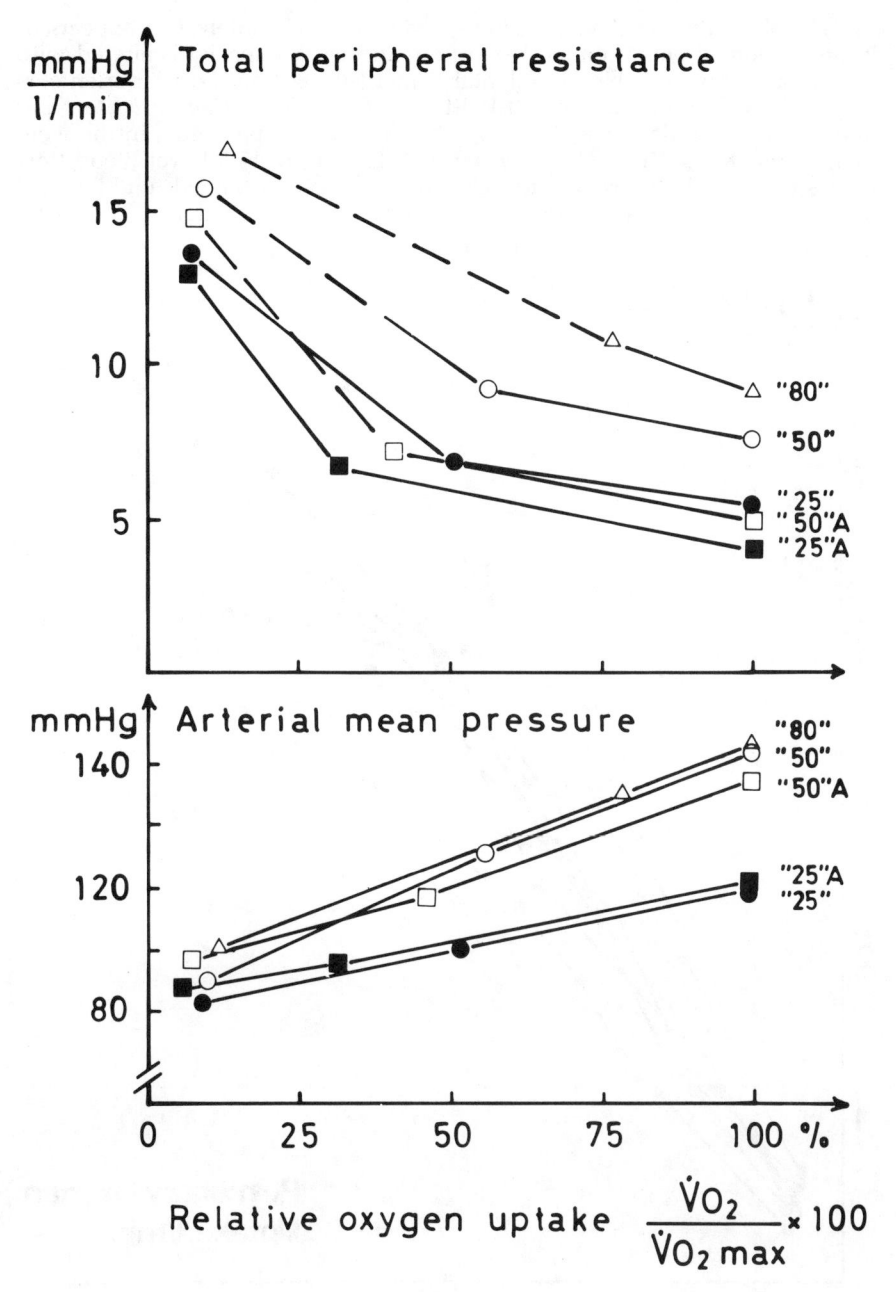

Fig. 6-7. *Mean arterial blood pressure and total peripheral resistance in the same groups as depicted in Fig. 6-6.*

Leg Blood Flow

The blood flow to the exercising limbs is of special interest. It appears as if the relationship between leg blood flow and work intensity is altered with age. Data are not available for sedentary older subjects, but exist for orienteers (Fig. 6-8). At a work load of 150 Watts, leg blood flow is about 5 liters per min^{-1} in young individuals, but "only" 4 to 4.5 liters, per min^{-1} in the well-trained orienteers. During peak exercise, at least 10 to 15% lower blood flow passes through the exercising muscles in the very well-trained, middle-aged orienteers, compared to young sedentary or trained individuals. The lower

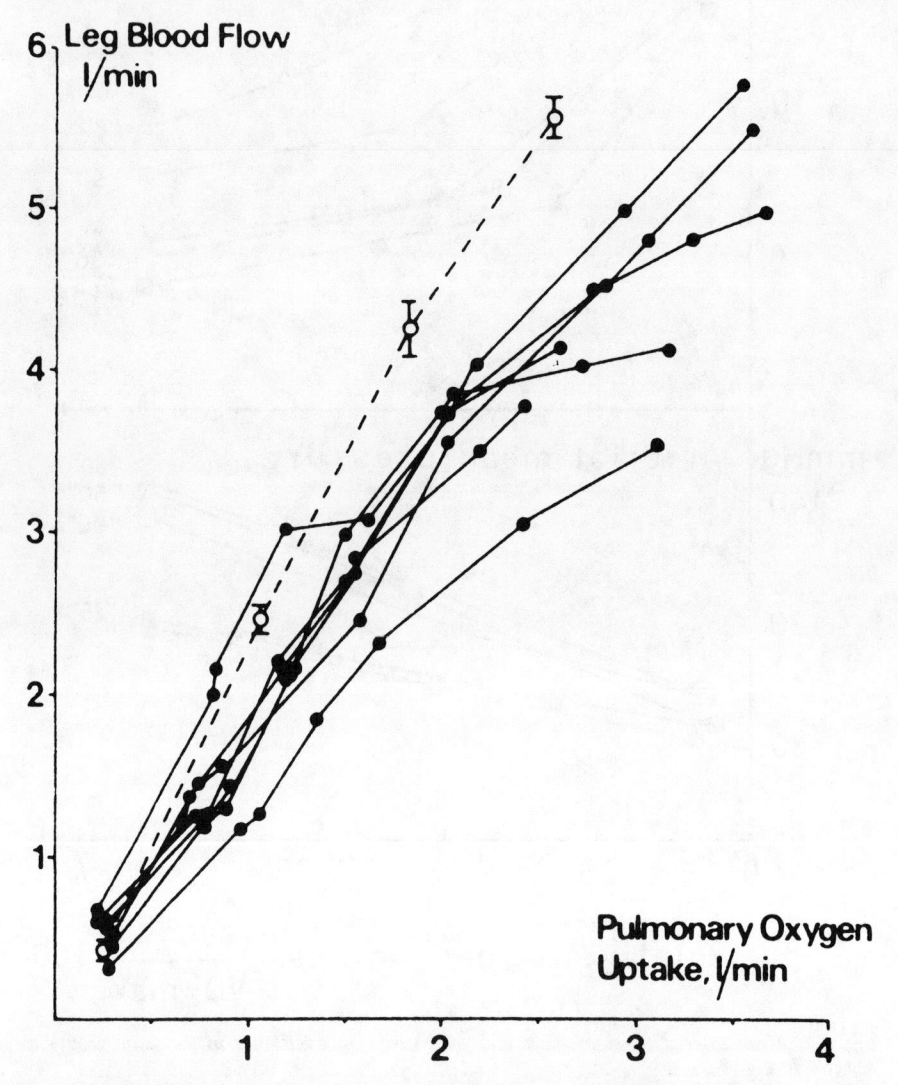

Fig. 6-8. *Leg blood flow during cycle exercise measured with the reversed dye dilution technique in young subjects (33) and middle-aged orienteers (62).*

TABLE 6-2. *Mean values for various variables obtained during maximal exercise in young and middle-aged sedentary (sed.) and trained (tr.) males.*

GROUP	Hb g × l^{-1}	S$_{o2}$ %	CaO$_2$ ml × l^{-1}	a-v$_{o2}$ diff ml × l^{-1} systemic	leg	C$_a$ pulm$_{o2}$ ml × l^{-1} estimated	ref.
young-sed.	159	94.0	201	154	162	47	7, 12, 45
young-tr.	152	93.5	188	159	175	29	11, 31, 45
middle-aged sed.	152	97.0	197	144	—	53	28
middle-aged tr.	145	97.2	184	134	170	50	22

leg blood flow in the middle-aged orienteers is compensated for by a larger O$_2$-extraction (a-v fem. difference for O$_2$ is wider). Thus the leg oxygen uptake is quite similar at a given work intensity in both age groups. These findings on leg blood flow give rise to several questions. One is related to the fact that the cardiac output/oxygen uptake relationship was unaltered in the middle-aged orienteers (Fig. 6-6). The first question is, then, to which tissues or organs is the flow distributed when less is directed to the exercising extremities?

Studies of the distribution of cardiac output in elderly athletes have not been performed. A direct answer to the question therefore cannot be given. The magnitude of flow which is not directed to the limbs may be in the order of 1.5 to 2.5 liters per min^{-1} during more intense submaximal work. This is too large a flow to be accounted for by an elevated blood flow, for example, to the liver. A possibility may be that older athletes, when exercising, shunt a larger fraction of the cardiac output to the skin. It would be interesting if this could be confirmed by studying thermoregulatory responses of elderly athletes.

Wherever the flow is distributed, it returns to the heart with a high oxygen content. Systemic a-v O$_2$ difference in the middle-aged orienteers at peak exercise is 134 ml l^{-1} and the a-v O$_2$ difference of the extremity is 170 ml l^{-1}. In Table 6-2, a collection of data is given to illustrate that older athletes oxygenate blood in the lungs to the same extent as other subjects and that their contracting muscles extract oxygen just as much as young, trained individuals. In fact, femoral venous oxygen content is only 18 ml l^{-1} in the middle-aged orienteers as compared to 25 ml l^{-1} in the young, trained orienteers and 40 ml l^{-1} or more in the untrained subjects.

The most important question in relation to the distribution of cardiac output in the elderly endurance athlete during exercise is why less is distributed to the exercising extremity. Several options to explain this finding are:

1. Reduced muscle mass.
2. Reduced capillary network per unit muscle mass.
3. Reduced elasticity and capacity for vasodilatation of arteries and arterioles.

It is true that the muscle mass is reduced with age (2, 61), but the finding of a reduced limb blood flow at submaximal work speaks against muscle mass playing a crucial role.

As is shown later, capillary density is maintained in aging muscle and appears to be as extensive in the older orienteers' trained muscles as in younger men. Finally, a reduced elasticity and vasodilatation of the arterial tree in the elderly is left as the explanation. In line with such a conclusion is the finding that blood pressure increased during exercise similarly in trained as well as untrained elderly men (Fig. 6-7). Further, it has been proposed that with an increased stiffness of the arterial wall, a less potent effect via the baroreceptors can be expected to contribute to a vasodilatation in older individuals (15).

OLDER ORIENTEERS VERSUS MASTER RUNNERS

Master runners in St. Louis and older orienteers in Sweden have very similar values for maximal oxygen uptake. It may then be of interest to compare in more detail the cardiovascular findings in the 2 groups although different techniques were used to measure some of the key variables (Table 6-3). Body size is about the same in the 2 groups, all athletes being shorter and leaner than the average. Resting systolic blood pressure is slightly higher in the Stockholm group (directly measured with a catheter in the brachial artery) but as the diastolic blood pressure is lower, mean blood pressure is quite similar in the two groups.

When the comparison is made at an exercise load representing 53 to 55% of maximal oxygen uptake, oxygen uptake being 2.02 and 2.08 liters per min^{-1}, the blood pressure response is much more marked in the orienteers than the runners. Mean blood pressure is 124 mmHg in the orienteers as compared to 100 mmHg in the runners. The other variables are more alike, although cardiac output and stroke volume (140 versus 133 ml) are higher in the orienteers. The estimated total peripheral resistance is also similar in the 2 groups, but the estimated stroke work of the heart is larger in the orienteers. This is true whether calculated either as the product of stroke volume and mean arterial blood pressure (26) or as the double product. Stroke volume, mean arterial pressure, and heart rate were all higher at the submaximal exercise level in the orienteers than in the master runners.

When comparisons are made between older and young endurance champion athletes, the findings and conclusions reached in the 2 studies differ on essential points. Most important is the blood pressure response. In the older orienteers there is a definite greater increase in systolic, diastolic, and mean arterial blood pressures during exercise than in the young orienteers. This is not apparent in the St. Louis runners. Stroke work of the heart was similar in the young and older runners, and the same conclusion is reached when

TABLE 6-3. *Mean values for some variables comparing middle-aged orienteers (22) with master-runners (26). The latter group was studied in St. Louis.*

	ORIENTEERS	MASTER-RUNNERS
Age, years	51	56
Height, cm	173	171
Weight, kg	69.3	66.1
Resting blood pressure Syst. mmHg	134	124
Dia. mmHg	78	84
MAXIMAL EXERCISE		
Oxygen uptake ml kg^{-1} min^{-1}	55.7	56.6
Heart rate, bpm	173	172
SUBMAXIMAL EXERCISE		
Oxygen uptake, 1 min^{-1}	2.08	2.02
Cardiac output, 1 min^{-1}	17.6	15.3
Heart rate, bpm	126	116
Mean arterial blood pressure, mmHg	124	100

comparing the young and older orienteers. However, in the latter study, stroke volume is reduced and mean arterial pressure is increased, whereas these variables are essentially the same in the young and master runners. The high exercise blood pressure (afterload) observed in the older orienteers probably is the reason why stroke volume is reduced. Thus, the overall conclusions as to why maximal oxygen uptake is reduced with age in well-trained older endurance athletes are different in the 2 studies. In the master runners, the whole reduction can be explained by the reduction in maximal heart rate. In the orienteers, a reduction in stroke volume and systemic a-v O_2 difference contribute as well (Tables 6-1 and 6-2). Cardiac output was not measured during maximal exercise in the master-runners, but estimations were made based on observed values for maximal heart rate and submaximal stroke volume. Although it is true that stroke volume does not always increase further during exercise beyond a relative work load of 50% of the maximal oxygen uptake, it is also true that most subjects reach their highest stroke volume at an exercise intensity close to one which elicits maximal oxygen uptake or at peak exercise (7, 11, 51). Thus the possibility exists that Hagberg et al. (26) have slightly underestimated the true maximal cardiac output in the master runners, which then has masked the fact that the systemic a-v O_2 difference may be slightly lower in their older runners than in their champion runners.

To explain why Hagberg et al. (26) found that a reduction in stroke volume contributed to a reduction in the master runners' maximal oxygen uptake, it must be reiterated that the maximal oxygen uptakes of the young champion runners studied in St. Louis were a little lower than the very highest values found in young endurance athletes.

If the competitive young runners in the St. Louis study had had a maximal aerobic power closer to 80 ml kg^{-1} min^{-1}, maximal stroke volume would have to have been close to 160 ml if the same body weight and maximal heart rate are assumed, as systemic a-v O_2 difference can hardly widen much above 170 ml^{-1} l^{-1}.

Heart Size in Older Endurance Athletes

In the study of orienteers it was found that heart size, determined with the biplane X-ray technique, was similar in the young and the older athletes and significantly larger than that found in sedentary men (21, 50). Heath et al. (29) give some more detailed information on this topic as they have made echocardiographic evaluations of the heart in their master runners. As anticipated, left ventricular end-diastolic volumes were larger in the trained (young and old) athletes when compared to sedentary men, but the body size-adjusted thickness index was similar and so were all measures of myocardial contraction indices. Of interest was the finding that left ventricular end-diastolic volume was slightly but significantly larger in the master runners than in the young athletes.

These findings support the notion that the stroke volume of older runners can be maintained well and that the afterload in the older orienteers is the factor which causes stroke volume to be reduced relative to that in the young champion orienteers.

Skeletal Muscle Capillarity and Enzyme Activities

Although total muscle mass is reduced in aging man, the quality of the remaining muscle mass is well maintained. This can be demonstrated in different ways.

TABLE 6-4. *Mean values for the capillarization of limb muscle (m. gastrocnemius (gas.) or vastus lateralis (v.l.)) in young and older men with different training back grounds (3, 13, 16, 32, 44, 53).*

	YOUNG MEN		OLDER MEN		
	control	orienteers	control	former orienteers	still active orienteers
n	26	6	8	8	12
age, years	25	24	61	66	66
maximal oxygen uptake ml kg^{-1} min^{-1}	48	78	28	36	49
muscle	v.l.	gas.	gas.	gas.	gas.
capillary density no per mm^2	333	628	315	385	503
capillary per fiber	1.4	2.7	1.3	2.0	2.5

The number of capillaries per unit area is very similar in limb skeletal muscles of man regardless of age (Table 6-4). Capillaries proliferate also in muscles of elderly men when they are used. Thus, both former and still-active older orienteers have a higher capillary density than sedentary men. Com-

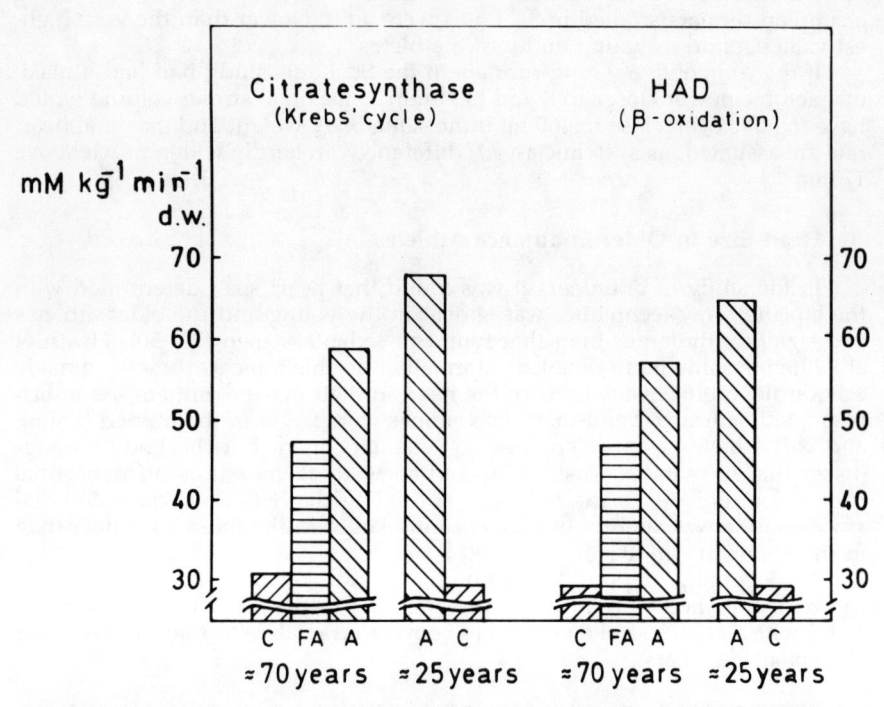

Fig. 6-9. *Mean values for maximal skeletal muscle citrate synthase (CS) and 3-hydroxy acyl CoA dehydrogenase (HAD) activities (V_{max}) in control subjects of young and older healthy sedentary men (unpublished material; 3, 16, 49), and in the present group of former (FA) and still active (A) orienteers (24, 52). Muscles samples were taken from the vestus lateralis of M. quadriceps femoris (n = 19 [A] and 9 [FA]).*

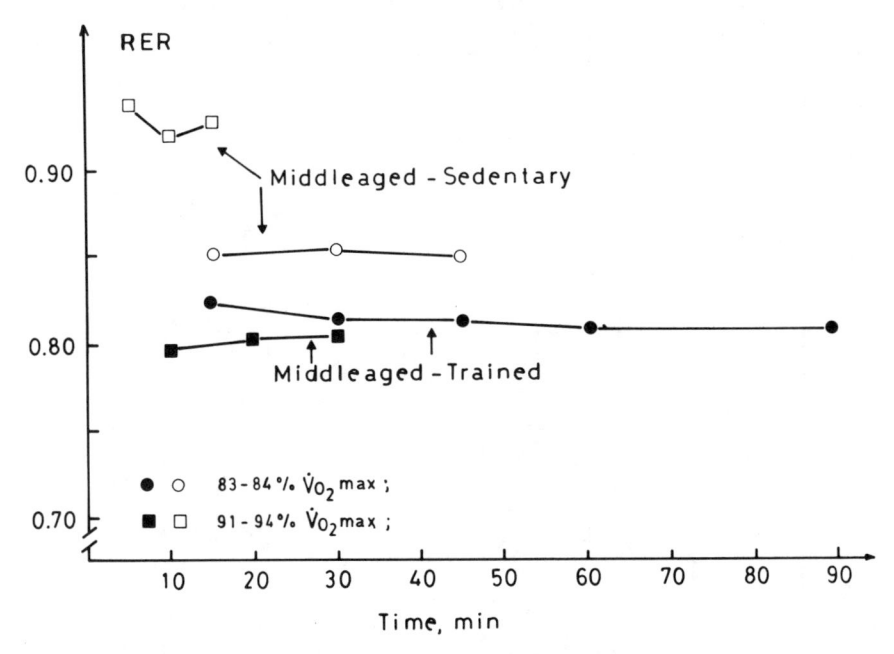

Fig. 6-10. Mean values for the respiratory exchange ratio (RER) observed during prolonged running on the treadmill to exhaustion at 2 relative work intensities in middle-aged sedentary men and very good marathon runners (<3 hours). Note the difference not only in RER values, but also in time to exhaustion (Nilsson, unpublished data).

pared with young top orienteers there is a difference, but not as large as could be anticipated from the notable difference in maximal oxygen uptake. This pattern, with higher than expected quality characteristics of the trained muscles in the older orienteers, relates also to the mitochondrial enzyme levels. Among older men there are higher maximal activities for both citrate synthase and 3-hydroxy acyl CoA dehydrogenase in relation to training status (Fig. 6-9). In the most trained older orienteers, these enzyme activities are only 10 to 15% lower than in the young orienteers in spite of at least a 50% difference in maximal oxygen uptake. Hexokinase and muscle lipoproteinlipase activities also follow the same pattern as the mitochondrial enzymes (22). The adaptations in the skeletal muscles of the elderly endurance-trained orienteers is then quite exceptional.

However, just like the aerobic fitness, the muscle adaptations vanish if the muscles are not used. A former Danish elite bicyclist who completely stopped training and competition revealed values for limb muscle capillarization and mitochondrial enzyme levels similar to those found in age-matched sedentary men (58).

There are several indications that the muscular adaptations have a functional significance. First, oxygen extraction by the contracting muscles was more complete than that observed in any other subjects studied (Table 6-2). Further, when middle-aged marathon runners covering the 42 km distance in less than 3 hours were compared with age-matched sedentary individuals, the respiratory exchange ratios were markedly lower, suggesting a greater utilization of fat than carbohydrate (Fig. 6-10). That older orienteers and runners

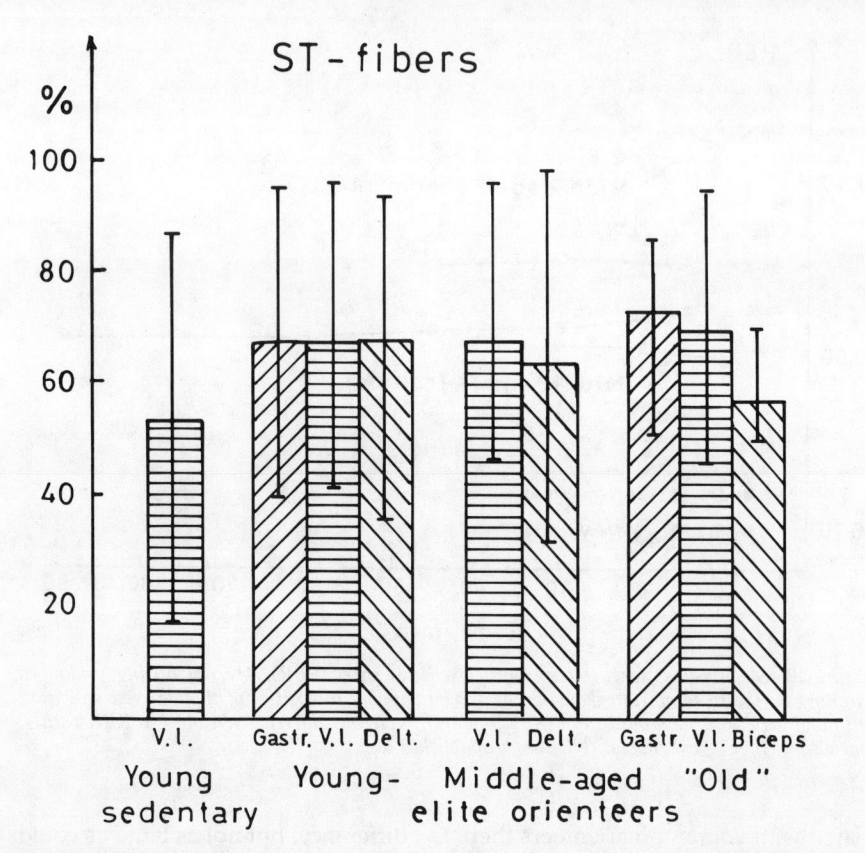

Fig. 6-11A and B. Mean values and range for A: relative percentage of slow-twitch (ST) fibers in various limb muscles of sedentary subjects (3, 30, 36), young (13), middle-aged (16), and old orienteers (24, 52). B: data corresponding to the data above, but the relative percentages of fast-twitch (FT) a and b fibers are illustrated in the same subjects as above.

can work at exceptionally high relative work loads without lactate accumulation in the blood has previously been demonstrated (21, 26, 29).

Skeletal Muscle Fiber Composition

One aspect of skeletal muscle adaptation which is intensely discussed today is whether the histochemical staining pattern for myofibrillar ATPase is altered with endurance training. Several reports suggesting this to be the case can now be found in the literature (20, 37, 54, 57). Muscle fiber composition has been studied in present and former, but still active, orienteers on the Swedish national team as well as in the present sample of still active and former orienteers. As not only leg muscles but also some upper limb muscles were sampled, some worthwhile comparisons can be made (22) (Fig. 6-11a, b). Regardless of age, the orienteers have a dominance of slow-twitch (ST; type I) fibers in their leg muscles, mean values being around 70% ST-fibers in young, middle-aged, and old orienteers. Of note is that the upper body

FT$_a$ and FT$_b$ fibers

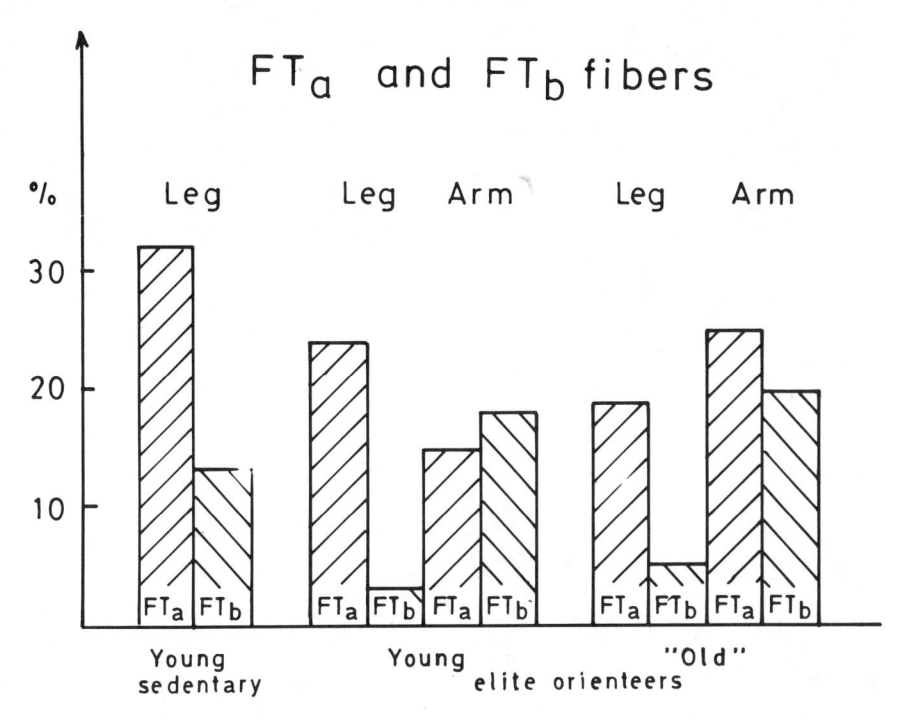

Fig. 6-11B (Continued).

muscles examined have an equally high percentage of ST fibers (32). The anticipated distribution of the subgroups of fast-twitch (FT) fibers is observed. In both the young and the old orienteers, very few FT$_b$ fibers are observed in the leg muscles, whereas they are numerous in the arm muscles (Fig. 6-11b).

In view of the huge difference in usage over the years of the leg as compared to the arm muscles in these orienteers, it is notable that the relative fiber composition is so similar. These findings argue then against any significant changes in myofibrillar staining pattern as the result of extreme endurance training. The findings on the former orienteers support this notion. In their leg muscles they have a percentage of ST fibers in the same range as the still-active orienteers and equal percentages of FT$_a$ and FT$_b$ fibers ($\approx 15\%$ each) are found. A pertinent question may be why there should be a need for a transformation of fiber types from FT to ST with endurance training. The question is raised as it is well documented that the capillarity and oxidative potential of FT fibers can be as high as observed in the ST fibers in human skeletal muscle (32). Further, when FT fibers are recruited in prolonged exercise, no signs of reduced mechanical efficiency are noted nor are there any obvious alterations in the metabolic response (17, 47).

Performance

In general, champion young orienteers have an average time of 5.5 to 6.0 minutes per km; middle-aged top orienteers may be close to 8 minutes per

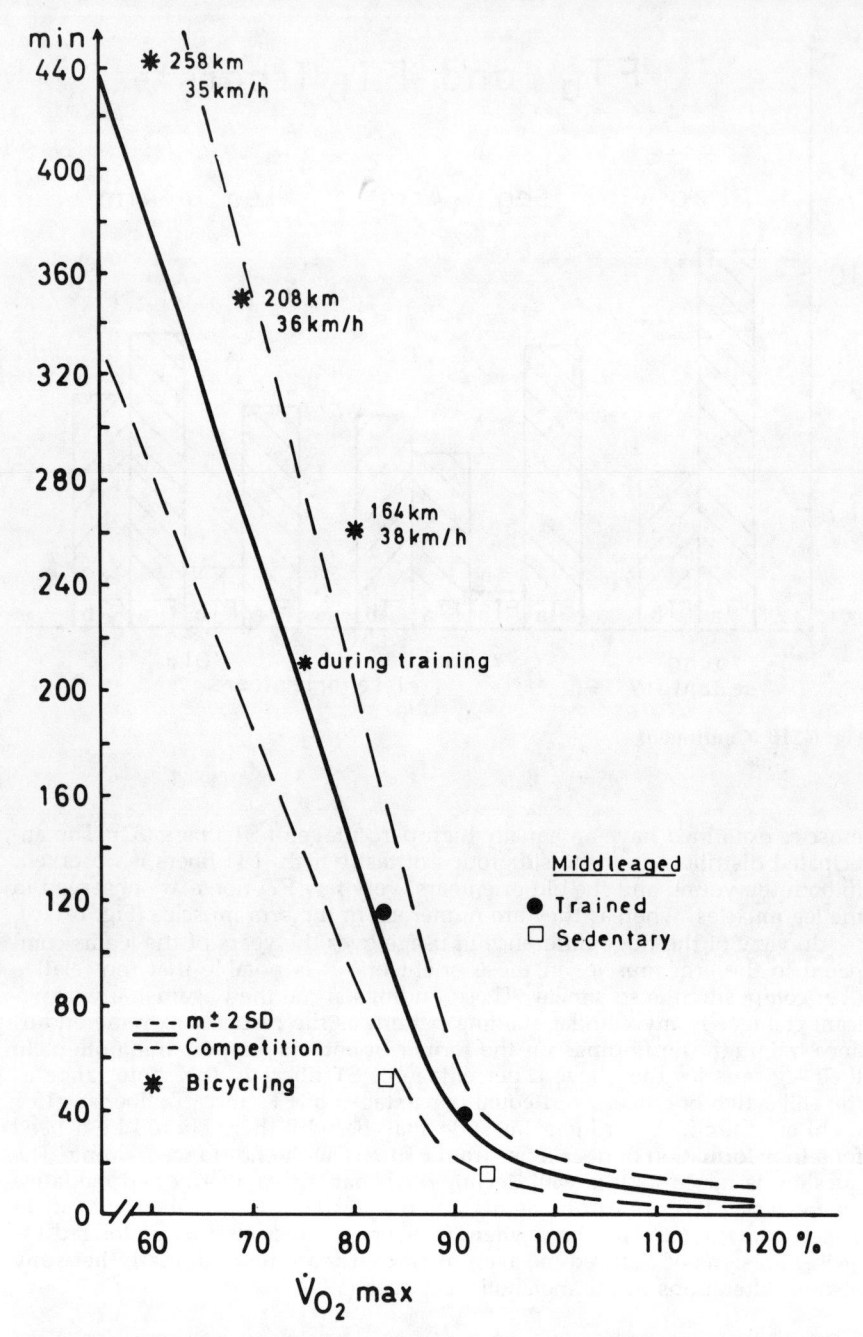

Fig. 6-12. Time to exhaustion is given at different relative work loads for young individuals (untrained-trained). Included are some mean values for young champion athletes as well as sedentary and trained middle-aged men. The data in the young people have been published earlier (58), and the data in the middle-aged runners and the sedentary men are from the same study as in Fig. 6-10.

km; and the elderly 9 to 10 minutes per km. The reduction in performance in orienteering cannot be more precisely estimated as type of terrain and distance vary between events. However, it appears that the reduction in performance, which amounts to 35 to 40% from the age of 20 to 25 to the age of 65 to 70 years in the orienteers, is quite similar to the observed relative change in maximal aerobic fitness over the same range of age.

In marathon running similar comparisons can also be made. Here very precise times are available for the best performers in each age category, but measurements of maximal oxygen uptake in these runners are lacking. However, if we assume that they follow the same age decline as that given for orienteers in Fig. 6-1, then performance would seem to be reduced to the same extent as maximal oxygen uptake. Thus, it appears that aging endurance athletes maintain the ability to utilize a high fraction of their aerobic capacity in prolonged exercise. That this in fact is the case is demonstrated in Fig. 6-12 in which data collected from young trained and untrained individuals are shown. Times to exhaustion at various relative work rates are given together with some results from young champion athletes during competition. The middle-aged men can perform as long as the young persons and at the same relative work load; the runners can perform longer than the sedentary men. These data and view are in contrast to the conclusion reached by Skinner (59).

As has been proposed (18), the endurance performance, which is the time a person can maintain a given relative work load, to a large extent is related to metabolic conditions including storage of muscle glycogen. Neither in orienteering nor in marathon running does glycogen storage need to be limiting, providing that the metabolism of the contracting muscles is geared to high relative usage of lipids and fat and that lactate production is minimized (17, 47, 49). This is exactly what was found in the highly trained endurance runners (Fig. 6-10, Fig. 6-12). As in the young individuals, the local training status of muscle is supposed to be the key factor for such an alteration of the metabolism (18). Thus, the rich capillarization and high oxidative potential of the leg muscles observed in endurance-trained older runners (orienteers) is not only important for complete oxygen extraction during exercise but also for an optimal metabolic response and fuel economy.

CONCLUDING REMARKS

The whole focus of this article has been on the aging athlete who tries to maintain a top performance and be placed high among fellow competitors. These athletes comprise a highly selected and extremely small group of men. One immediate reaction to the presented data could be that they are of little overall interest. This may not necessarily be true. Indeed, one of the very difficult problems encountered when evaluating biological effects of aging is to decide whether an alteration is age-related per se, a disease-related process, or simply due to physical inactivity. In these elderly endurance athletes, physical inactivity can definitely be ruled out as playing a role and very likely the same can be said about disease.

Thus the decline in top performance in these older athletes would seem to be age-related, something which cannot be overridden or compensated for by training. In addition to the age-induced reduction in maximal heart rate, increased stiffness of the arterial tree would also seem to contribute to the reduced maximal aerobic power. The higher resulting blood pressure (afterload) observed in the elderly endurance athlete during exercise then causes the stroke volume of the heart to be reduced, although the aging heart is as large and functioning as well as that of young men. Of note is that not only heart muscle but also skeletal muscles engaged in exercise maintain their adaptive responses to training surprisingly well. Thus, oxygen extraction and metabolic responses of cardiac and skeletal muscle are at least as effective in the old as in the young athlete and form the basis for the well maintained endurance performance of the elderly athlete.

REFERENCES

1. Adams, R. A. and B. Saltin. Maximal oxygen uptake in elite orienteers. 10F-report, *Doune*, Scotland, 1981.
2. Allen, T. H., E. C. Andersen, and W. H. Langham. Total body potassium and gross body composition in relationship to age. *J. Gerontol.* 15:348–357, 1960.
3. Aniansson, A., G. Grimby, E. Nygaard and B. Saltin. Muscle fibre composition and fibre area in various age groups, *Muscle Nerve* 2:271–272, 1980.
4. Asmussen, E., K. Fruensgaard and S. Nørgaard. A follow-up longitudinal study of selected physiological functions in former physical education students—after forty years. *J. Am. G. Soc.* 10:442–450, 1975.
5. Astrand, I. Aerobic work capacity in men and women with special reference to age. *Acta Physiol. Scand.* 49(Suppl. 169). 1960.
6. Astrand, P.-O. New records in human power. *Nature* 176:922–923, 1955.
7. Astrand, P.-O., T. E. Cuddy, B. Saltin, and J. Stenberg. Cardiac output during submaximal work. *J. Appl. Physiol.* 19:268–274, 1964.
8. Bergh, U. "Längdlöpning," *Idrottsfysiologi*, Rapport no. 11, Trygg-Hansa, Stockholm, 1974.
9. Dill, D. B. Marathoner DeMar: Physiological studies. *J. Nat. Cancer Inst.* 35:185–187, 1965.
10. Dill, D. B., S. Robinson, and J. C. Ross. A longitudinal study of 16 champion runners. *J. Sports Med.* 7:4–7, 1967.
11. Ekblom, B. and L. Hermansen. Cardiac output in athletes. *J. Appl. Physiol.* 25:619–625, 1968.
12. Ekblom, B., P.-O. Astrand, B. Saltin, J. Stenberg, and B. Wallström. Effects of training on the circulatory response to exercise. *J. Appl. Physiol.* 24:518–528. 1968.
13. Eklund, B., B. Hultén, A. Lundin, L. Nord, B. Saltin, and L. Silander. Orientering. *Idrottsfyiologi*. Rapport no. 10, Trygg Hansa, Stockholm 1973.
14. Eriksson, B. O., A. Lundin, and B. Saltin, Cardiopulmonary function in former girl swimmers and the effects of physical training. *Scand. J. Clin Lab. Invest*, 35:135–139, 1975.
15. Gerstenblick, G., E. G. Lakatta, and M. L. Weisfeldt. Age changes in myocardial function and exercise response. In: *Exercise and Heart Disease* (E. H. Sonnenblick & M. Lesch, eds.). 105–126. New York: Grune & Stratton, 1977.
16. Gollnick, P. D., R. B. Armstrong, W. Saubert, K. Piehl, and B. Saltin. Enzyme activity and fiber composition in skeletal muscle of untrained and trained men. *J. Appl. Physiol.* 33:312–319, 1972.
17. Gollnick, P. D., K. Piehl, and B. Saltin. Selective glycogen depletion pattern in human skeletal muscle fibres after exercise of varying intensity and at varying pedalling rates. *J. Physiol.* (Lond.). 241:45–57, 1974.
18. Gollnick, P. D. and B. Saltin. Hypothesis: Significance of skeletal muscle oxidative enzyme enhancement with endurance training. *Clin. Physiol.* 2:1–12, 1982.
19. Granath, A. and T. Strandell. Relationships between cardiac output, stroke volume and intracardiac pressures at rest and during exercise in supine position and some anthropometric data in healthy old men. *Acta Med. Scand.* 176:447–466, 1964.
20. Green, H. J., G. A. Klug, H. Reichmann, U. Seedorf, W. Wiehrer, and D. Pette. Exercise-induced fibre type transition with regard to myosin, parvalbumin, and sarcoplasmic reticulum in muscles of the rat. *Pflügers Arch.* 400:432–438, 1984.
21. Grimby, G. and B. Saltin. Physiological analysis of physically well-trained middle-aged and old athletes. *Acta Med. Scand.* 179:513–526, 1966.
22. Grimby, G., B. Danneskjold-Samsøe, K. Hvid, and B. Saltin. Morphology and enzymatic capacity in arm and leg muscles in 78–82 year old men and women. *Acta Physiol. Scand.* 115:125–134, 1982.
23. Grimby, G., N. J. Nilsson, and B. Saltin. Cardiac output during submaximal and maximal exercise in active middle-aged athletes. *J. Appl. Physiol.* 21:1150–1156, 1966.
24. Grimby, G., B. Saltin, L. Kaijser, and P. Renström. Aerobic power, muscle mophology and enzymatic capacity in a follow up study of very old still active endurance athletes. *Med. Sci. Sports Exerc.* 15:105 (abst.), 1983.
25. Grimby, G., L. Wilhelmsen, B. Ekström-Jodal, M. Aurell, J. Bjure, and G. Tibblin. Aerobic

power and related factors in a population study of men aged 54. *Scand. J. Clin. Lab. Invest.* 26:287–294, 1970.
26. Hagberg, J. M., W. K. Allen, D. R. Seals, B. F. Hurley, A. A. Ehsani, and J. O. Holloszy. A hemodynamic comparison of young and older endurance athletes during exercise. *J. Appl. Physiol.* 58:2041–2046, 1985.
27. Hanson, J., B. Tabakin, A Levy, and W. Nedde. Long-term physical training and cardiovascular dynamics in middle-aged men. *Circulation* 38:783–799, 1968.
28. Hartley, L. H., G. Grimby, A. Kilbom, N. J. Nilsson, I. Astrand, J. Bjure, B. Ekblom, and B. Saltin. Physical training in sedentary middle-aged and old men. III. Cardiac output and gas exchange during submaximal and maximal exercise. *Scand. J. Clin. Lab. Invest.* 24:335–349, 1969.
29. Heath, G. W., J. M. Hagberg, A. A. Ehsani, and J. O. Holloszy. A physiological comparison of young and older endurance athletes. *J. Appl. Physiol.* 51:634–640, 1981.
30. Hedberg, G. and E. Jansson. Skelettmuskelfiberkomposition. Kapacitet och interesse for olika fysiska aktiviteter bland elever i gymnasieskolan. Umeå, Sweden: Pedagogiska Inst., (Rep. 54). 1976.
31. Hermansen, L., B. Ekblom, and B. Saltin. Cardiac output during submaximal and maximal treadmill and bicycle exercise. *J. Appl. Physiol.* 29:82–86, 1970.
32. Jansson, E. and L. Kaijser. Muscle adaptation to extreme training in man. *Acta Physiol. Scand.* 100:315–324, 1977.
33. Jorfeldt, L. and J. Wahren. Leg blood flow during exercise in man. *Clin. Sci.* 41:459–473, 1971.
34. Kasch, F. and J. P. Wallace. Physiological variables during 10 years of endurance exercise. *Med. Sci. Sports* 8:5–8, 1976.
35. Lakatta, E. G. Alterations in the cardiovascular system that occur in advanced age. *Fed. Proc.* 38:163–167, 1979.
36. Lithell, H., F. Lindgård, K. Hellsing, G. Lundqvist, E. Nygaard, B. Vessby, and B. Saltin. Body weight, skeletal muscle morphology, and enzyme activities in relation to fasting serum insulin concentration and glucose tolerance in 48-year-old men. *Diabetes* 30:Jan. 19–25, 1981.
37. Pette, D. Activity-induced fast to slow transitions in mammalian muscle. *Med. Sci. Sports. Exerc.* 16:517–528, 1984.
38. Pollock, M. L., H. S. Miller Jr., and P. R. Ribsl. Effect of fitness on ageing. *Phys. Sportsmed.* 8:45–48, 1978.
39. Pollock, M. L., H. S. Miller, and J. Wilmore. Physiological characteristics of champion American track athletes 40 to 75 years of age. *J. Gerontol.* 29:645–649, 1974.
40. Reeves, T. J. and L. T. Sheffield. The influence of age and athletic training on maximal heart rate during exercise. In *Coronary Heart Disease and Physical Fitness*. (Eds. O. Andree-Larsen and R. O. Malmborg, 209–216. Munksgaard, Copenhagen. 1971.
41. Robinson, S., D. B. Dill, R. D. Robinson, S. P. Tzankoff, and J. H. Wagner. Physiological aging of champion runners. *J. Appl. Physiol.* 41:46–51, 1976.
42. Robinson, S., H. T. Edwards and D. B. Dill. New records in human power. *Science* 85:409–410, 1937.
43. Rowe, J. W. and B. R. Troen. Sympathetic nervous system and aging in man. *Endocr. Rev.* 1:167–179, 1980.
44. Saltin, B. Circulatory response to submaximal and maximal exercise after thermal dehydration. *J. Appl. Physiol.* 19:1125–1132, 1964.
45. Saltin, B. Tävlingsorientering. del II (in Swedish), SOFT, Idrottens Hus, Farsta, Sweden, 1968.
46. Saltin, B. Central circulation after physical conditioning in young and middle-aged men. In: *Coronary Heart Disease and Physical Fitness*. (Larsen, O. A., Malmborg, R. O., eds.) 21–26. Copenhagen: Munksgaard, 1971.
47. Saltin, B. Muscle fiber recruitment and metabolism in prolonged exhaustive dynamic exercise. In: *Human Muscle Fatigue: Physiological Mechanisms*. (R. H. T. Edwards, ed.) 41–58. London: Pitman Medical, 1981.
48. Saltin, B. and Astrand, P.-O. Maximal oxygen uptake in athletes. *J. Appl. Physiol.* 23:353–358, 1967.
49. Saltin, B. and P. D. Gollnick. Skeletal muscle adaptability. Significance for metabolism and performance. In: *Handbook of Physiology: Skeletal Muscle*. (Peachey L. D., Adrian, R. H., Geiger, S. R., eds.) 555–631. Bethesda: Am. Physiol. Soc., 1983.
50. Saltin, B. and G. Grimby. Physiological analysis of middle-aged and old former athletes. Comparison with still active athletes of the same age. *Circulation* 38:1104–1114, 1968.
51. Saltin, B., G. Blomqvist, J. H. Mitchell, R. L. Johansson Jr., K. Wildenthal, and C. P. Chapman, Response to exercise after bed rest and training. *Circulation* 38 (Suppl. 7), 1968.
52. Saltin, B., G. Grimby, L. Kaijser, P. Renström, and H. Lithell. Aerobic power, muscle morphology and enzyme capacity in a follow-up of still very active and former endurance athletes. *Clin. Physiol.* (In press).
53. Saltin, B., L. H. Hartley, A. Kilbom, and I. Astrand. Physical training in sedentary middle-aged and old men. II. Oxygen uptake, heart rate and blood lactate concentration at submaximal and maximal exercise. *Scand. J. Clin. Lab. Invest.* 24:323–334, 1969.
54. Schantz, P. and J. Henriksson. Increases in myofibrillar ATPase intermediate human skeletal

muscle fibers in response to endurance training. *Muscle and Nerve.* 6:553–557, 1983.
55. Schnohr, P. An investigation of previous athletes. *J. Sports Med.* 8:241–244, 1968.
56. Seals, D. R., J. M. Hagberg, B. F. Harley, A. A. Ehsani, and J. O. Holloszy. Endurance training in older men and women. I. Cardiovascular responses to exercise. *J. Appl. Physiol.* 57:1024–1029, 1984.
57. Simonau, J. A., G. Lortie, M. R. Boulay, M. Morcolte, M. C. Thiboult, and C. Bouchard. Human skeletal muscle fiber type alteration with high-intensity intermittent training. *Eur. J. Appl. Physiol.* 54:250–253, 1985.
58. Sjøgaard, G., B. Nielsen, F. Mikkelsen and B. Saltin. Etude Physiologique du cyclisme. Colloques Medico-Sportifs de Saint Etienne, 1982.
59. Skinner, J. S. Age and performance. In: *Limiting Factors of Physical Performance.* Ed. J. Keul. 271–282. Stuttgart: Georg Thieme Publ., 1973.
60. Strandell, T. Circulatory studies on healthy old men with special reference to the limitation of the maximal physical working capacity. *Acta Med. Scand.* 175 (Suppl. 414) 1964.
61. Tzankoff, S. P. and A. H. Norris. Effect of muscle mass decrease on age-related BMR changes. *J. Appl. Physiol.* 43:1001–1006, 1977.
62. Wahren, J., B. Saltin, L. Jorfeldt, and B. Pernow. Influence of age on the local circulatory adaptation to leg exercise. *Scand. J. Clin. Lab. Invest.* 33:79–86, 1974.

7
Heredity and Trainability

CLAUDE BOUCHARD, PH.D.

Laval University

INTRODUCTION

The effects of heredity on exercise capacity and exercise metabolism can be felt primarily a) by the heritability (i.e., the mean genetic effect for a given phenotype in the population), and b) by the importance of the genotype dependence of the adaptive response to training (i.e., the role of heredity in trainability) (5, 6). In the present paper only the latter component is considered. The question is whether the response to exercise training in mature and older individuals is heterogeneous in the population and whether this heterogeneity in trainability is related to the genotype.

Unfortunately, no studies dealing specifically with these issues in middle-aged and older subjects have been reported. We are therefore left with the option of discussing these questions assuming that the data available in young adults are applicable to older males and females. It appears that contemporary research on the response to training of older individuals supports the notion that this is a reasonable assumption, at least up to about 65 to 70 years of age.

THE EFFECTS OF TRAINING AND AGING

Several authors have discussed the topic of the response to training with aging (1–3, 8, 9, 19–22). Most of the data available suggest that the effects of age on trainability are minimal when direct measurements are obtained and training lasts about 20 weeks and is of sufficient frequency per week and intensity per session.

Table 7-1 illustrates changes in maximum oxygen uptake ($\dot{V}O_2$ max) in young adults and subjects into the 50s who trained for 20 weeks. In the study by Lortie et al. (12), $\dot{V}O_2$ max improved by 0.7 l O_2 (about 24%), while in the older subjects of Pollock et al. (15) gains reached 0.5 l O_2 in the group with a mean of 51 years (about 19%) and 0.4 l O_2 in the oldest subjects (about 16%). In general, training was less strenuous in the study of Pollock et al. (15) than

TABLE 7-1. *Comparison of maximal oxygen uptake changes with endurance training lasting a minimum of 20 weeks in young and older men.*[a]

Investigator	Mean age (years)	N cases	Duration of training (weeks)	$\dot{V}O_2$ max (l $O_2 \cdot$ min^{-1}) Pre	Post	% gain
Pollock et al. (1976)	58	11	20	2.38	2.75	16
Pollock et al. (1976)	51	11	20	2.56	3.05	19
Lortie et al. (1984)	27	11	20	2.90	3.60	24

a) Training was more frequent and more demanding in the study of Lortie et al.

in Lortie's group. In other words, these results along with some data reported with indirect or predictive measurements suggest that trainability of the oxygen transportation and utilization system remains quite good with age. This is probably true into the 60s, but whether this trend persists in the 70s and older remains to be determined with more convincing studies.

The effects of aging on skeletal muscle have been reviewed by Grimby and Saltin (8). An experimental training study conducted with 12 subjects, 69 to 74 years of age, who trained for 12 weeks has shown that the skeletal muscle remains trainable in terms of muscle strength, fiber type composition, and glycolytic and oxidative capacities (2, 3). The trainability of the skeletal muscle of these 70-year-old individuals was qualified as similar to that of young men. Moreover, Örlander and Aniansson (14) have suggested that in 70 to 75-year-old men, the adaptive response of the skeletal muscle to training may be slightly different in that the glycolytic potential may increase more relative to the oxidative capacity.

Little is known about the effects of aging on human adipose tissue metabolism. It has been suggested from studies on young and older rats that isolated fat cell catecholamine-stimulated lipolysis was progessively blunted with age (10, 13, 23). Recently, it has been shown that this decrement in hormone-stimulated lipolysis was not explained by a loss of β-adrenergic receptors (10), but appeared to be associated with an enhanced inhibitory effect of adenosine (11).

Human Variation in Trainability

To obtain acceptable estimates of the effects of training on $\dot{V}O_2$ max, skeletal muscle properties, and adipose tissue metabolism, it seems appropriate to rely on experiments which were specially designed to quantify human variation in response to training and to establish whether heredity was contributing to trainability. Such experiments have been undertaken in our laboratory with males and females ascertained as sedentary in the months prior to the study and with no history of participation in sports or training.

In one experiment designed to estimate the effects of training on $\dot{V}O_2$ max and endurance performance, 13 women and 11 men were subjected to a 20-week cycle ergometer training program (12). Subjects trained initially 4 times per week and then increased to 5 times per week. Each session lasted 40 and then 45 minutes, starting at 60% early in the program and progressively increasing the intensity to 85% of the heart rate reserve. Each training session was fully standardized and monitored for each subject. Table 7-2 summarizes some of the results reported by Lortie and co-workers (12). These sedentary males and females improved their $\dot{V}O_2$ max from 2.3 l O_2 to 2.9 l $O_2 \cdot$ min^{-1},

TABLE 7-2. *Influence of a 20-week aerobic program on $\dot{V}O_2$ max and endurance performance in 24 sedentary subjects of both sexes.*[a]

Variable	Pre-training $\bar{X}$	SD	Post-training $\bar{X}$	SD	Changes in % $\bar{X}$	SD	min	max
$\dot{V}O_2$ max (l $O_2 \cdot$ mi)	2.3	0.6	2.9	0.7	30	15	7	87
Max ml O_2/kg $\cdot$ min^{-1}	37	7	48	7	33	15	5	88
Endurance performance (kJ)[b]	562	129	836	215	49	21	16	91
Endurance performance (kJ/kg)	9.1	1.9	13.6	2.7	51	22	16	97

a) All training changes are significant at p $\leq$ 0.01 (Adapted from Lortie et al., 1984).
b) Endurance performance defined as the total work output during a 90-min. maximal cycle ergometer test.

a group gain of 0.6 l or about 26%. But when each individual's improvement was computed, a mean training change of 30% with a standard deviation of 15% was registered. Of the utmost interest was the observation that training response in $\dot{V}O_2$ max ranged from 7% to 87%. Similar individual differences were observed in endurance performance measured as the total work output in kJ during a 90-minute maximal cycle ergometer test. In the latter case, the range of training improvement in performance output was from 16% to 91%. In both cases, (i.e., $\dot{V}O_2$ max and endurance performance) considerable individual differences were seen equally in males and females (12).

Similar patterns of variation in skeletal muscle adaptation and adipose tissue metabolism to endurance training or high-intensity intermittent training in previously sedentary individuals have been found in our laboratory. Thus, changes in fiber type proportion and in skeletal muscle enzyme activities of marker enzymes of glycolytic and oxidative metabolism have been found with training, some individuals exhibiting sluggish response while others demonstrated high trainability (5, 17). The same observation was made on collagenase isolated fat cell basal and epinephrine-stimulated lipolysis after a 20-week endurance training program (4, 7). Individual changes with training reached about 70%, but the range of response was from about zero to 300%.

In summary, $\dot{V}O_2$ max, endurance performance, skeletal muscle properties, and adipose tissue metabolism are trainable phenotypes in young adults of both sexes and presumably also in middle-aged and older individuals. However, there are considerable individual differences in the response of these biological properties to exercise training, some exhibiting a high-responder pattern while others are clearly non-responders or at least low-responders. The next question is then, "What is (are) the factor(s) responsible for such human variation in adaptation to training?"

Heredity and Trainability

Fig. 7-1 describes the response to training in young adults for maximal oxygen uptake as it is commonly understood by sport scientists and coaches alike. In this schematic model, differences in $\dot{V}O_2$ max are associated with a genetic effect and training habits. Each of these effects is independent of one another and additive, however, which implies that all genotypes respond similarly to training. This model also assumes that all individuals have the same maximal trainability of $\dot{V}O_2$ max. Those are common beliefs or hidden assumptions which cannot be accepted any more due to recent findings. In other words, there are individual differences in the response to training and

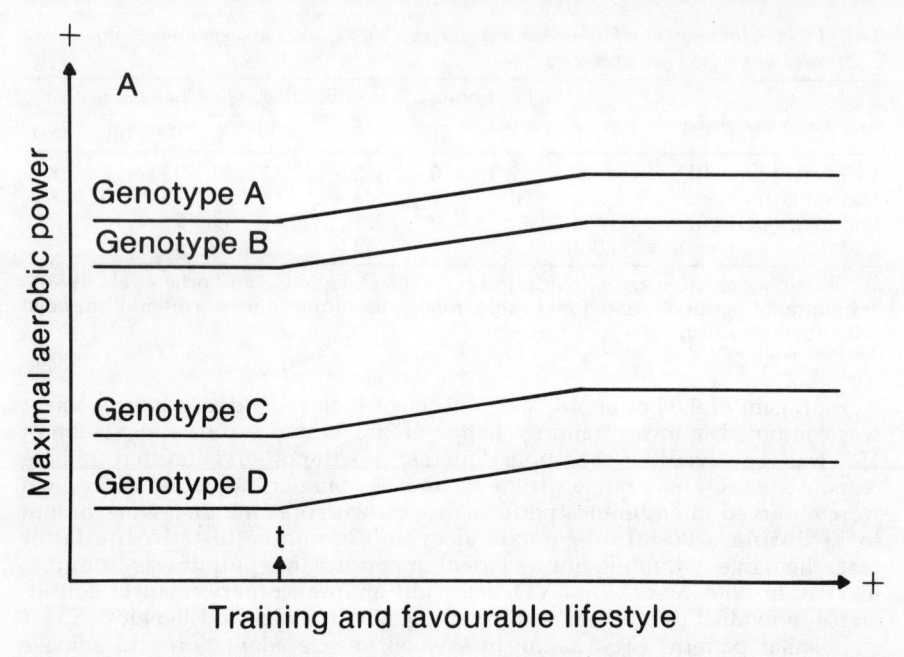

Fig. 7-1. *A schematic model of major causes of variation in $\dot{V}O_2$ max for individuals of given age and sex class assuming that heredity has no effect on trainability. t represents the initiation of training.*

maximal trainability as suggested by the data reported above.

The question then becomes, "What is responsible for these differences in adaptation to training?" We have reviewed this problem elsewhere in greater detail for maximal aerobic power and capacity (5). Briefly, age and sex of subjects as well as their prior training experience do not seem to contribute much to human variations in trainability. The major causes of human variation in the response to training are the current phenotype level (i.e., the pre-training status of the trait considered), and a genetically determined capacity to adapt to repeated exposure to exercise probably unique for each biological characteristic or family of characteristics. The latter represents this so-called role of heredity in trainability or, more rigorously, the genotype-training interaction. Let us review some of the evidence from our laboratory for a role of the genotype in the response to training.

Ten pairs of monozygotic (MZ) twins were subjected to a 20-week endurance training pogram initially meeting 4 and then increasing to 5 times per week, 40 minutes per session but increasing to 45 minutes, at an average intensity of 80% of the maximal heart rate reserve (starting at 60% and increasing to 85%). Under this program, $\dot{V}O_2$ max/kg improved by 14%. There were, however, considerable inter-individual differences in training gains as illustrated by a range of 0 to 41% for $\dot{V}O_2$ max per body weight. Differences in the response to training were not, however, distributed randomly among the twin pairs. Thus, intraclass correlations computed with the amount of training gain in liters of maximal oxygen uptake was 0.77 indicating that members of the same twin pair yielded a fairly similar response to training (i.e., 77% of the variance in the training response seemed to be genotype-dependent) (16).

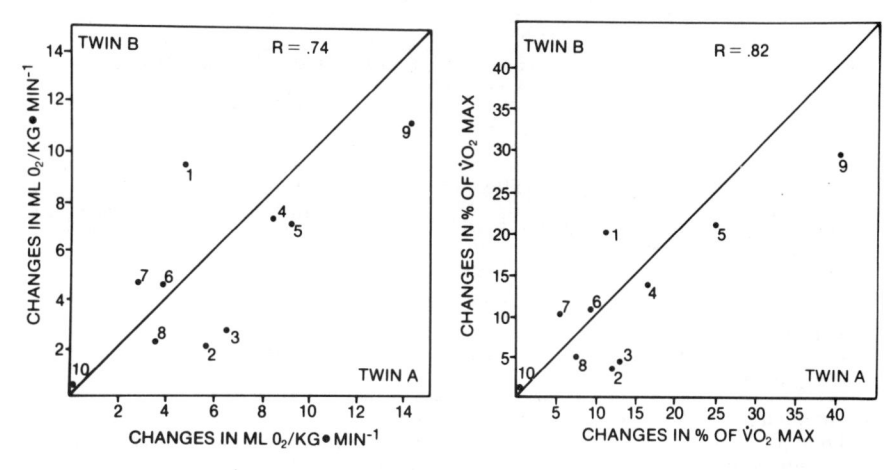

Fig. 7-2. Changes in V̇O₂ max with 20 weeks of training for each pair of MZ twins. R represents the intraclass coefficients. Both coefficients are significant at $p < 0.01$. Adapted from Prud'homme et al. (16) and unpublished data.

These results suggest that the sensitivity of maximal aerobic power to training is largely genotype-dependent (4, 5, 16). Fig. 7-2 illustrates the similarities in twin response to training in the experiment by Prud'homme et al. (16) for training gains in ml $O_2/kg \cdot min^{-1}$ (intraclass = 0.74; $p < 0.01$) and percent of V̇O₂ max (intraclass = 0.82, $p < .01$).

Because of the critical importance of these data for the topic of the role of the genes in adaptation to training, we decided to repeat the experiment to see whether these results would hold. In an as yet unpublished study, Hamel and co-workers submitted 6 pairs of MZ twins to a similar endurance training protocol lasting 15 weeks. In addition to V̇O₂ max, maximal aerobic capacity or endurance performance, defined as the maximal work output in a 90-minute cycle ergometer test, was monitored before and after training. The 12 subjects improved on the average from 2.6 to 2.9 l O_2, a gain of about 12%, and from 622 to 756 kJ in 90 minutes, an increase in endurance of about 21%. Data from Table 7-3 clearly show that there was a consistent genotype-training interaction effect. Intrapair resemblance for training response in maximal oxygen uptake was quite similar to the earlier findings of Prud'homme et al. (16) and in the same range as that for endurance performance. In other words, it seems that we have clearly demonstrated that unknown genetic factors are responsible for about three-quarters of the variation in aerobic performance with training. These results are quite compatible with those of previous studies from our laboratory and others which had established that the initial level of V̇O₂ max accounted for about 25% of the variance seen in response to training.

The role of heredity in the adaptation of the skeletal muscle to training was considered in an experiment by Simoneau et al. (18). Pairs of MZ twins were submitted to 15 weeks of high-intensity intermittent training consisting mainly of series of supramaximal 15 second and 90 second exercises on the cycle ergometer. The activity of several enzymes was determined before and after the training program from the biopsy of the vastus lateralis muscle. Significant within-pair similarity in the response of 12 pairs of MZ was found for creatine kinase (intraclass = 0.82, $p < 0.01$), hexokinase (intraclass = 0.59, p

TABLE 7-3. *Analysis of variance and intraclass coefficient for changes in maximal aerobic power and capacity following a 15-week aerobic training program in 6 pairs of MZ twins.*[a]

	F ratio[b]		Intrapair resemblance in response
Variable	Effect of training	Genotype-training interaction	
Maximal aerobic power			
l $O_2 \cdot$ min^{-1}	17.0**	4.6*	0.65
ml O_2/kg $\cdot$ min^{-1}	18.2**	5.3*	0.69[c]
Maximal aerobic capacity			
kJ in 90 min	38.0**	11.0**	0.83
kJ/kg in 90 min	66.4**	5.3*	0.68[c]

a) Adapted from Hamel et al., unpublished data.
b) From a two-way analysis of variance for repeated measurements on one factor (time).
c) In percent gain with training, coefficients are 0.82 and 0.83.
* For $p \leq 0.05$; ** for $p \leq 0.01$.

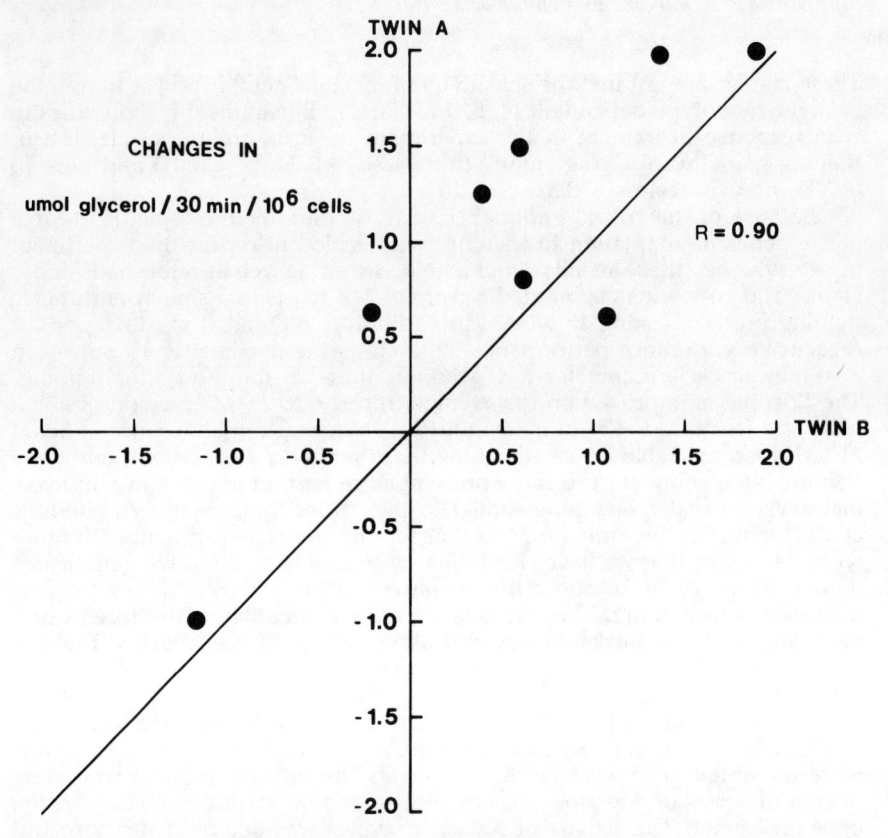

Fig. 7-3. *Changes in maximal epinephrine (10^{-3} M)-stimulated lipolysis of isolated fat cells with 20 weeks of training for each pair of MZ twins. R represents the intraclass coefficient ($p < 0.01$).*

< 0.05), lactate dehydrogenase (intraclass = 0.64, p < 0.01), malate dehydrogenase (intraclass = 0.50, p < 0.05), oxogluterate dehydrogenase (intraclass = 0.50, p < 0.05), and the ratio of phosphofructokinase to oxogluterate dehydrogenase activities (intraclass = 0.64, p < 0.01).

Recent data also support the contention that adaptive response of adipose tissue metabolism to endurance training is probably genotype-dependent. For instance, Després et al. (7) reported on the effects of 20 weeks of endurance training in 8 pairs of MZ twins. Basal and epinephrine submaximal and maximal stimulated lipolysis were determined before and after training on isolated fat cells. A genetically determined response to endurance training could not be found for basal lipolysis. The within-MZ pair resemblance in the sensitivity of maximal lipolysis was, however, very high, with an intraclass correlation of 0.90 (4, 7). It was concluded from these experiments that the sensitivity of stimulated lipolysis to endurance training is genotype-dependent. These results are illustrated in Fig. 7-3. Training increases maximal lipolysis in most pairs but causes a reduction in hormone-stimulated lipolysis in others.

All these studies clearly indicate that there are high (HR) and low (LR) responders to training found in association with certain genotypes. In addition, early and late responders were also identified, both types being found in the HR and in the LR categories (4, 5). Fig. 7-4 summarizes in a schematic way the general trends uncovered thus far concerning the response of maximal aerobic power to training. The same model would appear to be valid also for other performance, skeletal muscle, and adipose tissue phenotypes. The model integrates the contribution of three of the most potent causes of variation in human aerobic performance for individuals of a given sex and age

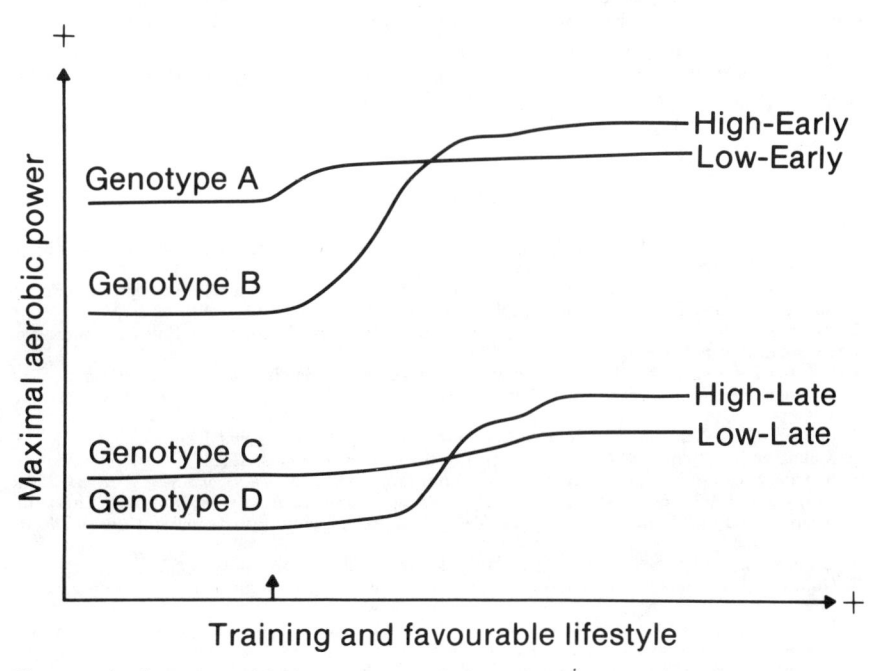

Fig. 7-4. *A schematic model of major causes of variation in $\dot{V}O_2$ max for individuals of given age and sex class incorporating the role of heredity in the response to training. Arrow represents the initiation of training.*

class; namely, a) the effect of training, b) the average genetic effect (heritability) for a given trait, and c) the role of the genotype in determining trainability.

An important avenue for research concerns the identification of those who happen to be HR or LR to training. There are at present no genetic markers that one could use to type an individual for sensitivity to training. In other words, at the present time, sensitivity to training is unpredictable. It can be ascertained only from past training experiences or as training progresses. Moreover, the question of the frequency of HR and LR phenotypes has not been addressed. On the basis of several training studies completed in our laboratory with sedentary individuals, we have attempted to obtain estimates of these frequencies (5). When defining LR individuals as those improving less than 5% in VO_2 max with a minimum of 15 weeks of training, we reported that about 5% of the population fell into that category. Similarly, with HR phenotypes, defined as those individuals increasing their VO_2 max by 60% or more, one could again conclude that their frequency reached about 5% of a sedentary population.

CONCLUSION

Aerobic performance is a multifactorial phenotype which is generally trainable in populations of young adults and older individuals. The average training effect is not sufficient, however, to account alone for the best performances of elite athletes of all ages. The elite performer has to be well endowed genetically, but he or she also has to be an innate high responder to the repeated stimulation of training. We believe that these concepts are applicable not only to the young athlete but also to the mature and older masters athletes.

REFERENCES

1. Adams, G. M., and H. A. DeVries. Physiological effects of an execise training regimen upon women aged 52 to 79. *J. Gerontol.* 28:50–55, 1973.
2. Aniansson, A., and E. Gustafsson. Physical training in elderly men with special reference to quadriceps muscle strength and morphology. *Clin. Physiol.* 1:87–98, 1981.
3. Aniansson, A., G. Grimby, Å. Rundgren, A. Svanborg, and J. Örlander. Physical training in old men. *Age and Ageing.* 9:186–187, 1980.
4. Bouchard, C. Human adaptability may have a genetic basis. In: *Health Risk Estimation, Risk Reduction and Health Promotion*, F. Landry (ed.). Ottawa: Canadian Public Health Association, 1983.
5. Bouchard, C. Genetics of aerobic power and capacity. In: *Sports and Human Genetics*, R. M. Malina and C. Bouchard (eds.). Champaign, Il.: Human Kinetics, 1985.
6. Bouchard, C., and G. Lortie. Heredity and endurancy performance. *Sports Med.* 1:38–64, 1984.
7. Després, J. P., C. Bouchard, R. Savard, D. Prud'homme, L. Bukowiecki, and G. Thériault. Adaptive changes to training in adipose tissue lipolysis are genotype-dependent. *Int. J. Obesity* 8:87–95, 1983.
8. Grimby, G., and B. Saltin. The ageing muscle. *Clin. Physiol.* 3:209–218, 1983.
9. Hodgson, J. L., and E. R. Buskirk. Physical fitness and age, with emphasis on cardiovascular function in the elderly. *J. Am. Geriatrics Soc.* 25: 385–392, 1977.
10. Hoffman, B. B., H. Chang, Z. Farahbakhsh, and G. Reaven. Age-related decrement in hormone-stimulated lipolysis. *Am. J. Physiol.* 247: E772–E777, 1984.
11. Hoffman, B. B., H. Chang, Z. Farahbakhsh, and G. Reaven. Inhibition of lipolysis by adenosine is potentiated with age. *J. Clin. Invest.* 74:1750–1755, 1984.
12. Lortie, G., J. A. Simoneau, P. Hamel, M. R. Boulay, F. Landry, and C. Bouchard. Responses of maximal aerobic power and capacity to aerobic training. *Int. J. Sports Med.* 5:232–236, 1984.

13. Miller, E. A., and D. O. Allen. Hormone-stimulated lipolysis in isolated fat cells from ⟨⟨young⟩⟩ and ((old)) rats. *J. Lipid Res.* 14:331–336, 1973.
14. Örlander, J. and A. Anianson. Effects of physical training on skeletal muscle metabolism and ultrastructure in 70- to 75-year-old men. *Acta Physiol. Scand.* 109:149–154, 1980.
15. Pollock, M. L., G. A. Dawson, H. S. Miller, A. Ward, D. Cooper, W. Headley, A. C. Linnerud, and M. M. Nomeir. Physiologic responses of men 49 to 65 years of age to endurance training. *J. Am. Geriatrics Soc.* 29:97–104, 1976.
16. Prud'homme, D., C. Bouchard, C. Leblanc, F. Landry, and E. Fontaine. Sensitivity of maximal aerobic power to training is genotype-dependent. *Med. Sci. Sports Exerc.* 16:489–493, 1984.
17. Simoneau, J. A., G. Lortie, M. R. Boulay, M. Marcotte, M. C. Thibault, and C. Bouchard. Human skeletal muscle fiber type alteration with high-intensity intermittent training. *Europ. J. Appl. Physiol.* (in press).
18. Simoneau, J. A., G. Lortie, M. R. Boulay, M. Marcotte, M. C. Thibault, and C. Bouchard. Inheritance of human skeletal muscle and anaerobic capacity adaptation to high-intensity intermittent training. *Int. J. Sports Med.* (revision pending review).
19. Skinner, J. S., C. M. Tipton, and A. C. Vailas. Exercise, physical training, and the ageing process. In: *Lectures on Gerontology*, Vol. 1B, A. Viidik (ed.). New York: Academic Press, 1982.
20. Stamford, B. A. Physiological effects of training upon institutionalized geriatric men. *J. Gerontol.* 27:451–455, 1972.
21. Suominen, H., E. Heikinnen, and T. Parkatti. Effects of eight weeks' physical training on muscle and connective tissue of the m. vastus lateralis in 69-year-old men and women. *J. Gerontol.* 32:33–37, 1977.
22. Suominen, H., E. Heikinnen, H. Liesen, D. Michel, and W. Hollmann. Effects of 8 weeks' endurance training on skeletal muscle metabolism in 56–70-year-old men. *Europ. J. Appl. Physiol.* 37:173–180, 1977.
23. Yu, B. P., H. A. Bertrand, and E. J. Masoro. Nutrition-aging influence of catecholamine-promoted lipolysis. *Metabolism* 29:438–444, 1980.

8

Testing The Elite Masters Athlete

JACK H. WILMORE, PH.D.

The University of Texas at Austin

INTRODUCTION

Over the past 15 years, close liaisons have developed among exercise and sport scientists, team physicians, athletic trainers, coaches, and athletes, helping to bridge the gap between the scientist, clinician, and practitioner. One major attraction pulling these diverse groups together has been a common interest in the concept of athletic profiling—comprehensive profiles developed to describe the qualities and characteristics of the athlete for any given sport or specific event. To date, detailed profiles have been established for athletes in almost all sports. These profiles have considerable application in developing a better understanding of the sport, and how to better train for that sport. They can also provide data on elite athletes against which data from aspiring athletes can be compared, allowing insight into those areas of training which should be emphasized, and providing guidance in placing athletes in positions or events where they will be most likely to excel.

This chapter is concerned with profiling in elite masters athletes. It provides only a general overview of the testing aspects of athletic profiling and is limited to a discussion of physiological testing. Three books have been published recently which address the topic of athletic profiling, and are recommended to the reader who is interested in pursuing this in much greater detail (21, 24, 31).

THE ATHLETIC PROFILE

When designing a test battery to determine profiles for specific athletic groups, several factors must be considered. First, the specific items in the test battery should be selected to reflect the unique nature of the sport or activity

---

Parts of this paper were adapted from: Wilmore, J. H. *Design Issues and Alternatives in Assessing Physical Fitness Among Apparently Healthy Adults in a Health Examination Survey of the General Population.* NHANES III, National Center for Health Statistics, Washington, D.C., 1985.

under study. In the sport of fencing, factors such as balance, general coordination and eye-hand coordination, reaction time, and movement time are obviously of importance to successful performance. Consequently, there should be test items in a fencing test battery designed specifically to measure or evaluate these factors. In the sport of American football, factors such as strength, power, muscular endurance, speed, and agility are important, and a football test battery should include an evaluation of these specific factors. In looking at the entire spectrum of sport, it is apparent that there are general factors common to most sports and specific factors which are unique to one or several sports. Discussion in this chapter will be limited to those general factors which are common to most test batteries for determining profiles of elite athletes in individual, dual, and team sports.

What specific components are evaluated in a general test battery for elite masters athletes? From the available literature, most general test batteries include items to evaluate cardiorespiratory endurance capacity or aerobic power, anaerobic power and anaerobic threshold, muscular strength, power, and endurance, flexibility, and body composition. Each of these will be discussed relative to standard measurement procedures, and representative values will be provided, where available, for different athletic populations.

Cardiorespiratory Endurance Capacity

Cardiorespiratory endurance can be defined as the ability to perform high intensity activity for a prolonged period of time without experiencing fatigue or exhaustion (31). It differs from muscular endurance in that it involves total body activity which is limited by cardiovascular and respiratory factors. Muscular endurance, on the other hand, refers to the ability of a single muscle or muscle group to sustain prolonged exercise, either of a rhythmical and repetitive nature, or of a static nature (e.g., sustained isometric contraction). A highly developed cardiorespiratory endurance capacity is typified by the marathon or cross-country runner, or cross-country skier, who is able to run or ski long distances at a fast pace.

Exercise scientists agree that the best measure of cardiorespiratory endurance capacity is one's maximal oxygen uptake (23). In the research laboratory, oxygen uptake is measured directly while the individual exercises are measured at increasing intensities on either the treadmill or cycle ergometer. While other types of ergometers can be used, the treadmill and cycle ergometer are by far the most common. As the intensity of exercise increases, the oxygen uptake increases in direct proportion. Eventually, the individual will reach his or her maximum ability to deliver oxygen to the active tissue (i.e., the oxygen uptake will plateau as the rate of work continues to increase). This is illustrated in Fig. 8-1 using two examples, a highly fit athlete and an unfit individual. Both individuals are at or near exhaustion at that time when oxygen uptake plateaus. The value achieved at the point of the plateau is referred to as the maximal oxygen uptake ($\dot{V}O_2$ max). With respect to the two examples in Fig. 8-1, the higher $\dot{V}O_2$ max allows the trained athlete to run on the treadmill at substantially higher speeds than the untrained individual. This is an important point, for several of the field tests used to estimate $\dot{V}O_2$ max are based on this linear relationship between speed and oxygen uptake capacity.

Since oxygen uptake represents the product of cardiac output and arteriovenous oxygen difference, $\dot{V}O_2$ max represents the ability of the individual to maximize both oxygen delivery (i.e., cardiac output) and oxygen extraction

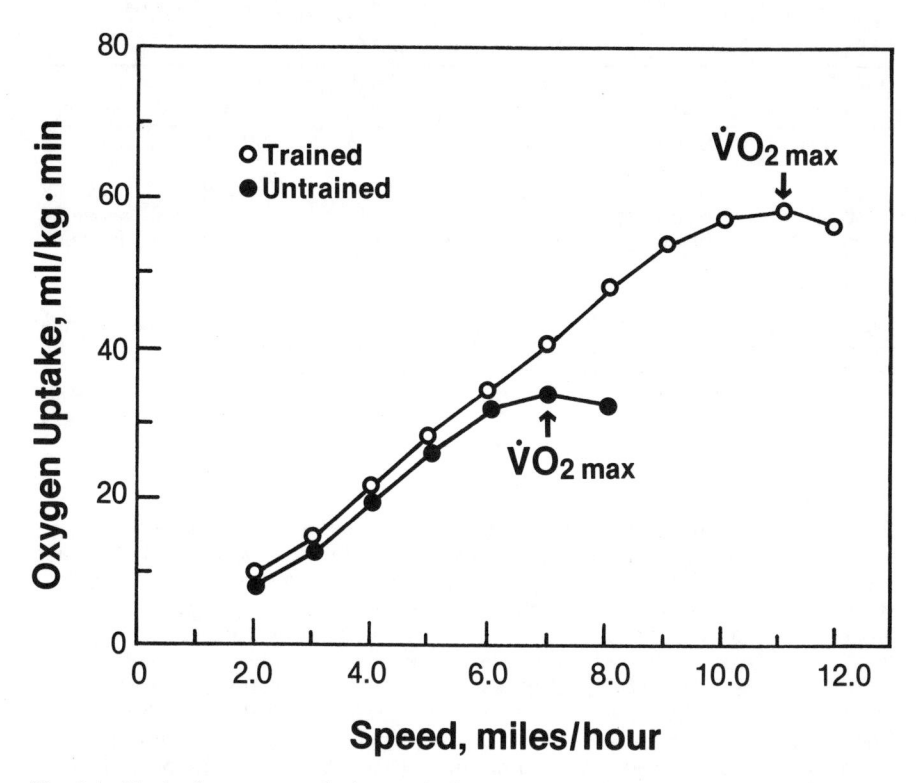

Fig. 8-1. *Maximal oxygen uptake in a trained and an untrained individual, determined on a treadmill using increases in speed with the grade held constant at 0.0%.*

(i.e., arteriovenous oxygen difference). Maximal cardiac output is determined by the interaction of heart rate and stroke volume. Maximal heart rates do not usually differ significantly between highly fit and unfit individuals of the same age. In fact, highly fit individuals tend to have slightly lower maximal heart rates compared to relatively unfit individuals (31). Highly fit individuals have, however, considerably higher stroke volumes at the point of maximal exercise than unfit individuals. Arteriovenous oxygen difference is determined by one's ability to extract oxygen at the active site of muscular contraction and reflects not only local enzyme activity within the cell, but also the ability to perfuse more blood through the active muscle bed. Again, the more fit individual appears to have achieved adaptations through training which increase the perfusion of blood through the active tissue and increase enzyme levels at the cellular level, allowing greater extraction of oxygen at the tissue level. The combination of a higher stroke volume and an increased ability to extract oxygen in the muscles provides a highly trained individual with a greater cardiorespiratory capacity which is reflected in a higher $\dot{V}O_2$ max compared to the untrained individual.

Maximal oxygen uptake values relative to fitness category and age are presented in Table 8-1. Values for athletes trained in different sports are presented in Table 8-2. $\dot{V}O_2$ max is a particularly good index of cardiorespiratory endurance capacity as it is highly responsive to changes in the activity level of the individual. With endurance training, $\dot{V}O_2$ max will increase in propor-

TABLE 8-1. *Maximal oxygen uptake values by age and fitness level*[a,b]

Age Group Years	Maximal Oxygen Uptake, ml·kg^{-1}·min^{-1}				
	Low	Fair	Average	Good	High
10–19	below 38	38–46	47–56	57–66	above 66
20–29	below 33	33–42	43–52	53–62	above 62
30–39	below 30	30–38	39–48	49–58	above 58
40–49	below 26	26–35	36–44	45–54	above 54
50–59	below 24	24–33	34–41	42–50	above 50
60–69	below 22	22–30	31–38	39–46	above 46
70–79	below 20	20–27	28–35	36–42	above 42

[a] Since females are generally 20% lower on the average compared to males, normal values for females can be obtained by shifting over one category to the right (e.g., the "fair" category for males would be considered "good" for females).
[b] This table was adapted from, Wilmore, J. H. *Training for Sport and Activity: The Physiological Basis of the Conditioning Process*, 2nd ed. Boston: Allyn and Bacon, 1982, p. 274.

tion to the training stimulus (i.e., intensity, duration and frequency of exercise) (25). Likewise, with physical inactivity or bed rest, $\dot{V}O_2$ max will decrease accordingly (12). A word of caution must be raised at this point. There is a strong genetic component that influences one's $\dot{V}O_2$ max. This was first demonstrated by the work of Klissouras (18), who concluded that 93.4% of variation in $\dot{V}O_2$ max was genetically determined. In a recent review of literature on the genetics of physiological fitness, Bouchard and Malina (4) indicate that the genetic component is not as dominant as was initially proposed by Klissouras. They concluded, on the basis of their analysis of the literature in this area, that heredity accounts for not more than 40 to 60% of the overall variability in $\dot{V}O_2$ max.

When selecting an ergometer for testing an athletic population, it is important to recognize the concept of test specificity. Most individuals will normally attain the highest $\dot{V}O_2$ max when tested on a treadmill. This is not always the case, however, with highly trained athletes. Stromme et al. (29) tested 14 female and 10 male cross-country skiers, 8 elite male rowers, and 8 elite male cyclists while running to exhaustion on the treadmill, and during maximal performance on their specific sport activity (i.e., uphill roll skiing, rowing in a single sculler, and uphill cycling on a treadmill). The $\dot{V}O_2$ max values were higher in almost every case when the athletes were tested on the sport-specific activity (Fig. 8-2), with an average of 3.5, 4.6, and 5.8% higher $\dot{V}O_2$ max while skiing, rowing, and cycling, respectively, compared to uphill running. These results underscore the specific local adaptations which occur in response to training. For the average untrained individual, this would not be a factor. This point is further illustrated by Magel et al. (22), who studied alterations in $\dot{V}O_2$ max with swim training (1 hour a day, 3 days a week, for 10 weeks), with subjects performing maximal treadmill running and tethered swimming tests, both before and after training. The initial $\dot{V}O_2$ max while swimming was 15% lower than the $\dot{V}O_2$ max during running. Following 10 weeks of swim training, the swimming $\dot{V}O_2$ max increased by 11.2% while the treadmill $\dot{V}O_2$ max increased by only 1.5% (non-significant). Had the treadmill been used as the only mode of testing, the authors would have concluded that swim training had no influence on $\dot{V}O_2$ max when, in fact, major changes were realized. The results of this study were recently confirmed by Gergley et al. (11), who reported no change in $\dot{V}O_2$ max as determined on the

TABLE 8-2. *Maximal oxygen uptake of male and female athletes*

Athletic group or sport	Sex	Age (years)	Height (cm)	Weight (kg)	$\dot{V}O_2$ max (ml·kg^{-1}·min^{-1})	References[a]
Baseball/softball	M	21	182.7	83.3	52.3	Novak[55]
	M	28	183.6	88.1	52.0	Wilmore[95]
	F	19–23	—	—	55.3	Rubal[70]
Basketball	F	19	167.0	63.9	42.3	Conger[14]
	F	19	169.1	62.6	42.9	Sinning[79]
	F	19	173.0	68.3	49.6	Vaccaro[90]
Centers	M	28	214.0	109.2	41.9	Parr[57]
Forwards	M	25	200.6	96.9	45.9	Parr[57]
Guards	M	25	188.0	83.6	50.0	Parr[57]
Bicycling (competitive)	M	24	182.0	74.5	68.2	Gollnick[32]
	M	24	180.4	79.2	70.3	Hermansen[38]
	M	25	180.0	72.8	67.1	Burke[8]
	M	—	180.3	67.1	74.0	Burke[6]
	M	—	—	—	74.0	Saltin[73]
	M	—	—	—	69.1	Strømme[85]
	F	20	165.0	55.0	50.2	Burke[8]
	F	—	167.7	61.3	57.4	Burke[6]
Canoeing/paddlers	M	19	173.0	64.0	60.0	Sidney[77]
	M	22	190.5	80.7	67.7	Hermansen[38]
	M	24	182.0	79.6	66.1	Rusko[72]
	M	26	181.0	74.0	56.8	Gollnick[32]
	F	18	166.0	57.3	49.2	Sidney[77]
Dancing, ballet	M	24	177.5	68.0	48.2	Cohen[13]
	F	24	165.6	49.5	43.7	Cohen[13]
general	F	21	162.7	51.2	41.5	Novak[56]
Football	M	19	186.8	93.1	56.5	Smith[80]
	M	20	184.9	96.4	51.3	Novak[55]
Defensive backs	M	25	182.5	84.8	53.1	Wilmore[96]
Offensive backs	M	25	183.8	90.7	52.2	Wilmore[96]
Linebackers	M	24	188.6	102.2	52.1	Wilmore[96]
Offensive linemen	M	25	193.0	112.6	49.9	Wilmore[96]
Defensive linemen	M	26	192.4	117.1	44.9	Wilmore[96]
Quarterbacks/kickers	M	24	185.0	90.1	49.0	Wilmore[96]
Gymnastics	M	20	178.5	69.2	55.5	Novak[55]
	F	15	159.7	48.8	49.8	Hermansen[38]
	F	19	163.0	57.9	36.3	Conger[14]
Ice hockey	M	11	140.5	35.5	56.6	Cunningham[23]
	M	22	179.0	77.3	61.5	Rusko[72]
	M	24	179.3	81.8	54.6	Seliger[75]
	M	26	180.1	86.4	53.6	Wilmore[95]
Jockey	M	31	158.2	50.3	53.8	Wilmore[95]
Orienteering	M	25	179.7	70.3	71.1	Hermansen[38]
	M	31	—	72.2	61.6	Knowlton[42]
	M	52	176.0	72.7	50.7	Gollnick[32]
	F	23	165.8	60.0	60.7	Hermansen[38]
	F	29	—	58.1	46.1	Knowlton[42]
Pentathlon	F	21	175.4	65.4	45.9	Krahenbuhl[44]
Racketball/handball	M	24	183.7	81.3	60.0	Hermansen[38]
	M	25	181.7	80.3	58.3	Pipes[61]
Rowing	M	—	—	—	65.7	Strømme[85]
	M	23	192.7	89.9	62.6	Mickelson[50]
	M	25	189.9	86.9	66.9	Hermansen[38]
Heavyweight	M	23	192.0	88.0	68.9	Hagerman[34]
Lightweight	M	21	186.0	71.0	71.1	Hagerman[34]
	F	23	173.0	68.0	60.3	Hagerman[34]

TABLE 8-2. (continued)

Athletic group or sport	Sex	Age (years)	Height (cm)	Weight (kg)	$\dot{V}O_2$ max (ml·kg^{-1}·min^{-1})	References[a]
Skating, speed	M	20	175.5	73.9	56.1	Maksud[47]
	M	21	181.0	76.5	72.9	Rusko[72]
	M	25	183.1	82.4	64.6	Hermansen[38]
	F	20	168.1	65.4	52.0	Hermansen[38]
	F	21	164.5	60.8	46.1	Maksud[47]
Figure	M	21	166.9	59.6	58.5	Niinimaa[53]
	F	17	158.8	48.6	48.9	Niinimaa[53]
Skiing, Alpine	M	16	173.1	65.5	65.6	Song[81]
	M	21	176.0	70.1	63.8	Rusko[72]
	M	22	177.8	75.5	66.6	Haymes[37]
	M	26	176.6	74.8	62.3	Sprynarova[83]
	F	19	165.1	58.8	52.7	Haymes[37]
Cross-country	M	21	176.0	66.6	63.9	Niinimaa[54]
	M	25	180.4	73.2	73.9	Hermansen[38]
	M	26	174.0	69.3	78.3	Rusko[72]
	M	23	176.2	73.2	73.0	Haymes[37]
	M	—	—	—	72.8	Strømme[85]
	F	20	163.4	55.9	61.5	Haymes[37]
	F	24	163.0	59.1	68.2	Rusko[72]
	F	25	165.7	60.5	56.9	Hermansen[38]
	F	—	—	—	58.1	Strømme[85]
Nordic	M	23	176.0	70.4	72.8	Rusko[72]
	M	22	181.7	70.4	67.4	Haymes[37]
Ski jumping	M	22	174.0	69.9	61.3	Rusko[72]
Soccer	M	26	176.0	75.5	58.4	Raven[67]
Swimming	M	12	150.4	41.2	52.5	Cunningham[21]
	M	13	164.8	52.1	52.9	Cunningham[21]
	M	15	169.6	59.8	56.6	Cunningham[21]
	M	15	166.8	59.1	56.8	Vaccaro[89]
	M	20	181.4	76.7	55.7	Magel[45]
	M	20	181.0	73.0	50.4	Charbonnier[11]
	M	21	182.9	78.9	62.1	Novak[55]
	M	21	181.0	78.3	69.9	Gollnick[32]
	M	22	182.3	79.1	56.9	Sprynarova[83]
	M	22	182.3	79.7	55.9	Cunningham[21]
	F	12	154.8	43.3	46.2	Cunningham[21]
	F	13	160.0	52.1	43.4	Cunningham[21]
	F	15	164.8	53.7	40.5	Cunningham[21]
Sprint	M	19	181.1	75.0	58.3	Shephard[76]
Middle-distance	M	22	178.0	74.6	55.4	Shephard[76]
Long-distance	M	21	179.0	74.9	65.4	Shephard[76]
	F	19	168.0	63.8	37.6	Conger[14]
Tennis	M	42	179.6	77.1	50.2	Vodak[92]
	F	39	163.3	55.7	44.2	Vodak[92]
Track and field	M	21	180.6	71.6	66.1	Novak[55]
Runners	M	22	177.4	64.5	64.0	Sprynarova[83]
	M	23	177.0	69.5	72.4	Gollnick[32]
Sprint	M	17–22	—	—	51.0	Thomas[88]
	M	46	177.0	74.1	47.2	Barnard[3]
Middle-distance	M	25	180.1	67.8	70.1	Costill[18]
	M	25	179.0	72.3	69.8	Rusko[72]
Distance	M	10	144.3	31.9	56.6	Mayers[49]
	M	17–22	—	—	65.5	Thomas[88]
	M	26	176.1	64.5	72.2	Hermansen[38]
	M	26	178.9	63.9	77.4	Costill[18]

96 SPORTS MEDICINE FOR THE MATURE ATHLETE

TABLE 8-2. (continued)

Athletic group or sport	Sex	Age (years)	Height (cm)	Weight (kg)	$\dot{V}O_2$ max (ml·kg^{-1}·min^{-1})	References[a]
	M	26	177.0	66.2	78.1	Rusko[72]
	M	27	178.7	64.9	73.2	Costill[17]
	M	32	177.3	64.3	70.3	Costill[19]
	M	35	174.0	63.1	66.6	Costill[18]
	M	36	177.3	69.6	65.1	Hagan[33]
	M	40–49	180.7	71.6	57.5	Pollock[64]
	M	55	174.5	63.4	54.4	Barnard[3]
	M	50–59	174.7	67.2	54.4	Pollock[64]
	M	60–69	175.7	67.1	51.4	Pollock[64]
	M	70–75	175.6	66.8	40.0	Pollock[64]
	M	—	—	—	72.5	Davies[24]
	F	16	162.2	48.6	63.2	Burke[7]
	F	16	163.3	50.9	50.8	Butts[9]
	F	21	170.2	58.6	57.5	Hermansen[38]
	F	32	169.4	57.2	59.1	Wilmore[97]
	F	44	161.5	53.8	43.4	Vaccaro[91]
	F	—	—	—	58.2	Davies[24]
Race walking	M	27	178.7	68.5	62.9	Franklin[28]
Jumpers	M	17–22	—	—	55.0	Thomas[88]
Shot/discus	M	17–22	—	—	49.5	Thomas[88]
	M	26	190.8	110.5	42.8	Wilmore[95]
	M	27	188.2	112.5	42.6	Fahey[27]
	M	28	186.1	104.7	47.5	Fahey[27]
Volleyball	M	25	187.0	84.5	56.4	Conlee[15]
	M	26	192.7	85.5	56.1	Puhl[66]
	F	19	166.0	59.8	43.5	Conger[14]
	F	20	172.2	64.1	56.0	Kovaleski[43]
	F	22	183.7	73.4	41.7	Spence[82]
	F	22	178.3	70.5	50.6	Puhl[66]
Weightlifting	M	25	171.0	81.3	40.1	Gollnick[32]
	M	25	166.4	77.2	42.6	Sprynarova[83]
Power	M	26	176.1	92.0	49.5	Fahey[27]
Olympic	M	25	177.1	88.2	50.7	Fahey[27]
Bodybuilder	M	27	178.8	88.1	46.3	Pipes[60]
	M	29	172.4	83.1	41.5	Fahey[27]
Wrestling	M	21	174.8	67.3	58.3	Stine[84]
	M	23	—	79.2	50.4	Taylor[86]
	M	24	175.6	77.7	60.9	Nagel[52]
	M	26	177.0	81.8	64.0	Fahey[27]
	M	27	176.0	75.7	54.3	Gale[30]

[a]First author only.
From: Wilmore, J. H. The Assessment of and Variation in Aerobic Power in World-Class Athletes as Related to the Specific Sport. *Am. J. Sport Med.* 12:12:–127, 1984. Refer to original publication for references.

treadmill following swim training, while $\dot{V}O_2$ max during tethered swimming improved by 18%. Thus, with certain groups of athletes, mode selection may be an important issue.

In addition to the proper selection of ergometers, selecting an appropriate exercise test protocol is equally important. An inappropriate protocol may provide erroneous data and lead to inaccurate interpretations. For most applications, the protocol selected should not exceed 8 to 12 minutes. The se-

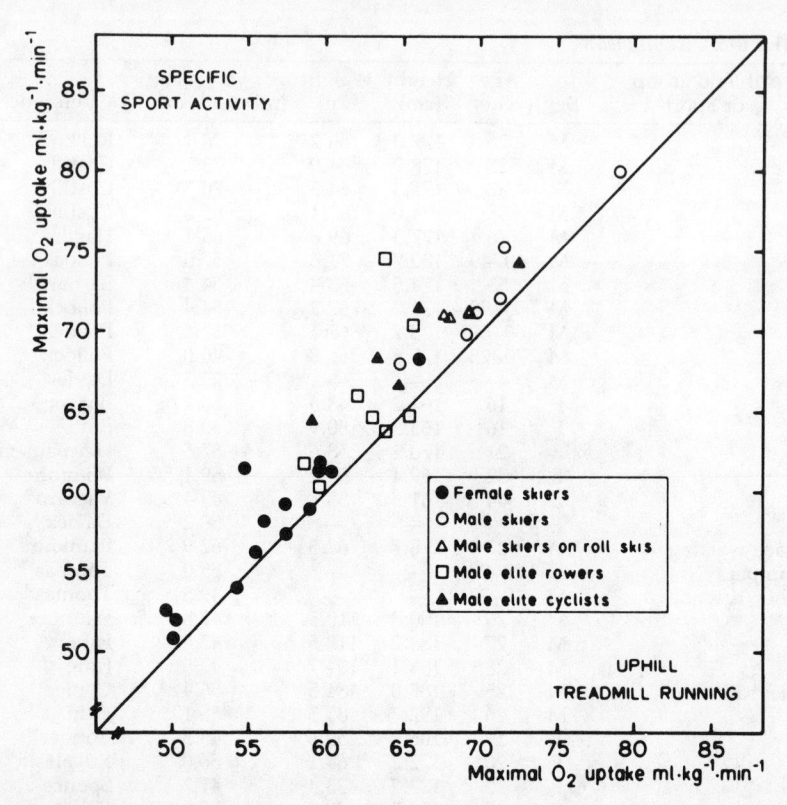

Fig. 8-2. *Maximal oxygen uptake values during uphill treadmill running vs. sport-specific activities in selected groups of athletes. (adapted from Stromme, S. B., et al., J. Appl. Physiol:REEP 42:833–837, 1977.)*

lected protocol should be of approximately the same length for all subjects to avoid the comparison of data collected under different physiological conditions. The selected protocol should provide increments in power output which do not exceed 1.0 to 2.0 METS, and the length of the work periods should be at least 3 minutes if steady state data are desired. However, much shorter periods should be used for non-steady state tests. Finally, it is recommended that protocols be designed which are customized to the problem under study. Existing protocols can be used as guidelines, but a customized protocol meets the needs of the specific athletic population being tested and should result in more representative data.

Anaerobic Power and Anerobic Threshold

For many athletes in certain sports or events within a sport, the aerobic power demands are low, but the anaerobic power demands are high. Bouchard et al. (5) have recently proposed a new conceptual framework for the assessment of aerobic power based on those metabolic events which occur within a certain time frame. This classification includes: a) alactacid anaerobic capacity (total energy output during a maximal effort of 10 to 15 seconds); b) alactacid anaerobic power (maximal rate of energy output during an all-out

10-to-15-second bout of work); c) lactacid anaerobic capacity (total energy output during a maximal effort lasting 60 to 120 seconds); and d) lactacid anaerobic power (maximum rate of energy output during a maximal effort of 60 to 120 seconds). The alactacid assessment attempts to evaluate the ATP/CP energy system, while the lactacid assessment attempts to evaluate the glycolytic energy system.

While several tests of anaerobic power have been proposed, the two most popular are the Margaria-Kalamen Power Test and the Wingate Anaerobic Power Test. In the Margaria-Kalamen Power Test, the athlete runs up a staircase at full speed, taking 3 steps at a time. A switchmat is placed on the 3rd and 6th steps, and the time necessary to go from the 3rd to the 6th step is recorded. The weight of the subject, the vertical height between the 3rd and 6th steps, and the time to cover the distance between the 3rd and 6th steps are used to compute anaerobic power. Unfortunately, the test is greatly influenced by the weight of the subject. The Wingate Anaerobic Power Test is administered on a cycle ergometer, with the athlete attempting to complete as many pedal revolutions as possible in a 30-second period of time at a resistance predetermined on the basis of the individual's body weight. The number of pedal revolutions is recorded every 5 seconds, and the maximal power output for any one 5-second period and the total work performed in 30 seconds is determined. Unfortunately, a large data base is presently unavailable for athletes in a wide variety of sports for either test. Other tests of anaerobic power have been proposed (5), but have not received as wide acceptance as these 2 tests.

Anaerobic threshold refers to that point during a graded exercise test at which blood lactate levels begin to increase above pre-exercise resting levels. This point has also been referred to as the lactate threshold and the onset of plasma lactate accumulation, among others. For most individuals, this occurs at a work rate which represents 40 to 60% of their $\dot{V}O_2$ max. While the concept of anaerobic threshold has been openly debated over the past few years (6, 9), there is good evidence that this breakpoint in blood lactate levels has considerable significance with respect to performance. Farrell et al. (10) found that the speed of the treadmill corresponding to the lactate breakpoint in a group of trained distance runners was highly correlated to their race pace. In fact, this was the most significant factor differentiating variations in the runners' race pace. The treadmill speed at which the lactate breakpoint occurred was remarkably close to the race pace for the runner's fastest marathon. Others have confirmed these findings (9).

The assessment of lactate threshold requires multiple blood samples at various steady state paces, which necessitates a venous catheter and considerable work to analyze the lactate concentration in these multiple samples. This has led investigators to search for alternative, non-invasive techniques to estimate this lactate breakpoint. While the use of respiratory/metabolic parameters such as the ventilatory equivalent for oxygen ($\dot{V}E/\dot{V}O_2$) and the ventilatory equivalent for carbon dioxide ($\dot{V}E/\dot{V}CO_2$), have demonstrated validity in the prediction of this breakpoint (9), these non-invasive techniques are also very indirect and have come under considerable criticism (6). As with anaerobic power, there is not a large data base on lactate thresholds of athletes in different sports.

Muscular Strength, Power, and Endurance

There are three different types of muscular contraction: isometric, in which the muscle length remains unchanged; eccentric, in which muscle performs a lengthening contraction (e.g., a controlled lowering of the weight in a two-arm curl), and concentric, in which the muscle performs a shortening contraction. Isometric contractions are also referred to as static contractions; eccentric and concentric contractions are referred to as dynamic contractions.

Strength refers to the ability of the muscle or a group of muscles to exert or apply force. Usually, the term "strength" is used in the context of one's maximum force-producing capabilities. The individual who can successfully bench press a maximum of 200 pounds is twice as strong as the individual who can bench-press a maximum of only 100 pounds. In the purest sense, however, this illustration is not totally accurate, as the result of a bench press is work (i.e., work = force × distance), not just force alone. A static or isometric contraction provides a more precise estimation of strength. In fact, Atha (2), in his extensive review of the strength literature, defines strength very specifically as the ability to develop force against an unyielding resistance in a single contraction of unrestricted duration. However, dynamic tests of functional strength are generally considered acceptable.

For the masters athlete, and possibly for the average person as well, power is the key component for most physical activity. Power is defined as work per unit time (i.e., power = (force × distance)/time). Two individuals who can bench press a maximum of 200 pounds have identical functional strength. However, if one individual is able to execute his or her maximum bench press strength in half of the time (e.g., 1.0 seconds compared to 2.0 seconds), he or she would have twice the power of the other individual. While absolute strength is important for many activities, power is probably of even greater functional significance.

Muscular endurance refers to the ability of the muscle or a group of muscles to sustain repeated contractions or to sustain a fixed or static contraction for an extended period of time. Muscular endurance is frequently equated with resistance to local muscular fatigue and is not to be confused with cardiorespiratory endurance associated with total body fatigue.

There is no universally accepted standard measure which is considered representative of muscular strength in the same manner that $\dot{V}O_2$ max is considered representative of cardiorespiratory endurance capacity. First, there appears to be a high degree of specificity associated with strength. A person with a high level of grip strength does not necessarily have high levels of upper or lower body strength. Clarke (8) has conducted possibly the most extensive analysis of the specificity vs. generality of muscular strength. Reporting the results of extensive testing on males and females, from fourth grade through college, he concluded that generally the strength of various muscle groups throughout the body did not correlate highly with one another. While one intercorrelation reached $r = 0.91$, seldom did intercorrelations reach $r = 0.80$. Using cable-tension, static strength testing procedures on 25 selected sites, he reported that the highest correlations among strength tests were between muscle groups in the same joint area, frequently antagonists. Using the average of all 25 strength tests as the strength criterion, shoulder extension strength had the highest correlation with the strength criterion in the upper elementary and junior high school ages for both boys and girls, and for boys in senior high school.

As a result of the high degree of specificity of strength, some test batteries will include several estimates of strength, representing different regions of the body. Clarke (8), using factor analysis, reported 5 cluster areas including arm-shoulder strength, leg-back lift strength, lower-leg strength, grip strength, and general strength. Jackson et al. (15) conducted a similar factor analysis study using one-repetition maximum strength assessments of 12 selected sites. They identified 3 factors which included upper and lower extremity, as well as trunk strength. Thus, strength assessment in at least 3 areas (i.e., upper body, trunk, and lower body) would seem highly desirable for most athletic performance profiles of specific sports.

Muscular power, while probably of greater functional significance than the single component of strength, has received relatively little attention. While most scientists, clinicians, and practitioners would agree on the importance of muscular power, the inability to obtain simple measurements of power has greatly restricted the development of an adequate data base. With advancements in technology, new testing systems interfaced with dedicated computers have recently provided the researcher with accurate and rapid means of power assessment. Within the next several years it should be possible to define a representative power testing battery which then will be followed logically by testing of the general and athletic populations to establish normative data.

Muscular endurance appears to be highly specific to the muscle or muscle group tested. In addition, there are few pure tests of muscular endurance that have been used to test the general population. Most testing of muscular endurance has been through field tests. In fact, many of these field tests could be classified as combination strength-muscular endurance tests. Examples from existing test batteries would include the pull-up, flexed arm hang, and sit-up from the AAHPERD Youth Fitness Test (1) and the President's Council on Physical Fitness and Sports' Youth Physical Fitness Test (26). Use of laboratory test equipment, such as the Cybex II isokinetic test device, allows much more accurate assessments of muscular endurance as a distinct component. As an example, the Cybex II test device allows the expression of maximal force on each repetition. Having the individual perform a series of maximal contractions at a constant rate (e.g., one contraction every 2 seconds) for a set time period (e.g., 1 minute) allows the calculation of the total work performed during the test period, the decrement in power output from the initial few contractions to the final few contractions, the variation in performance at varying speeds of contraction, or other measurements that would reflect the muscular endurance of that muscle or muscle group. Since the use of these more advanced laboratory testing devices has been greatly limited, normative data is not available.

Flexibility

Flexibility refers to the range of motion, or to the looseness or suppleness of the body or specific joints, and reflects the interrelationships between muscles, tendons, ligaments, and the joint itself (31). Most young people have relatively high levels of flexibility, but this is rapidly lost with aging. Too much flexibility can lead to joint laxity, which is associated with joint instability and increased susceptibility to injury. At the other extreme, joint tightness also predisposes one to increased risk for injury, particularly sports-related injuries. Several factors limit the range of motion at a joint, including the structure of the joint, the interface between 2 articulating surfaces, soft tissues surrounding the joint (e.g., muscles, tendons, ligaments, fascia, and skin) and certain pathologies or previous injuries (14).

Flexibility is not an easy component to measure accurately. In the laboratory, flexibility is typically assessed by an electrogoniometer or flexometer. Both of these devices are used to measure the degrees of rotation through the range of joint motion. The Leighton flexometer has a weighted 360-degree dial and a weighted pointer mounted in a case. The dial and pointer move independently and both are controlled by gravity. Both can be locked in position independently of each other. The segment to be measured is usually positioned at one extreme in the range of motion, the dial locked in position, and then the segment is moved through the full range of motion. The pointer follows the movement of the segment, thus indicating the extent of movement or degrees of movement. The electrogoniometer is a protractor-like device which is used to measure the joint angle at both extremes in the range of movement. A potentiometer provides an electrical signal proportional to the angle of the joint. Most of the major joints in the body can be measured using either of these devices.

Field testing of flexibility has generally been limited to the sit-and-reach test. In this test, the individual sits on the floor with the legs extended forward. Bending forward at the waist with the knees locked and pressed against the floor, the individual reaches forward as far as possible, attempting to touch the toes, or as far beyond the toes as possible. The extent of forward reach is then measured. This test is used as an index of lower back and hamstrings flexibility.

Unfortunately, similar to strength as discussed previously, flexibility is highly specific to the joint and joint action (14). Harris (13) investigated the structure of certain measures of flexibility by the technique of factor analysis in 147 college women. Using 42 joint action measures of flexibility and an additional 13 composite measures of flexibility, it was concluded that no one composite test or no one joint action measure provides a satisfactory index of individual flexibility. Thus, to develop an appropriate battery to test flexibility, it would be necessary first to define those joints or composite movements considered important to the athletic population being evaluated.

Body Composition

The body is composed of a number of different components which can be categorized into chemically or anatomically-defined compartments. Possibly the simplest, and probably the most widely used classification system differentiates total body weight into two components: fat weight and lean weight. Fat weight is defined as the weight of the body's total fat stores, and includes what some have termed the "essential fat." Lean weight, or fat-free body weight, is composed of the skeletal mass, muscle mass, and organs of the body including the skin. By using such a classification system, it is possible to differentiate between overweight and obesity. Overweight is defined as exceeding the range of values established from general population norms for a given height and frame size. Obesity refers to the state of being overfat (i.e., the weight of fat expressed as a percentage of one's total body weight exceeds that value which is considered to represent the upper limit of normal). For men, values ranging from 20 to 25% body fat are considered borderline obesity, and values exceeding 25% are considered frank obesity. For women, the values are 30 to 35% for borderline obesity and 36% or above for frank obesity.

The major problem associated with the use of standardized height/weight tables is that these tables do not take into consideration the composition of the body. This was clearly demonstrated by Welham and Behnke (30) in their study of professional football players reported in 1942. The players were found to be grossly overweight, yet they had high levels of lean body weight and low levels of body fat. This illustrates the important point that one can be overweight but of normal body composition. Likewise, it is possible to be excessively fat, yet fall within the normal range for height and frame size.

A number of procedures have been devised to assess body composition. In the laboratory, the densitometric technique has been regarded as the "gold standard," or the criterion technique. Other laboratory techniques include helium dilution to determine total body volume; isotopic dilution to determine total body water; ^{40}K to determine lean body weight; radiography of the extremities to determine proportions of bone, muscle and fat; computer-assisted tomography to observe cross sections of extremity segments; nuclear magnetic resonance; total body electrical conductivity; and electrical impedance. The densitometric technique was used in dogs in the early 1930s, and in humans beginning with the early work of Behnke and his colleagues in the late 1930s and early 1940s (3, 30). Since that time, body composition by the densitometric technique has become widely used in both research and clinical practice.

Although the underwater weighing technique is the most accurate laboratory test available to determine the total density of the body and its subsequent composition, it does have limitations. For those individuals undergoing changes in bone mineral (i.e., increasing bone mineral in the youngster as he or she matures, or decreasing bone mineral in the aging individual), the equations used to estimate relative fat from body density will be inaccurate, providing an overestimation of the actual fat percentage. For those individuals with a larger preponderance of bone, or bone that is denser than the population average, the estimate of relative fat will also be inaccurate, with an underestimation of the actual fat percentage. These inaccuracies occur infrequently, but they do occur. The primary reason for these inaccuracies relates to the fact that for the several equations available for translating body density to relative body fat, only a single constant is used to represent the density of all body fat, and a single constant is used to represent the density of all of the body's lean tissue.

There is little disagreement as to the appropriate value to use for the density of the fat tissue, since there appears to be consistency in the density of fat among different sites on the same individual, and consistency between individuals. The value typically selected to represent the density of fat is 0.9007 gm/cm^3 (7). There is, however, considerable variation in the density of the lean body mass among individuals. While the value 1.100 gm/cm^3 has been used in most equations (7), this assumes a chemically mature individual who has not undergone substantial changes in lean tissue associated with inactivity and aging. Lohman (19) argues that for certain groups of individuals, the density of lean tissue should be less than the assumed value of 1.100 gm/cm^3. These groups would include children, females, certain athletic groups, and the aged. For other groups such as blacks and lean athletes, it appears that the density of lean tissue would be higher than that presently used (27). Schutte et al. (27) have recently presented convincing data which support the use of a higher value for the density of lean tissue in a population of blacks (i.e., 1.113 vs. 1.100 gm/cm^3). While this may seem like an inconsequential difference, for a body density of 1.075, the relative body fat calculated from the standard formulae would be 10.5% using a constant of 1.100 gm/cm^3, and 14.1% using a constant of 1.113 gm/cm^3. Lohman et al. (20) have reported a similar finding for children, but in the opposite direction. They reported that a constant of 1.085 gm/cm^3 is much more appropriate for prepubescent children who have not achieved the density of adult lean tissue.

This variability in the density of lean tissue leads to a violation of the basic assumptions underlying the derivation of a specific density value for the conversion equation. To derive a single value for a specific equation, it must be assumed that each component of the lean body mass has a constant density which does not vary among individuals. In addition, the assumption must be made that each of these components makes a constant proportional contribution to the density of the lean tissue. It is now recognized that neither of these assumptions is based on a solid foundation, and that there are individuals and entire populations that violate these basic assumptions (32).

The underwater weighing technique, despite the above limitations, is still considered the criterion method to evaluate body composition. However, the procedure is time-consuming, requires considerable space and equipment, and must be conducted by someone who is highly trained. As a result, most body composition evaluations, particularly in non-research, clinical settings, are derived through anthropometric techniques. Using skinfold thickness measurements, girths, and diameters, either singly or in combination, it is possible to derive accurate estimates of body composition. For many years, data were reported which suggested that equations to predict body composition were highly specific to the population from which they were derived. Jackson and Pollock (16) and Jackson, Pollock, and Ward (17) derived a series of equations for men and women, respectively, that are generalized (i.e., applicable to all men and women of varying age and body composition). Sinning and Wilson (28) recently confirmed the validity of these equations in groups of women athletes.

Relative body fat values vary by sex and level of physical activity. While there is a substantial difference in relative fat between college-age males and females (i.e., mean values of 13 to 16% for males and 20 to 25% for females), differences between the sexes are much less when comparing equally trained athletes. This is illustrated in Table 8-3. The larger differences in the non-athletic population are probably the result of a more active male being compared with a relatively sedentary female (33). Thus, true sex-specific differ-

TABLE 8-3. *Body Composition Values of Selected Athletes*

Athletic Group or Sport	Sex	Age (yr)	Height (cm)	Weight (kg)	Relative Fat %	Reference
Baseball	male	20.8	182.7	83.3	14.2	Novak et al., 1968 (58)
	male	—	—	—	11.8	Forsyth and Sinning, 1973 (18)
	male	27.4	183.1	88.0	12.6	Wilmore, unpublished
Basketball	female	19.1	169.1	62.6	20.8	Sinning, 1973 (82)
	female	19.4	167.0	63.9	26.9	Conger and MacNab, 1967 (12)
Centers	male	27.7	214.0	109.2	7.1	Parr et al., 1978 (68)
Forwards	male	25.3	200.6	96.9	9.0	Parr et al., 1978 (68)
Guards	male	25.2	188.0	83.6	10.6	Parr et al., 1978 (68)
Canoeing	male	23.7	182.0	79.6	12.4	Rusko et al., 1978 (80)
Football	male	20.3	184.9	96.4	13.8	Novak et al., 1968 (58)
	male	—	—	—	13.9	Forsyth and Sinning, 1973 (18)
Defensive backs	male	17–23	178.3	77.3	11.5	Wickkiser and Kelley, 1975 (100)
	male	24.5	182.5	84.8	9.6	Wilmore et al., 1976 (110)
Offensive backs	male	17–23	179.7	79.8	12.4	Wickkiser and Kelley, 1975 (100)
	male	24.7	183.8	90.7	9.4	Wilmore et al., 1976 (110)
Linebackers	male	17–23	180.1	87.2	13.4	Wickkiser and Kelley, 1975 (100)
	male	24.2	188.6	102.2	14.0	Wilmore et al., 1976 (110)
Offensive linemen	male	17–23	186.0	99.2	19.1	Wickkiser and Kelly, 1975 (100)
	male	24.7	193.0	112.6	15.6	Wilmore et al., 1976 (110)
Defensive linemen	male	17–23	186.6	97.8	18.5	Wickkiser and Kelly, 1975 (100)
	male	25.7	192.4	117.1	18.2	Wilmore et al., 1976 (110)
Quarterbacks, kickers	male	24.1	185.0	90.1	14.4	Wilmore et al., 1976 (110)
Gymnastics	male	20.3	178.5	69.2	4.6	Novak et al., 1968 (58)
	female	19.4	163.0	57.9	23.8	Conger and MacNab, 1967 (12)
	female	20.0	158.5	51.5	15.5	Sinning and Lindberg, 1972 (84)
	female	14.0	—	—	17.0	Parizkova, 1972 (66)
	female	23.0	—	—	11.0	Parizkova, 1972 (66)
	female	23.0	—	—	9.6	Parizkova and Poupa, 1963 (67)

TABLE 8-3. *(continued)*

Athletic Group or Sport	Sex	Age (yr)	Height (cm)	Weight (kg)	Relative Fat %	Reference
Ice hockey	male	26.3	180.3	86.7	15.1	Wilmore, unpublished
	male	22.5	179.0	77.3	13.0	Rusko et al., 1978 (80)
Jockeys	male	30.9	158.2	50.3	14.1	Wilmore, unpublished
Orienteering	male	31.2	—	72.2	16.3	Knowlton et al., 1980 (40)
	female	29.0	—	58.1	18.7	Knowlton et al., 1980 (40)
Pentathlon	female	21.5	175.4	65.4	11.0	Krahenbuhl et al., 1979 (44)
Racketball	male	25.0	181.7	80.3	8.1	Pipes, 1979 (69)
Lightweight	male	21.0	186.0	71.0	8.5	Hagerman et al., 1979 (28)
	female	23.0	173.0	68.0	14.0	Hagerman et al., 1979 (28)
Skiing	male	25.9	176.6	74.8	7.4	Sprynarova and Parizkova, 1971 (88)
Alpine	male	21.2	176.0	70.1	14.1	Rusko et al., 1978 (80)
	male	21.8	177.8	75.5	10.2	Haymes and Dickinson, 1980 (29)
	female	19.5	165.1	58.8	20.6	Haymes and Dickinson, 1980 (29)
Cross-country	male	21.2	176.0	66.6	12.5	Niinimaa et al., 1978 (57)
	male	25.6	174.0	69.3	10.2	Rusko et al., 1978 (80)
	male	22.7	176.2	73.2	7.9	Haymes and Dickinson, 1980 (29)
	female	24.3	163.0	59.1	21.8	Rusko et al., 1978 (80)
	female	20.2	163.4	55.9	15.7	Haymes and Dickinson, 1980 (29)
Nordic combination	male	22.9	176.0	70.4	11.2	Rusko et al., 1978 (80)
	male	21.7	181.7	70.4	8.9	Haymes and Dickinson, 1980 (29)
Skijumping	male	22.2	174.0	69.9	14.3	Rusko et al., 1978 (80)
Soccer	male	26.0	176.0	75.5	9.6	Raven et al., 1976 (78)
Speed skating	male	21.0	181.0	76.5	11.4	Rusko et al., 1978 (80)
Swimming	male	21.8	182.3	79.1	8.5	Sprynarova and Parizkova, 1971 (88)
	male	20.6	182.9	78.9	5.0	Novak et al., 1968 (58)
	female	19.4	168.0	63.8	26.3	Conger and MacNab, 1968 (12)
Sprint	female	—	165.1	57.1	14.6	Wilmore et al., 1977 (106)
Middle distance	female	—	166.6	66.8	24.1	Wilmore et al., 1977 (106)
Distance	female	—	166.3	60.9	17.1	Wilmore et al., 1977 (106)
Tennis	male	—	—	—	15.2	Forsyth and Sinning, 1973 (18)
	male	42.0	179.6	77.1	16.3	Vodak et al., 1980 (98)
	female	39.0	163.3	55.7	20.3	Vodak et al., 1980 (98)
Track and field	male	21.3	180.6	71.6	3.7	Novak et al., 1968 (58)
	male	—	—	—	8.8	Forsyth and Sinning, 1973 (18)
Runners	male	22.5	177.4	64.5	6.3	Sprynarova and Parizkova, 1971 (88)
Distance	male	26.1	175.7	64.2	7.5	Costill et al., 1970 (13)
	male	26.2	177.0	66.2	8.4	Rusko et al., 1978 (80)
	male	40–49	180.7	71.6	11.2	Pollock et al., 1974 (74)
	male	55.3	174.5	63.4	18.0	Barnard et al., 1974 (3)
	male	50–59	174.7	67.2	10.9	Pollock, et al., 1974 (74)
	male	60–69	175.7	67.1	11.3	Pollock et al., 1974 (74)
	male	70–75	175.6	66.8	13.6	Pollock et al., 1974 (74)
	male	47.2	176.5	70.7	13.2	Lewis et al., 1975 (45)
	female	19.9	161.3	52.9	19.2	Malina et al., 1971 (47)
	female	32.4	169.4	57.2	15.2	Wilmore and Brown, 1974 (104)
Middle distance	male	24.6	179.0	72.3	12.4	Rusko et al., 1978 (80)
Sprint	female	20.1	164.9	56.7	19.3	Malina et al., 1971 (47)
	male	46.5	177.0	74.1	16.5	Barnard et al., 1979 (3)
Discus	male	28.3	186.1	104.7	16.4	Fahey et al., 1975 (17)
	male	26.4	190.8	110.5	16.3	Wilmore, unpublished
	female	21.1	168.1	71.0	25.0	Malina et al., 1971 (47)
Jumpers and hurdlers	female	20.3	165.9	59.0	20.7	Malina et al., 1971 (47)
Shot put	male	27.0	188.2	112.5	16.5	Fahey et al., 1975 (17)
	male	22.0	191.6	126.2	19.6	Behnke and Wilmore, 1974 (4)
	female	21.5	167.6	78.1	28.0	Malina et al., 1971 (47)
Volleyball	female	19.4	166.0	59.8	25.3	Conger and MacNab, 1968 (12)
	female	19.9	172.2	64.1	21.3	Kovaleski et al., 1980 (43)
Weight lifting	male	24.9	166.4	77.2	9.8	Sprynarova and Parizkova, 1971 (88)
Power	male	26.3	176.1	92.0	15.6	Fahey et al., 1975 (17)
Olympic	male	25.3	177.1	88.2	12.2	Fahey et al., 1975 (17)
Body builders	male	29.0	172.4	83.1	8.4	Fahey et al., 1975 (17)
	male	27.6	178.8	88.1	8.3	Pipes, 1979 (70)
Wrestling	male	26.0	177.8	81.8	9.8	Fahey et al., 1975 (17)
	male	27.0	176.0	75.7	10.7	Gale and Flynn, 1974 (20)
	male	22.0	—	—	5.0	Parizkova, 1972 (66)
	male	23.0	—	79.3	14.3	Taylor et al., 1979 (92)
	male	19.6	174.6	74.8	8.8	Sinning, 1974 (81)
	male	15–18	172.3	66.3	6.9	Katch and Michael, 1971 (35)
	male	20.6	174.8	67.3	4.0	Stine et al., 1979 (90)

*Adapted from J. H. Wilmore et al., Body physique and composition of the female distance runner. *Ann. NY Acad. Sci.* 301:764–776, 1977.

ences in relative body fat, independent of the level of physical activity, are more likely between 4 and 6 percentage units. Once full maturity is reached, relative body fat tends to increase with age. Again, this appears to be more related to reduced levels of physical activity and inappropriate dietary intake as opposed to a natural response to aging.

REFERENCES

1. AAHPERD Youth Fitness Test Manual. Reston, VA: American Alliance for Health, Physical Education, Recreation, and Dance, 1976.
2. Atha, J. Strengthing muscle. *Exerc. Sport Sci. Rev.* 9:1–73, 1982.
3. Behnke, A. R., and J. H. Wilmore. *Evaluation and Regulation of Body Build and Composition.* Englewood-Cliffs, NJ: Prentice-Hall, 1974.
4. Bouchard, C., and R. M. Malina. Genetics of physiological fitness and motor performance. *Exerc. Sports Sci. Rev.* 11:306–339, 1983.
5. Bouchard, C., A. W. Taylor, and S. Dulac. Testing maximal anaerobic power and capacity. In: *Physiological Testing of the Elite Athlete*, J. D. MacDougall, H. A. Wenger, and H. J. Green (eds.) Ottawa: Canadian Association of Sport Sciences, Mutual Press Ltd., 1982.
6. Brooks, G. A. Anaerobic threshold: Review of the concept and directions for future research. *Med. Sci. Sports Exerc.* 17:22–31, 1985.
7. Brozek, J., F. Grande, J. T. Anderson, and A. Keys. Densitometric analysis of body composition: Revision of some quantitative assumptions. *N.Y. Acad. Sci.*, 110:113–140, 1963.
8. Clarke, H. H. Toward a better understanding of muscular strength. *Phys. Fitness Res. Digest* 3:1–20, 1973.
9. Davis, J. A. Anaerobic threshold: Review of the concept and directions for future research. *Med. Sci. Sports Exerc.* 17:6–18, 1985.
10. Farrell, P. A., J. H. Wilmore, E. F. Coyle, J. E. Billing, and D. L. Costill. Plasma lactate accumulation and distance running performance. *Med. Sci. Sports* 11:338–344, 1979.
11. Gergley, T. J., W. D. McArdle, P. DeJesus, M. M. Toner, S. Jacobowitz, and R. J. Spina. Specificity of arm training on aerobic power during swimming and running. *Med. Sci. Sports Exerc.* 16:349–354, 1984.
12. Greenleaf, J. E., and S. Kozlowski. Physiological consequences of reduced physical activity during bed rest. *Exerc. Sport Sci. Rev.*, 10:84–119, 1982.
13. Harris, M. L. A factor analytic study of flexibility. *Res. Quart.* 40:62–70, 1969.
14. Hubley, C. Testing flexibility. In: *Physiological Testing of the Elite Athlete*. J. D. MacDougall, H. A. Wenger, and H. J. Green (eds.) Ottawa: Canadian Association of Sports Sciences, Mutual Press Limited, 1982.
15. Jackson, A., M. Watkins, and R. W. Patton. A factor analysis of twelve selected maximal isotonic strength performances on the Universal Gym. *Med. Sci. Sports Exerc.* 12:274–277, 1980.
16. Jackson, A. S., and M. L. Pollock. Generalized equations for predicting body density of men. *Br. J. Nutr.* 40:497–504, 1978.
17. Jackson, A. S., M. L. Pollock, and A. Ward. Generalized equations for predicting body density of women. *Med. Sci. Sports Exerc.* 12:175–182, 1980.
18. Klissouras, V. Heritability of adaptive variation. *J. Appl. Physiol.* 31:338–344, 1971.
19. Lohman, T. G. Skinfolds and body density and their relation to body fatness: A review. *Human Biol.* 53:181–225, 1981.
20. Lohman, T. G., R. A. Boileau, and M. H. Slaughter. Body composition in children and youth. In: *Advances in Pediatric Sport Sciences*, R. A. Boileau (ed.) Champaign, IL: Human Kinetics Publishers, Inc., 1984.
21. MacDougall, J. D., H. A. Wenger, and H. L. Green (eds.) *Physiological Testing of the Elite Athlete*. Ottawa: Canadian Association of Sport Sciences, Mutual Press, Ltd., 1982.
22. Magel, J. R., G. F. Foglia, W. D. McArdle, B. Gutin, G. S. Pechar, and F. I. Katch. Specificity of swim training on maximum oxygen uptake. *J. Appl. Physiol.* 38:151–155, 1975.
23. Mitchell, J. H., and G. Blomqvist. Maximal oxygen uptake. *N. Engl. J. Med.* 284:1018–1022, 1971.
24. Nicholas, J. A., and E. B. Hershman. Profiling. In: *Clinics in Sports Medicine*, Vol. 3, #1, January, 1984. Philadelphia: W. B. Saunders, 1984.
25. Pollock, M. L. The quantification of endurance training programs. *Exerc. Sport Sci. Rev.* 1:155–188, 1973.
26. President's Council on Physical Fitness. *Youth Physical Fitness*. Washington, D.C., U.S. Government Printing Office, 1967.
27. Schutte, J. E., E. J. Townsend, J. Hugg, R. F. Shoup, R. M. Malina, and C. G. Blomqvist. Density of lean body mass is greater in Blacks than in Whites. *J. Appl. Physiol.: REEP* 56:1647–1649, 1984.

28. Sinning, W. E., and J. R. Wilson. Validity of "generalized equations" for body composition analysis in women athletes. *Res. Quart. Exerc. Sports.* 55:153–160, 1984.
29. Stromme, S. B., F. Ingjer, and H. D. Meen. Assessment of maximal aerobic power in specifically trained athletes. *J. Appl. Physiol.: REEP* 42:833–837, 1977.
30. Welham, W. C., and A. R. Behnke. The specific gravity of healthy men; body weight divided by volume and other physical characteristics of exceptional athletes and of naval personnel. *J.A.M.A.* 118:498–501, 1942.
31. Wilmore, J. H. *Training for Sport and Activity: The Physiological Basis of the Conditioning Process*, 2nd ed. Boston: Allyn and Bacon, 1982.
32. Wilmore, J. H. Body composition in sport and exercise: Directions for future research. *Med. Sci. Sports Exerc.* 15:21–31, 1983.
33. Wilmore, J. H., C. H. Brown, and J. A. Davis. Body physique and composition of the female distance runner. *Ann. NY Acad. Sci.*, 301:764–776, 1977.

9

The Canadian Association Of Sport Sciences' Guidelines For the Physiological Testing Of the Elite Athlete

HOWARD A. WENGER

University of Victoria

The Canadian Association of Sport Sciences developed in 1982 a manual, "Physiological Testing of the Elite Athlete." The project grew from concerns of scientists, coaches, administrators and athletes that:

1. Test batteries were composed of general tests of fitness which were not tailored to the specific needs of the elite athlete.
2. Coaches and athletes were unable to interpret the test results.
3. Many testing programs were designed for research and data collection rather than directed toward assisting the athlete in training program design.
4. Testing protocols to assess the same physiological functions varied from laboratory to laboratory, making comparisons and interpretations difficult, if not impossible.

The manual outlines the importance of a sound testing program, suggests appropriate tests and standardized protocols, and presents the rationale behind the tests and the importance of the component tested for performance. It is intended for use by coaches and technical directors as well as the technicians and scientists involved in testing and counseling elite athletes.

The manual devotes a chapter each to the evaluation of strength and power, aerobic power, anaerobic power, flexibility, body composition, and anthropometry. These chapters include a rationale for testing that component, its relevance to various sports, the validity and reliability of the tests, interpretation guidelines, and a suggested fee structure. As well, there is a chapter on the use of field tests to evaluate the health status of the athlete and suggestions on monitoring training progress. The authors are both knowledgeable scientists and experienced in the testing of athletes. The manual has the following outline:

THE PURPOSE OF PHYSIOLOGICAL TESTING
  J. D. MacDougall, H. A. Wenger
  Introduction
  What the Athlete Gains
  What Testing Will Not Do
  What Constitutes an Effective Testing Program

OVERVIEW OF THE ENERGY DELIVERY SYSTEMS
  H. J. Green
  Introduction
  Utilization of Energy Systems During Exercise
  Considerations in Measurement of Strength, Power, and Energy Potential

TESTING STRENGTH AND POWER
  D. G. Sale, R. W. Norman
  Introduction
  Relevance and Relative Importance of Strength and Power to Sport Performance
  Purposes of Testing Strength and Power
  Methods of Measuring Strength and Power
  Recommended Procedures
  Interpretation of Results
  Fee Structure

TESTING AEROBIC POWER
  J. S. Thoden, J. D. MacDougall, B. A. Wilson
  Introduction
  Purposes of Testing Aerobic Power
  Relevance
  Interpretation of Test Results
  Testing Procedures
  Recommended Testing Procedures
  Fee Structure

TESTING MAXIMAL ANAEROBIC POWER AND CAPACITY
  C. Bouchard, A. W. Taylor, S. Dulac
  Introduction
  A Conceptual Framework
  Recommended Testing Procedures
  Existing Laboratory and Field Tests
  Conducting the Tests

KINANTHROPOMETRY
  W. D. Ross, M. J. Marfell-Jones
  Introduction
  Measurement of Status and Change
  Anthropometry
  Data Management
  Somatotypes
  Proportionality
  Body Composition
  Maturation
  Size and Performance Expectation
  Competency of Personnel
  Fee Structure

TESTING FLEXIBILITY
C. Hubley
　Introduction
　Purpose of Testing Flexibility
　Relevance
　Testing Procedures
　Recommended Testing Procedures
　Interpretation of Results
　Fee Structure

FIELD TESTS
　A. Reed
　　Introduction
　　Criteria for Evaluation of Field Tests

EVALUATING THE HEALTH STATUS OF THE ATHLETE
　R. Backus
　　Introduction
　　Sport Medicine Council of Canada Forms
　　Standardized Procedures for Assessing the Health Status of Athletes

MONITORING TRAINING
　E. W. Banister, H. A. Wenger
　　Rationale for Monitoring Training
　　Measures Required to Monitor Training
　　Data Storage, Formatting, and Display

I would like to focus on our deliberations into the purpose of physiological testing. An ongoing program of properly selected and administered tests can benefit both the coach and the athlete. Strengths and weaknesses can be determined in order to prescribe optimal training programs. Performance in many sports involves the effective use of a number of different physiological components. The performance itself is the sum result which can often mask the operation of a specific component. Laboratory testing can isolate these components to identify strengths and weaknesses and be the basis for the design of an optimal training program.

In any successful management system, there must be a means to evaluate whether programs have met the desired objectives. Tests which bracket specific programs can be an effective tool to evaluate success of training. As well, physiological tests can flag health problems associated with overuse or abnormalities not detected by standard physical examinations. And test results can be an integral part of the educational process to help the athlete better understand his or her body in relation to training and sport performance.

Although there are many benefits to a sound testing program, there are also some cautions. It is not a magical tool for predicting future stars. It has severe limitations for identifying potential since the determination of genetic limits still eludes us. The ultimate performance is a composite of many different factors of which physiological function is only one.

An effective testing program is one in which:

1. *The variables which are tested are relevant to that sport.*
   Although this might appear to be an obvious statement, it has not been unusual in the past for the coach, athlete, and scientist to waste considerable time testing physiological components which have little application to a particular sport or its problems.

2. *The tests that are selected are valid and reliable.*
   A test is valid only when it actually measures what it claims to measure. It is reliable when the results are consistent and reproducible. The scientist may administer what he considers to be a valid test, but if the reliability of the test is not sufficiently high to reflect the slight changes which might occur in the elite athlete over a given training period, it is of little value.
3. *The test protocols are as sport-specific as possible.*
   For the test results to have optimal practical significance, the exercise mode must be specific to the sport. For example, a maximal aerobic or anaerobic capacity test which uses a treadmill-running protocol, when administered to a swimmer, will give very little information regarding his state of training for swimming. Ideally, the swimmer should be tested in a swimming flume, or "swimming treadmill." Since such a facility does not yet exist in Canada, the next best choice is to test him or her on a simulated swimming task, or exercise on a swim bench. In such cases, despite the fact that results may be highly reliable, their validity declines as the motor pattern becomes more and more removed from that of swimming.
4. *Test administration is rigidly controlled.*
   Once test items are selected, they must be administered consistently at all times. This necessitates standard instructions to the athletes, standard practice or warm-up procedures, standard order of test items and recovery time between items, standard environmental temperature and humidity, and standard equipment and equipment calibration procedures. In addition, all intra-athlete variables which might affect test results should be carefully recorded. These include details such as the stage of training, the time of the most recent competition, the time of day in relation to previous tests, the nutritional status of the athlete, and other interventions such as sleep, injury or illness, hydration, drugs, or anxiety.
5. *The athlete's human rights are respected.*
   Ethical criteria which must be met before administering a test include: a thorough explanation of the purpose of the test, a realistic statement of the possible physical or psychological risks involved in the test, and provision for ensuring that confidentiality of test results will be maintained.
6. *Testing is repeated at regular intervals.*
   Since one of the main purposes of testing is to monitor training effectiveness, it is apparent that the tests must be repeated following different phases of training. "One-shot" testing, or even once-per-year testing, although of potential interest to the scientist, is of little practical value to the athlete.
7. *Results are interpreted to the coach and athlete directly.*
   This final crucial step often is the one which is most poorly handled by the scientist. Not only must test results be reported promptly to the athlete, but also they must be interpreted in language which he and his coach understand.

Our association is presently doing a revision of its manual with expected completion in September 1986. We hope it will continue to offer direction and guidance for the development of elite athletes at all ages.

10

Special Cardiovascular Precautions For the Masters Athlete

ROBERT S. MCKELVIE, M.D., F.R.C.P.(C)

McMaster University Health Sciences Centre

ABSTRACT

This review examines the risk of cardiovascular morbidity and mortality in the mature athlete. The literature suggests that coronary artery disease represents the major cause of risk in this age group. The review also discusses the risks and benefits of exercise. The significance and investigation of asymptomatic coronary artery disease for this group is examined. Exercise in this group appears to reduce the risks related to coronary heart disease. During exercise there seems to be an increased risk of a cardiovascular event (morbidity or mortality). The overall risk appears to be reduced in the group who habitually perform vigorous physical activity. Guidelines are presented to assess the risk of coronary artery disease in the masters athlete.

INTRODUCTION

Recently people over the age of 30 years have become more involved in exercise. The type of exercise performed is varied, but often involves some degree of distance running. As stated by Rennie and Hollenberg (31), "We run for fun and for reasons ranging from the transcendental through the esthetic to competitive." Studies have also indicated a lower risk of morbidity and mortality from coronary artery disease when some degree of regular vigorous exercise is maintained over a period of years (19, 22, 26, 28, 33).

James Fixx was the stereotype of many mature athletes seen today. In his younger years he smoked, was overweight, had a stressful lifestyle, did not exercise, and had a family history of coronary artery disease (13, 29). He then became interested in long-distance running and achieved a high level of physical fitness. Totally convinced of the benefit of long-distance running, he shared his belief with the rest of the running world. James Fixx died suddenly during a training run. A short time preceding his death, he had developed symptoms of chest pain. He neither reported to a doctor nor underwent exercise testing to determine the etiology of these symptoms. His untimely death emphasizes that the risk of exercise should be seriously considered in this group of athletes.

There are studies that suggest risk is associated with exercise and this appears to be related most frequently to coronary artery disease (20, 23, 38, 39). It is important to consider this factor in the masters athlete despite the level of physical fitness.

This review will examine the benefits and risks of vigorous exercise in the age group of the masters athlete. The focus is on the problem of coronary artery disease, the most common cause of death during exercise in adults (36, 39). The review will also examine the problem of asymptomatic or minimally symptomatic coronary artery disease. Finally, guidelines to assess the risk of coronary artery disease in this group of athletes will be presented.

Benefits of Exercise

Many studies have indicated that subjects engaged in regular vigorous physical activity have a reduced risk of mortality related to coronary artery disease (2, 19, 22, 26, 28, 33). Bassler and Scaff (1, 2, 3), strong proponents of this theory, feel that marathon running and the associated life style confer virtual immunity to coronary artery disease (2, 3). This statement is based on anecdotal information and not on data from well-designed studies.

Paffenbarger and Hale (26) examined different levels of physical activity and the risk of coronary mortality in 6,351 longshoremen between the ages of 35 and 74 years. Heavy work was defined as using 5.2 to 7.5 kilocalories per minute (Kcal/min), an average 1,876 Kcal over basal output per 8-hour work day; moderate work required 2.4 to 5.0 Kcal/min (1,473 Kcal. above basal output); and light work required 1.5 to 2.0 Kcal/min (865 Kcal over basal output). They found the age-adjusted coronary death rate for the heavy work category was 26.9 per 10,000 work years, and the moderate and light work categories had rates of 46.3 and 49.0, which were little different from each other. This protective threshold was especially apparent in the sudden death syndrome in which the death rate for heavy workers was 5.6 compared to 19.9 for moderate and 15.7 for light workers. The authors felt these results indicated that repeated bursts of high energy output established a plateau of protection against coronary mortality.

An editorial by Paffenbarger and Hyde (27) suggested various ways that exercise may protect against coronary artery disease. Exercise may produce enhanced fibrinolytic activity stimulated by thrombotic occlusion, a reduction in low density lipoprotein cholesterol, and an increase in high density lipoprotein cholesterol. The influence of exercise on cardiovascular fitness is at least partly independent of other risk factors, with the added benefit of influencing these factors (reducing weight, lowering blood pressure slightly, and discouraging the wish to smoke). In their opinion, therefore, physiologic evidence exists which bolsters the case for exercise as an essential protective element in human health (27).

Another study examined middle-aged marathon runners, joggers, and inactive men to determine the effect of their activity level on coronary risk factors (11). The researchers found both active groups weighed less and had higher high density lipoprotein levels. Their main conclusions were that physical activity reduces coronary heart disease risk and that running as little as 6 miles per week would be sufficient activity. They felt a reduction in coronary heart disease risk could be achieved by most individuals through exercise because it does not seem to require an undue amount of activity.

Morris et al. (22) followed 17,944 male office workers for an average of 8.5 years to ascertain if activity level, as determined by a standard questionnaire, influenced the morbidity and mortality from coronary heart disease. The subjects participated in a wide range of activities including swimming, tennis, hill climbing, running or jogging, cycling, digging, and moving heavy objects. There were 1,138 first clinical episodes of coronary heart disease in this group of subjects. Men engaged in vigorous sports or activities had somewhat less than half the incidence of coronary heart disease (both fatal and non-fatal manifestations), compared to the non-vigorous exercise group. The authors felt their results supported the theory that vigorous activity helps to protect the aging heart against ischemia and its consequences (22).

Siscovick et al. (33) employed a retrospective study to examine the relationship between vigorous physical activity and primary cardiac arrest. A group of 163 subjects was chosen because of a documented absence of cardiac disease. Their spouses were interviewed to quantify leisure time activity during the prior year. Energy expenditure during leisure time requiring 60% of maximum oxygen intake was considered high-intensity. This study demonstrated the risk of primary cardiac arrest was 55 to 65% lower in persons involved in high-intensity leisure time activity. The researchers felt that, because this association was demonstrated in a clinically healthy population without prior morbidity, their data supported the hypothesis that high-intensity leisure time activity protects against primary cardiac arrest.

In Puerto Rico a study (8) documented all forms of work and leisure time activity to assess the effects of physical activity on the risk of developing coronary heart disease in men 45 to 64 years old. This prospective study involved 2,585 rural men and 6,208 urban men who were free of clinically recognized coronary disease and followed them for 8.25 years. The study demonstrated that subjects having a more physically active life style had a lower incidence of coronary heart disease. Physical activity was inversely associated with most known coronary risk factors, but multivariate analyses indicated that a significant independent inverse relationship existed with the incidence of coronary heart disease. Based on these data the authors felt increased physical activity appears to be an independent protective factor against heart attacks.

A study by Lie and Erikssen (19) examined 122 middle-aged and elderly long-time active, well-trained male cross-country skiers. In this study, 117 subjects were followed for 5 years after the initial examination, and the incidence of new coronary disease was determined. This was found to be 2.4% in the group of skiers compared to 9% in the general population. Therefore, this study suggests that training over a long period of time is protective against coronary artery disease.

In 1984 Paffenbarger et al. (28) published a report which examined the physical activity level of 16,936 Harvard alumni and their risk of developing coronary artery disease. They found habitual post-college exercise indicative of low coronary heart disease risk. The more vigorous the activity, the greater the reduction in risk. Sedentary ex-athlete alumni were found to have a high risk, whereas previously sedentary students becoming physically active alumni acquired low risk. It was also shown that exercise benefit was independent of contrary life style elements (e.g., smoking, obesity, weight gain, hypertension, and adverse parenteral disease history) in affecting coronary heart disease. This study suggests risk reduction is on a continuum related to physical activity level; therefore, a threshold activity level may not have to be achieved before some reduction in risk occurs.

Risk of Exercise

Although many studies have suggested there is decreased risk from coronary artery disease when people exercise regularly, there has been some concern that there is risk involved in vigorous activity. Noakes et al. (23) presented 6 cases of well-trained athletes who had suffered myocardial infarction; 4 of these cases had angiographically demonstrated coronary artery disease. All these subjects were well trained at the time of their infarction. Some of them had been fit all their lives; others had only started training in the 10 years or so previous to their infarctions. This paper indicates that even well-trained subjects are susceptible to the development of coronary artery disease despite, in some cases, high levels of physical activity throughout their lives.

A study by Waller and Roberts (39) made clinical and autopsy observations on 5 while male runners 40 to 53 years old who ran 22 to 176 kilometers (km) per week. These subjects all died while running, although none had clinical evidence of cardiac disease when they became habitual runners. When studied, 4 of the runners had hypercholesterolemia; 2 had systemic hypertension; 1 had angina pectoris, but none had clinical evidence of acute myocardial infarction. The single symptomatic patient had an abnormal resting electrocardiogram and a positive exercise test. At autopsy, all 5 men had significant three-vessel coronary artery disease. Four of the 5 subjects had healed myocardial infarctions at autopsy. In this report coronary artery disease was found to be the major killer of conditioned runners aged 40 years and over who die while running. The fact that these men had coronary artery disease despite their running history is not so surprising, as they all started habitual running later in life and they had other risk factors for coronary artery disease. It may be that habitual vigorous physical activity should be initiated earlier in life and maintained throughout the years in order to derive benefit from its effects.

Another report by Waller et al. (40) discusses the case of a 51-year-old man who died suddenly following an early morning 5-km run. This subject had run habitually for about 5 years and initially had hypertension which required treatment with a diuretic. The autopsy demonstrated the presence of significant coronary artery disease. This case further emphasizes that habitual exercise initiated in middle age does not necessarily protect against coronary artery disease or its progression, as this subject undoubtedly had subclinical coronary disease before initiating his regular exercise habit.

Noakes et al. (24) published a report of 5 cases of marathon runners with documented coronary artery disease. Each subject had run regularly for about 1 year or more before his death. Three of the 5 men died accidentally; the other 2 died because of problems related to their cardiovascular systems. Two of the 3 who died accidentally and both subjects who died suddenly had coronary artery disease. As in previous reports, these men had relatively short histories of habitual vigorous exercise. The presence of coronary artery disease was not surprising given the relatively short duration of the habitual exercise. This suggests exercise does not completely prevent progression of coronary disease once it begins.

Virmani et al. (38) examined autopsy results of 30 joggers who died suddenly or shortly after experiencing chest pain. The average age was 36 years and the running history was from 1 to 28 years and 7 to 105 miles per week. Over 50% of the patients had risk factors for coronary artery disease, and 8 patients had a previous history of coronary heart disease. The autopsy results showed 73% of the patients had coronary artery disease and 47% had evidence of an acute and/or healed myocardial infarction. It was also of note that 1 patient had been running vigorously for 23 of his 38 years and at autopsy severe 4-vessel disease was found. There were also a high number of healed infarctions found at autopsy but only three patients gave a history of previous myocardial infarction. As discussed in other studies (20, 23, 39, 40), this report raises the issue of silent myocardial infarctions in runners. At the present time, it is unclear whether they occur more frequently in this group compared to the general population.

The case of a 47-year-old male marathon runner who died suddenly while running was reviewed in a clinical pathological conference report published in 1984 (20). This patient had started running during middle age, but other than asymptomatic hypertension he had been well. The report states there are obvious health benefits to regular exercise; however, in patients not active all their lives and with risk factors for heart disease, consideration should be given to the possibility of the presence of coronary artery disease.

Northcote et al. (25) published a study of 30 squash players who had died suddenly within 6 hours of playing squash. In their report, autopsies were performed on 27 of these patients. The average age was 46.7 years and the most common abnormality felt to be responsible for sudden death was coronary artery disease. A number of patients had prodromal symptoms before death. There was concern on the part of the authors that coronary artery disease had already developed in these people before they took up the game and the exercise was unable to protect against or reverse existing atheroma. In fact, it may even have rendered the individual more susceptible to cardiac complications.

It appears there may be some risk involved in exercise training, and it is not absolutely clear whether the benefits outweigh the risk. To assume that habitual exercise provides absolute protection is wrong because there are examples of men exercising for many years, starting in their early 20s, who have developed coronary artery disease. In the age group of the masters athlete, it appears that coronary artery disease is the most common cause for sudden death. The problem is to determine if the benefit outweighs the risk of exercise.

Benefit versus Risk of Exercise

The death of well-known long distance runner James Fixx (13, 29) has generated further concern about the hazards of vigorous physical exercise. The various reports previously discussed have also increased awareness that there may be definite risks involved in vigorous physical activity even when initiated early in life, and exercise does not confer absolute protection against coronary artery disease.

Gibbons et al. (9) followed 2,935 volunteers from an exercise facility (mean age 37 years) over a 65-month period. A total of 374,789 person-hours of exercise, including 2,726,272 kilometers of running and walking, was recorded. Over this period, one subject had an episode of ventricular tachycardia-fibrillation with a successful reversion and another had an inferior wall myocardial infarction. When the rate of risk was determined, based on exercising 30 minutes per session 3 times a week, it was found to be 0.002 to 0.027 events per person-year for men and 0.005 to 0.05 events per person-year for women. The participants did not record all their activity time, but all cardiac events were recorded so the actual risk was lower than calculated. This study demonstrates a very small acute risk of cardiovascular events associated with exercise. The study does not indicate if this is greater than expected for this population of people; also, it is unclear if any benefit is derived from exercise.

Thompson et al. (35) examined the number of deaths occurring in subjects while jogging over a 6-year period in Rhode Island. They compared this death rate with the death rate during less vigorous activities. This study demonstrated the hourly death rate for jogging of 1 per 396,000 hours was 7 times the hourly death rate of 1 in 3 million hours for non-vigorous activity. The death rate was 1 in 7,620 joggers per year. This was considered a low risk in the absolute sense despite being much higher than the rate in non-vigorous activity. This report suggests the death rate is higher during exercise compared to less vigorous activity.

Siscovick et al. (32) examined the cardiovascular risk of sedentary subjects and of subjects who exercised to varying degrees regularly. Compared to rest, they found the risk of sudden death was greater during exercise. There was an inverse relationship between the level of habitual activity and the magnitude of the increased risk during exercise (e.g., the greater the habitual activity, the lower the increased risk). When the overall risk was examined, the men maintaining the higher level of activity had a lower risk than either men maintaining lower habitual activity levels or those with a sedentary lifestyle.

These reports indicate there is a small but definite increased risk associated with vigorous activity. However, as one study demonstrates (32), despite the increased risk during exercise, the overall risk from sudden death is reduced in subjects who exercise vigorously and regularly.

Asymptomatic Coronary Artery Disease

Studies have demonstrated that coronary artery disease appears to be the major cause of cardiovascular risk in the age group of the masters athlete (20, 23, 25, 36, 38, 39, 40). Reports have also demonstrated (20, 23, 38, 39, 40) areas of healed myocardial infarction in subjects who have died suddenly, even in the presence of extensive running histories. Furthermore, there is often no previous complaint related to coronary artery disease before the death of these patients.

Asymptomatic coronary artery disease is gaining more attention and it remains a difficult problem in terms of management (5, 37). The prognosis in these patients is not well understood because of the relatively small number who undergo coronary angiography (5). A few studies have provided some prognostic data on this group of patients (6, 10, 12, 17, 18). Hickman et al. (12) followed (for up to 90 months) 78 asymptomatic airmen who had angiographically proven coronary artery disease. In this group there was a 1% per year mortality and 29% developed either angina or myocardial infarction, or died during the follow-up.

A series by Langou et al. (18) of 12 industrial workers, identified by a combination of positive exercise tests and coronary artery calcification on fluoroscopy, were followed for 3 years. During this time, 33% developed either angina or a myocardial infarction.

Another group of studies examined patients who were asymptomatic or mildly symptomatic (6, 10, 17). In the National Institutes of Health Study (17) 147 asymptomatic or mildly symptomatic patients were followed for 6 to 67 months (mean 25). A number of these patients had previous infarctions (in both the symptomatic and asymptomatic groups). The overall mortality was 3% per year and the mortality for 3-vessel disease was 4% per year. In a study by Hammermeister et al. (10), 619 patients were followed for a mean of 66 months. They found an annual mortality of 2% per year in patients with 3-

vessel disease and ejection fraction greater than 50%. In contrast, mortality was nearly 5% per year in patients with an ejection fraction of 31 to 50%. The Duke-Harvard Collaborative Artery Disease Data Bank (6) also examined prognosis. Thirty-two of their 44 patients had a previous myocardial infarction, but all were asymptomatic. The overall mortality for the group was 2.7% per year. The subgroup with 3-vessel disease had the highest mortality of 5% per year. It was found that 30% of the patients suffered a cardiac event over the mean follow-up of 42 months. Bruce et al. (4) have also found the group with 2- or 3-vessel coronary disease is the most likely to suffer a coronary event. These studies would suggest asymptomatic patients have a better prognosis than symptomatic patients. The study of the Cleveland Clinic (30) reported an annual mortality of 4% in patients with 1-vessel, 7% in patients with 2-vessel and 12.5% in patients with 3-vessel disease. A recent report from the Coronary Artery Surgery Study (CASS) (21) gives an annual mortality for 1-, 2-, and 3-vessel disease as 2%, 4%, and 8% respectively. It may be that the population with asymptomatic coronary artery disease forms the pool from which a certain number of persons will surface each year as victims of sudden death or non-fatal myocardial infarction (5). These patients with silent myocardial ischemia and a defective anginal warning system may theoretically be at increased risk during strenuous exertion (5). In view of this, it would be important to screen subjects in the age group of the masters athlete before they undertake vigorous physical activity in an attempt to determine who might be at increased risk of a cardiac event. A study by Hopkirk et al. (14) examined whether clinical or exercise test variables could reliably detect coronary disease in asymptomatic men. All 225 men in the study had coronary angiography performed. The researchers found the combination of any single clinical risk factor (e.g., smoking, hypertension) and any two of the exercise risk predictors (at least 3 mm ST depression, persistent ST depression 6 minutes after exercise, and total exercise duration of less than 7 minutes of the Bruce protocol) was highly predictive (89%) but relatively insensitive (37%) for detecting any coronary disease. In patients with 2-vessel and 3-vessel disease, these criteria have a sensitivity of 55% and an 84% predictive value. This is important as patients with 2-vessel and 3-vessel disease are the ones at greatest risk for morbidity and mortality.

Guidelines to Assess Cardiovascular Risk in the Masters Athlete

The data in the literature indicate that although the risk is low, there is a definite cardiovascular risk associated with vigorous exercise. This risk seems to be related mainly to coronary artery disease; very often this disease is occult and presents as sudden death. It is important to remember this risk can exist despite many years of vigorous physical activity. Therefore, coronary artery disease should be considered in any mature athlete despite the level of fitness.

A 3-step approach to screening asymptomatic subjects about to commence or who have been participating in vigorous physical activity can be followed (37). This approach would be recommended for athletes who are 35 years or older. The first step would be to obtain a history of angina, risk factor analysis (including level of high-density lipoprotein cholesterol), and a resting electrocardiogram (Table 10-1). For a subject with symptoms suggestive of angina, risk factors, or an abnormal resting ECG, the second step would be a symptom-limited maximal exercise test.

An awareness of Bayesian analysis is required to properly interpret the results of the exercise test. Bayes' theorem of conditional probability deals

TABLE 10-1. *Three-step approach to screening asymptomatic subjects*

Step 1.
  History—chest pain

			Relative Risk
—risk factors	—increased blood pressure	(16*)	2.14
	—smoking history	(16*)	1.59
	—family history	(34*)	1.5
	—impaired glucose tolerance	(16*)	1.25
	—increased serum cholesterol	(16*)	2.1
	—obesity	(15*)	2.0

  Physical examination
  Resting 12 lead ECG
Step 2. —(If indicated by Step 1.)
      Symptom-limited maximal incremental progressive exercise test
Step 3. —(If indicated by Steps 1 and 2.)
    —thallium exercise test
    —coronary arteriography—if indicated by the thallium exercise test

*references.

with the predictive value of the test result. It states that the prevalence of the disease in the population being studied determines the predictive value of the test result (7). Therefore, the pre-test likelihood of disease must be taken into consideration when interpreting the results of the test (Fig. 10-1). Exercise testing a subject with a very low pre-test risk (e.g., absence of chest pain history, risk factors, and resting ECG changes; young age; and female) (Table 10-1) of having coronary artery disease would not be very useful according to Bayes' theorem. A negative test result would reduce the risk from 5% to 2%, whereas a positive test would only increase the risk to 27% (Fig. 10-1). Therefore, the exercise test would not significantly increase the subject's risk of coronary artery disease, and there would be many false positive test results. If there is a history of chest pain or risk factors present, the subject is in a subgroup (50% risk) that is at higher risk for coronary artery disease. A posi-

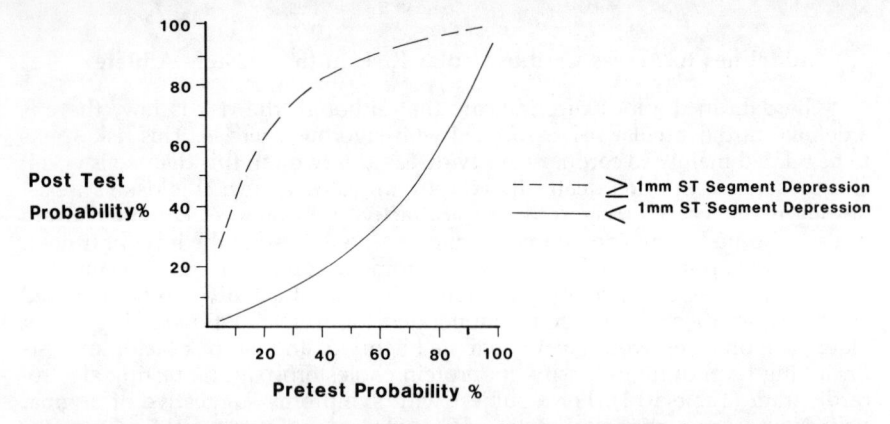

Fig. 10-1. *Subject with a pretest probability of 5% for coronary artery disease has a post-test probability of 2% if the test is negative and 27% if the test is positive. A subject with a 50% pretest probability for coronary artery disease has a post-test probability of 25% if the test is negative and an 88% probability if the test is positive.*

tive exercise test in this case would be useful as the risk of the presence of coronary artery disease would be significantly (88% risk) increased in this individual, whereas a negative test would significantly reduce the risk (25% risk) (7). Recently a study has suggested (14) the combination of any single clinical risk factor and any two exercise risk predictors accurately identifies a group with 2-vessel or 3-vessel coronary disease, which is the group most likely to suffer a coronary event.

The third step, if indicated by the initial findings, would include thallium scintigraphy and coronary arteriography if indicated by the thallium study (37). Finally, it should be impressed upon the athlete in this age group that coronary artery disease can develop despite maintaining a high level of physical activity and that prodromal symptoms such as vague or definite chest pain should not be ignored but should be reported to a physician (38).

REFERENCES

1. Bassler, T. J. Previous health and longevity of male athletes (letter). *Lancet* 1:863–864, 1974.
2. Bassler, T. J. Marathon running and immunity to atherosclerosis. *Ann. N.Y. Acad. Sci.* 301:579–592, 1977.
3. Bassler, T., and J. Scaff. Can I avoid heart-attack? (letter). *Lancet* 1:863–864, 1974.
4. Bruce, R. A., T. A. DeRouen, and K. F. Hossack. Value of maximal exercise test in risk assessment of primary coronary heart disease events in healthy men. Five years experience of the Seattle Heart Watch Study. *Am. J. Cardiol.* 46:371–378, 1980.
5. Cohen, P. F. Prognosis and treatment of asymptomatic coronary artery disease. *J. Am. Coll. Cardiol.* 1:959–964, 1983.
6. Cohen, P. F., P. Harris, W. H. Barry, R. A. Rosati, P. Rosenbaum, and C. Waternaux. Prognostic importance of anginal symptoms in angiographically defined coronary artery disease. *Am. J. Cardiol.* 47:233–237, 1981.
7. Diamond, G. A., and J. S. Forrester. Analysis of probability as an aid in the clinical diagnosis of coronary artery disease. *N. Engl. J. Med.* 300:1350–1358, 1979.
8. Garcia-Palimieri, M. R., P. Costas, M. Cruz-Vidal, P. D. Sorlie, and R. J. Havlik. Increased physical activity: A protective factor against heart attacks in Puerto Rico. *Am. J. Cardiol.* 50:749–755, 1982.
9. Gibbons, L. W., K. H. Cooper, B. M. Meyer, and C. Ellison. The acute cardiac risk of strenuous exercise. *J.A.M.A.* 244:1799–1801, 1980.
10. Hammermeister, K. E., T. A. DeRouen, and H. T. Dodge. Effect of coronary surgery on survival in asymptomatic and minimally symptomatic patients. *Circulation* 62 (Suppl. I):98–102, 1980.
11. Hartung, G. H., E. J. Farge, and R. E. Mitchell. Effects of marathon running, jogging and diet on coronary risk factors in middle-aged men. *Prev. Med.* 10:316–323, 1981.
12. Hickman, J. R., G. S. Uhl, R. L. Cook, P. J. Engel, and A. Hopkirk. A natural history study of asymptomatic coronary artery disease (Abstr.). *Am. J. Card.* 45:422, 1980.
13. Higdon, H. Jim Fixx: How he lived, why he died. *The Runner*, November, 1984, 32–38.
14. Hopkirk, J. A. C., G. S. Uhl, J. R. Hickman, J. Fisher, and A. Medina. Discriminant value of critical and exercise variables in detecting significant coronary artery disease in asymptomatic men. *J. Am. Coll. Cardiol.* 3:887–894, 1984.
15. Hubert, H. B., M. Feinleib, P. M. McNamara, and W. P. Castelli. Obesity as an independent risk factor for cardiovascular disease: A 26-year follow-up of participants in the Framingham Heart Study. *Circulation* 67:968–977, 1983.
16. Kannel, W. B. Role of blood pressure in cardiovascular disease: The Framingham Study. *Angiology* 26:1–14, 1975.
17. Kent, K. M., D. R. Rosing, C. J. Ewels, L. Kipson, R. Bonow, and S. E. Epstein. Prognosis of asymptomatic or mildly symptomatic patients with coronary artery disease. *Am. J. Cardiol.* 49:1823–1830, 1982.
18. Langou, R. A., E. K. Huang, M. J. Kelley, and L. S. Cohen. Predictive accuracy of coronary artery calcification and abnormal exercise test for coronary artery disease in asymptomatic men. *Circulation* 62:1196–1203, 1980.
19. Lie, H., and J. Erikssen. Five year follow-up of ECG aberrations, latent coronary heart disease and cardiopulmonary fitness in various age groups of Norwegian cross-country skiers. *Acta. Med. Scand.* 216:377–383, 1984.
20. Ludmerer, K. M., and J. M. Kissane. Sudden death in a 47-year-old runner. *Am. J. Med.* 76:517–526, 1984.

21. Mock, M. B., I. Ringvist, L. D. Fisher, K. B. Davis, B. R. Chaitman, N. T. Kouchoukos, G. C. Kaiser, E. Alderman, T. J. Ryan, R. O. Russell, Jr., S. Mullin, D. Fray, and T. Killip, III. Survival of medically treated patients in the coronary artery surgery study (CASS) registry. *Circulation* 66:562–568, 1982.
22. Morris, J. N., R. Pollard, M. G. Everitt, and S. P. W. Chave. Vigorous exercise in leisure-time: Protection against coronary heart disease. *Lancet* 2:1207–1210, 1980.
23. Noakes, T., L. Opie, and W. Beck. Coronary heart disease in marathon runners. *Ann. N.Y. Acad. Sci.* 301:593–619, 1977.
24. Noakes, T. D., L. H. Opie, A. G. Rose, and P. H. T. Kleynhans. Autopsy-proved coronary atherosclerosis in marathon runners. *N. Engl. J. Med.* 301:86–89, 1979.
25. Northcote, R. J., A. D. B. Evans, and D. Ballantyne. Sudden death in squash players. *Lancet* 1:148–150, 1984.
26. Paffenbarger, R. S., and W. E. Hale. Work activity and coronary heart mortality. *N. Engl. J. Med.* 292:545–550, 1975.
27. Paffenbarger, R. A., and R. T. Hyde. Exercise as protection against heart attack. *N. Engl. J. Med.* 302:1026–1027, 1980.
28. Paffenbarger, R. S., R. T. Hyde, A. L. Wing, and C. H. Steinmetz. A natural history of athleticism and cardiovascular health. *J.A.M.A.* 252:491–495, 1984.
29. Pietschmann, R. J. Probing death on the run. *Runner's World*, November, 1984, 38–44 and 90–94.
30. Proudfit, W. L., A. V. G. Bruschke, and F. M. Sones Jr. Natural history of obstructive coronary artery disease: ten-year study of 601 nonsurgical cases. *Prog. Cardiovasc. Dis.* 21:53–78, 1978.
31. Rennie, D. and N. K. Hollenberg. Cardiomythology and marathoners. *N. Engl. J. Med.* 301:103–104, 1979.
32. Siscovick, D. D., N. S. Weiss, R. H. Fletcher, and T. Lasky. The incidence of primary cardiac arrest during vigorous exercise. *N. Engl. J. Med.* 311:874–877, 1984.
33. Siscovick, D. S., N. S. Weiss, A. P. Hallstrom, T. S. Inui, and D. R. Peterson. Physical activity and primary cardiac arrest. *J.A.M.A.* 248:3113–3117, 1982.
34. Snowden, C. B., D. M. McNamara, R. J. Garrison, M. Feinleib, W. B. Kannel and F. H. Epstein. Predicting coronary heart disease in siblings—a multivariate assessment. *Am. J. Epidemiol.* 115:217–222, 1982.
35. Thompson, P. D., E. J. Funk, R. A. Carlton, and W. Q. Sterner. Incidence of death jogging in Rhode Island from 1975 through 1980. *J.A.M.A.* 247:2535–2538, 1982.
36. Thompson, P. D., M. P. Stern, P. Williams, K. Duncan, W. L. Haskell, and P. D. Wood. Death during jogging or running. A study of 18 cases. *J.A.M.A.* 242:1265–1267, 1979.
37. Uhl, G. S., and V. Froelicher. Screening for asymptomatic coronary artery disease. *J. Am. Coll. Cardiol.* 1:946–955, 1983.
38. Virmani, R., M. Robinowitz, and H. A. McAllister. Nontraumatic death in joggers. A series of 30 patients at autopsy. *Am. J. Med.* 72:874–882, 1982.
39. Waller, B. F., and W. C. Roberts. Sudden death while running in conditioned runners aged 40 years or over. *Am. J. Cardiol.* 45:1292–1301, 1980.
40. Waller, B. F., R. S. Csere, W. P. Baker, and W. C. Roberts. Structure-function correlations in cardiovascular and pulmonary diseases (CPC). Running to death. *Chest* 79:346–349, 1981.

Section IV
Environmental Stresses

11

Thermal Problems In Masters Athletes

JOHN R. SUTTON, M.D.

McMaster University Medical Centre

With mass participation in fun runs, marathons, triathlons, and ultramarathons at an all-time high, a significant number of entrants will belong to the masters age class. In these events thermal problems, especially hyperthermia, are important. The more enterprising seek their adventure in the hostile environments of mountains, rivers, and remote wilderness areas in all seasons of the year. In such environments, the risk of hypothermia is ever present. *Are masters athletes at special risk?* (Figure 11-1)

Dr. Carl Gisolfi will examine the specific effects of age on thermal regulation, and subsequent chapters will focus on the problems associated with hyperthermia, its prevention and management, in fun runs and marathons in Australasia, Europe, and North America. Other special problems associated with mass participation include the following.

Logistics

Of all mass participation events, the annual pilgrimage to Mecca has the greatest number of participants of all ages who are at risk (Fig. 11-2). It represents enormous logistic problems for those responsible for providing medical care for the large numbers of heat stroke victims (1). On a considerably smaller scale, fun runs and marathons with a few hundred to 80,000 participants also present major logistic problems. From our first experience with fun run casualties, it became clear that to be effective in preventing complications from heat stroke, treatment, especially rehydration and cooling, must begin immediately on site (10).

Hyperthermia or Hypothermia?

Although most thermal casualties of fun runs will suffer hyperthermia, in the longer runs with slow runners or cold wet days or in hostile environments, hypothermia may be more common (8). However, it is possible that

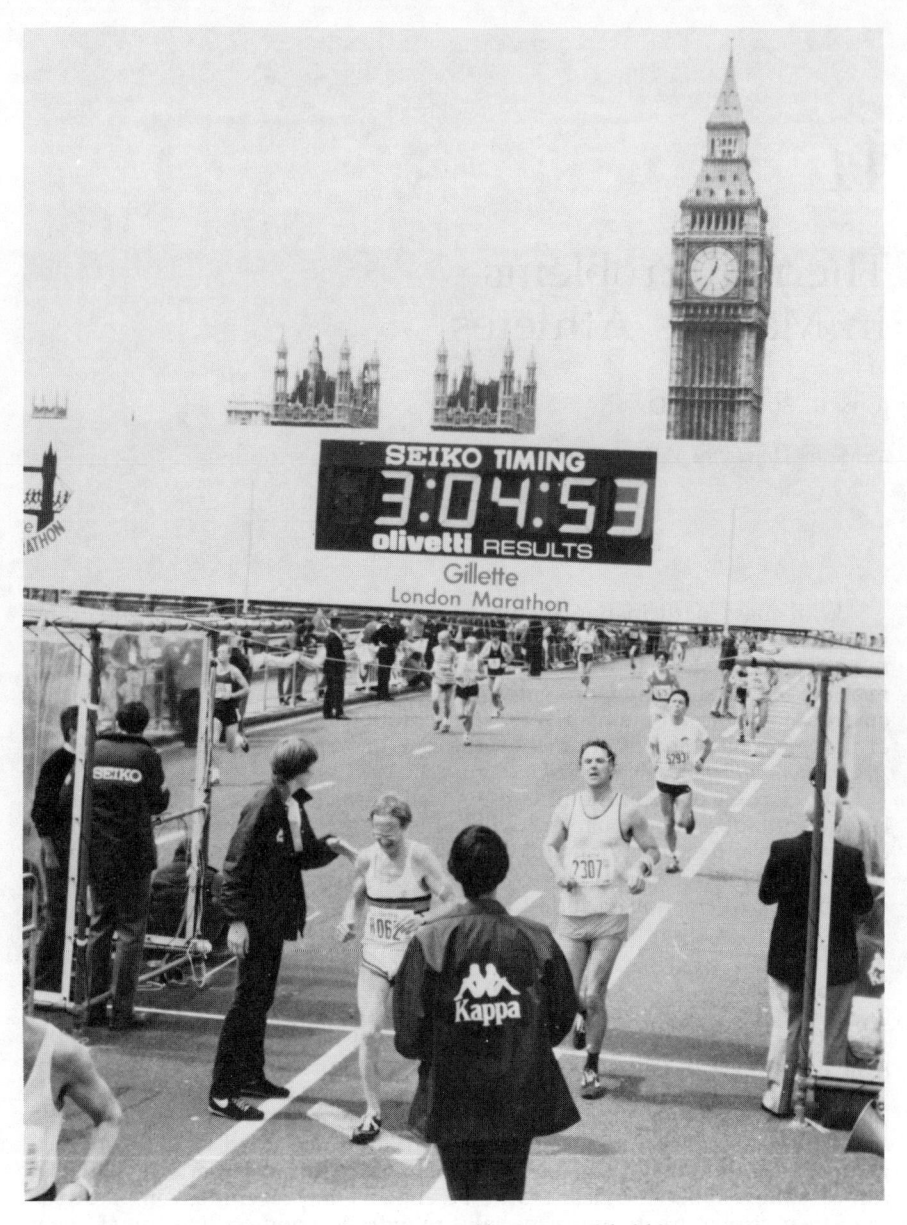

Fig. 11-1. *Are masters athletes at special risk?*

hyperthermia goes unrecognized. Since it usually presents differently from the classical heat stroke (Table 11-1), diagnosis may be delayed (4). This in turn will delay commencement of treatment—a critical factor in determining outcome.

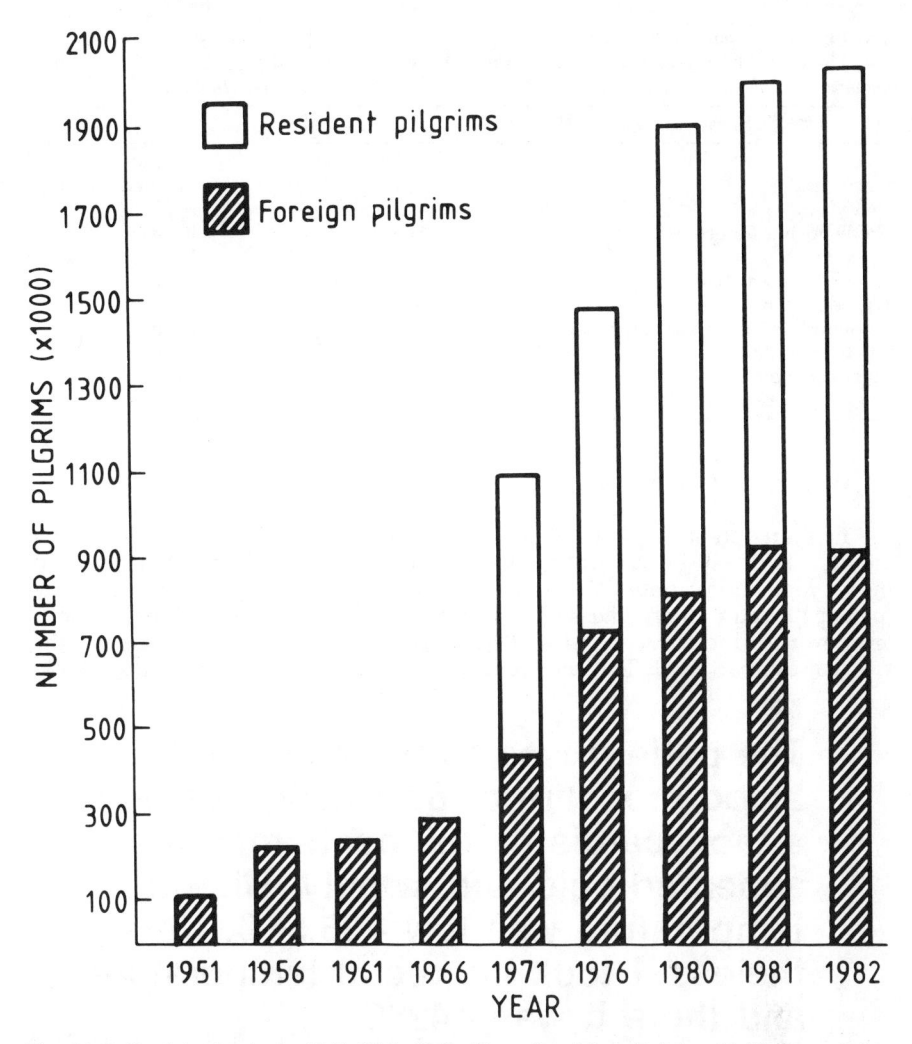

Fig. 11-2. *Participation in the Hajj, 1951–1982. (Reproduced from Ref. 1, with kind permission of the authors and editors).*

Even when hyperthermia is suspected, unless body core temperature is measured with a rectal thermometer, a spurious reading may be obtained. An oral or axillary temperature can be very misleading (Fig. 11-3) and may be several degrees lower than core temperature (8). There may be many core temperatures; rectal temperature may be different from tympanic temperature and from esophageal. It is interesting that, for a person in the dehydrated state, forehead sweating will continue normally whereas back sweating and total sweat rate will decrease. This results in increased esophageal temperature in the dehydrated state while tympanic temperature remains relatively normal, presumably maintaining brain function (Fig. 11-4).

TABLE 11-1. *Characteristics of "classical" and "exertion-induced" heat stroke. (Reproduced from* Heat Stroke and Temperature Regulation, *M. Khogali, and J. R. S. Hales (eds.), p.3, Sydney: Academic Press Australia, 1983, with kind permission of the authors and editors.)*

Characteristics	Classical	Exertional
Age	Older	Young
Occurrence	Epidemic form	Isolated cases
Pyrexia	Very high	High
Predisposing illness	Frequent	Rare
Sweating	Often absent	Usually present
Acid-base disturbance	Resp. Alkalosis	Lactic acidosis
Rhabdomyolysis	Rare	Common
Disseminated intravascular coagulation	Rare	Common
Acute renal failure	Rare	Common
Hyperuricemia	Mild	Marked
Enzymes elevation	Mild	Marked

Dehydration or Overhydration?

In short fun runs of less than 10 kilometers (km), it seems unlikely that enough fluid will be lost from sweating to impair circulatory function and thermoregulation, unless the athlete begins in an already dehydrated state (perhaps because of an illness like gastroenteritis). Nevertheless, even in short-term exercise there is a significant hemoconcentration with fluid leaving the vascular compartment. This may reduce circulating plasma volume up to 20%.

The patient was hypotensive, with a blood pressure of 60 mmHg systolic, a tachycardia of 180 beats/min and appeared cold and sweaty. His oral temperature was low - 35.5°C. Nevertheless, I took his rectal temperature and there it was - 42°C.

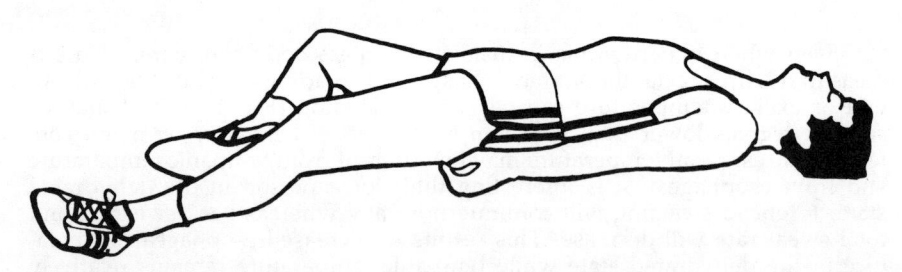

Fig. 11-3. *Oral and rectal temperature discrepancies. (Reproduced from Ref. 8, with kind permission of the editor.)*

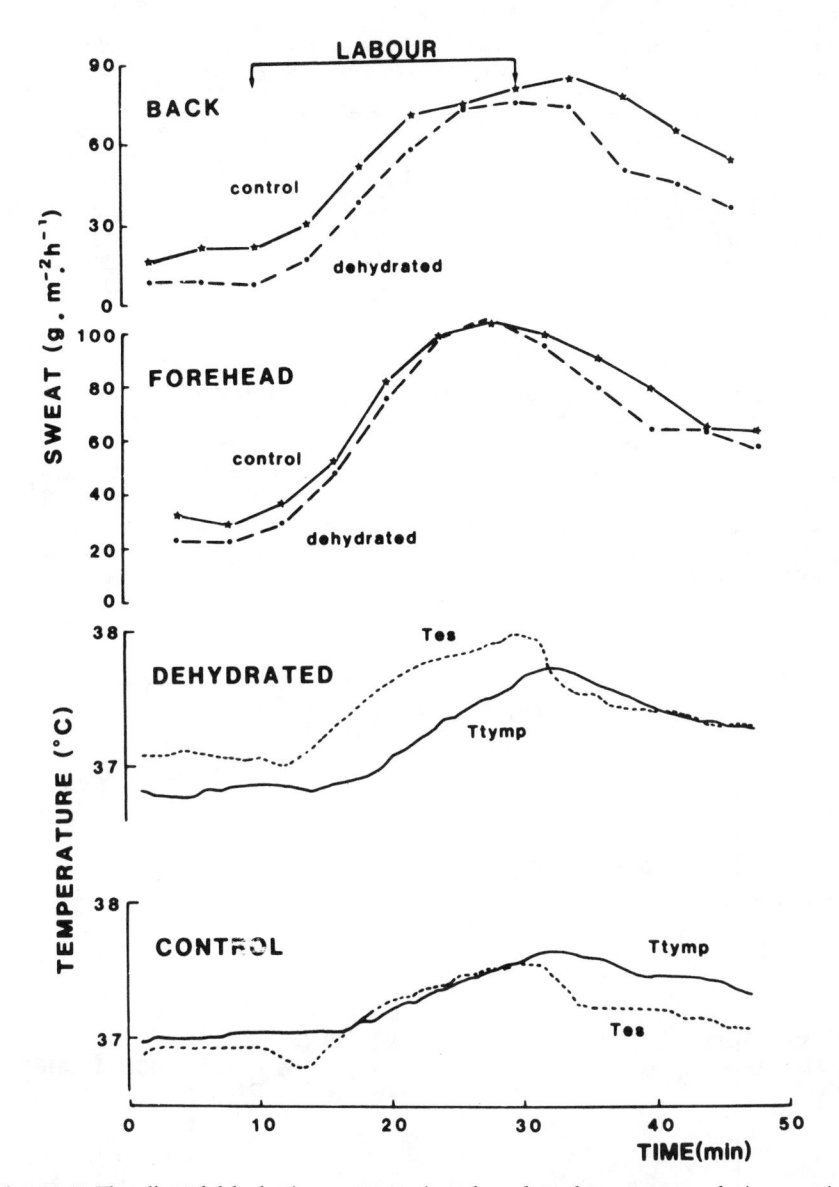

Fig. 11-4. *The effect of dehydration on tympanic and esophageal temperatures during exercise. (Reproduced from Ref. 2 with kind permission of the author and editors.)*

In longer races, dehydration is the rule and in a marathon, fluid losses of 5 to 8 liters are not uncommon. Even now that the need for fluid and electrolyte replacement has been widely publicized, rarely is more than a small proportion of the fluid replenished. Probably uncommon but only recently recognized is the problem of overhydration, reported in ultramarathons (Table 11-2) (6) and triathlons (5). This unusual situation of overhydration with hyponatremia occurred in slower athletes who, over several hours, consumed excess

TABLE 11-2. *Estimated water and sodium chloride balance in four athletes who developed water intoxication during prolonged exercise. (Reproduced from Ref. 6, p. 373, with kind permission of the authors and editors.)*

Age	Sex	Body Wt. (kg)	Exercise Duration (h:min)	Post-Race Serum Sodium Concentration (mmol.l^{-1})
46	F	49	±7:00	115
37	M	75	10:10	118
20	M	73	±9:00	124
29	F	57	9:56	125

fluids that did not contain electrolytes. However, with the tendency for greater participation in ultramarathons, trail runs, and triathlons, voluntary overhydration and hyponatremia will be recognized more often. The cerebral effects of hyponatremia and cerebral edema may be expected earlier in masters athletes, many of whom may have asymptomatic cerebral vascular disease. Thus, a good case can be made for replenishing body fluid with solutions containing electrolytes, and monitoring body weight during long races to help assess fluid balance.

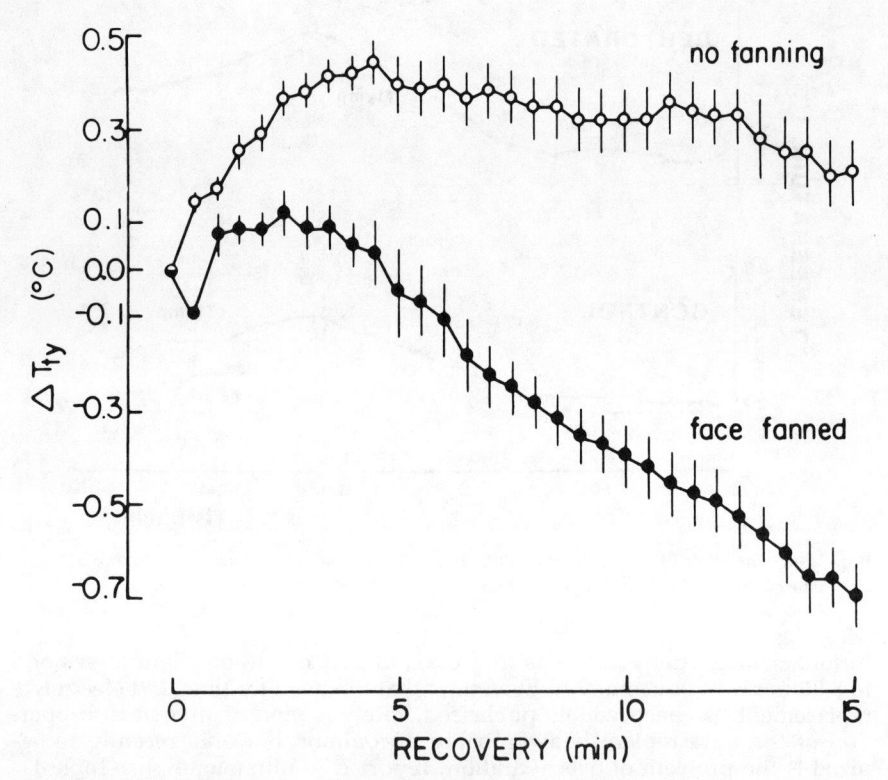

Fig. 11-5. *The effect of face fanning on change in tympanic temperature. (Reproduced from Ref. 2 with kind permission of the author and editors.)*

COOLING STRATEGIES

When a diagnosis of hyperthermia is made, immediate cooling is vital to the prevention of serious sequelae (brain, blood, renal, liver, and cardiac complications). However, the methods of cooling vary considerably and there is no widespread agreement as to which is the more effective approach. Regional cooling has received little attention but face fanning will lower tympanic temperature and, presumably, brain temperature (Fig. 11-5). Such an effect may be particularly relevant in reversing brain malfunction (2).

Total body cooling using the Makkah body cooling unit is effective but expensive (12). Furthermore, the combination of rehydration and the use of cool packs on axillae and groin appears to be at least as effective in the rate of lowering body core temperature (7).

We now have a clear understanding of the physiology of thermoregulation and its alteration with age. The pathophysiological states associated with disordered thermoregulation are also understood in biological terms. However, logistical difficulties to date have prevented more than simple descriptive analyses of predisposing factors and evaluation of treatment regimens. Formal epidemiological tools must be applied to this clinical arena before we can advance our understanding of the causal factors (3) and most effective methods for prevention and treatment of exercise-induced thermal illness as it occurs in mass participation events (9, 11).

REFERENCES

1. Al-Marzoogi, A., M. Khogali, and A. El-Ergesus. Organizational set-up: Detection, screening, treatment and follow-up of heat disorders. In: *Heat Stroke and Temperature Regulation,* M. Khogali and J. R. S. Hales (eds.) 31–39. Sydney: Academic Press Australia, 1983.
2. Cabanac, M. Face fanning: A possible way to prevent or cure brain hyperthermia. In: *Heat Stroke and Temperature Regulation,* M. Khogali and J. R. S. Hales (eds.) 213–221. Sydney: Academic Press Australia, 1983.
3. England, A. C. III, D. W. Fraser, A. W. Hightower, R. Tirinnanzi, D. J. Greenberg, K. E. Powell, C. M. Slovis, and R. A. Varsha. Preventing severe heat injury in runners: Suggestions from the 1979 Peachtree Road Race experience. *Ann. Int. Med.* 97:196–201, 1982.
4. Hart, G. R., R. J. Anderson, C. P. Crumpler, A. P. Shulkin, G. Reed, and J. P. Knochel. Epidemic classical heat stroke: Clinical characteristics and course of 28 patients. *Medicine* 61:189–197, 1982.
5. Hiller, W. D. B., M. L. O'Toole, F. Massimino, R. E. Hiller, and R. H. Laird. Plasma electrolyte and glucose changes during the Hawaiian Ironman Triathlon. *Med. Sci. Sports Exerc.* 17:219, 1985 (abstract).
6. Noakes, T. D., N. Goodwin, B. L. Rayner, T. Branken, and R. K. N. Taylor. Water intoxication: a possible complication during endurance exercise. *Med. Sci. Sports Exerc.* 17:370–375, 1985.
7. Richards, D., R. Richards, P. J. Schofield, V. Ross, and J. R. Sutton. Management of heat exhaustion in Sydney's *The Sun* City-to-Surf fun runners. *Med. J. Aust.* 457–461, 1979.
8. Sutton, J. R. Heat illness. In: *Sports Medicine,* R. H. Strauss (ed.) 307–322. Philadelphia: W. B. Saunders, 1984.
9. Sutton, J. R. Not so fun run. *Med. J. Aust.* 141:782–783, 1984.
10. Sutton, J., M. J. Coleman, A. P. Millar, L. Lazarus, and P. Russo. The medical problems of mass participation in athletic competition. The "City-to-Surf" Race. *Med. J. Aust.* 2:127–133, 1972.
11. Walter, S. D., J. R. Sutton, J. M. McIntosh, and C. Connolly. The aetiology of sports injuries. A review of methodologies. *Sports. Med.* 2:47–58, 1985.
12. Weiner, J. S. and M. Khogali. A physiological body cooling unit for treatment of heat stroke. *Lancet* I:507–509, 1980.

12

Thermal Regulation: Effects Of Exercise And Age

M. J. Kenney, Carl V. Gisolfi

University of Iowa

ABSTRACT

The rise in central body temperature during exercise is proportional to exercise intensity or percentage of maximum oxygen uptake (%VO_2 max) and independent of ambient temperature over a wide range. This rise is not associated with a set-point shift and is reduced by physical training and heat acclimation. Old age is associated with heat intolerance, but it is unclear whether thermoregulation is impaired by age per se or related to other factors such as disease processes or a decrement in cardiovascular fitness. Evidence indicating reduced responsiveness of the sweating mechanism with advancing age is controversial, and reported changes in skin blood flow in older persons compared with young adults are not independent of changes in core and/or mean skin temperatures. The ability to acclimatize to work in the heat is unaffected in men up to 60 years of age. This review of the pertinent literature indicates there is insufficient evidence to support the notion that age per se results in a dysfunction of the temperature regulatory system.

INTRODUCTION

This chapter deals with temperature regulation during exercise and the influence of age on thermoregulatory function and heat tolerance. Consequently, it focuses on heat dissipation mechanisms and how they are affected by physical training and heat acclimation. Old age has been associated with reduced sensitivity and capacity of the sweating mechanism (14, 15, 21, 23-

---

Acknowledgements

The authors are grateful to Ms. Joan Seye for the preparation of the manuscript. This research was supported by NIH Grant HL 32731.

TABLE 12-1. *Analysis of heat related deaths during recent heat waves in the United States*

Investigator	Date & Location	Heat-Related Illness*	Heat Related Deaths Total No.	Patients ≥60 yrs	Percent ≥60 yrs
Henschel, A. (1969)	July 1966 St. Louis	—	246	192	78.0%
†MMWR	July 11–Aug. 15, 1983 St. Louis	348	35**	23	65.7%
†MMWR	July–August 1983 Georgia	804	35**	20	57.0%

†*Morbidity and Mortality Weekly Report*-Ref. 66.
*Defined as any hospital admission with a body temperature higher than 40.6° C.
**Defined as any death related to excessive heat, either directly or indirectly through exacerbation of a preexisting medical condition.

25, 34, 44, 55, 61) and increased cutaneous blood flow (35, 36, 44, 68). Moreover, there is considerable evidence that during heat waves, older individuals are more susceptible to fatal thermal injuries than their younger counterparts (Table 12-1). However, old age is also associated with varying patterns of disease (18) and decreased cardiovascular functional capacity, as indicated by reduced aerobic power (53). Thus, are the observed changes in temperature regulation with age due to aging per se, age-related disease processes, and/or changes in cardiovascular fitness? It is well documented that physical training can markedly improve thermal tolerance (30, 49, 50) and temperature regulatory function (4, 48). Can older persons improve their ability to regulate their core body temperature (T_c) through physical training or through the process of heat acclimation?

Basic Concepts

With the start of exercise, heat produced within working muscles is transferred primarily to the body core by convective blood flow (Fig. 12-1). The consequent rise in T_c is proportional to exercise intensity and stimulates thermodetectors located in the preoptic anterior hypothalamus and spinal cord (8, 65). This input combines with afferent signals from cutaneous thermoreceptors to provide a weighted sum (T_{ws}) of thermal input to the central controller (29). T_{ws} is compared with a set condition of the controller (T_{set}) to produce a thermal command signal to the thermoregulatory effectors. A positive difference in $T_{ws} - T_{set}$ (or load error) drives heat loss mechanisms (sweating and cutaneous vasodilatation), while a negative difference drives heat gain mechanisms. When heat dissipation balances heat production, T_c reaches a plateau reflecting the proportional nature of the control system (11, 32, 33, 63, 64).

The demonstration that steady-state T_c is proportional to %$\dot{V}O_2$ max (2, 58) probably reflects the influence of training on the sweating response. After training, sweating is initiated at a lower T_c (4), and a unit increase in T_c elicits a greater sweating response (48). Thus, at a given absolute heat load, a trained person reaches thermal equilibrium faster and at a lower T_c than his or her untrained counterpart. Training shifts the threshold of the T_c:skin blood flow (SkBF) relation to a lower T_c (52).

The observation that T_c is maintained relatively constant independent of ambient temperature (T_a) over a wide range is explained by alterations in heat

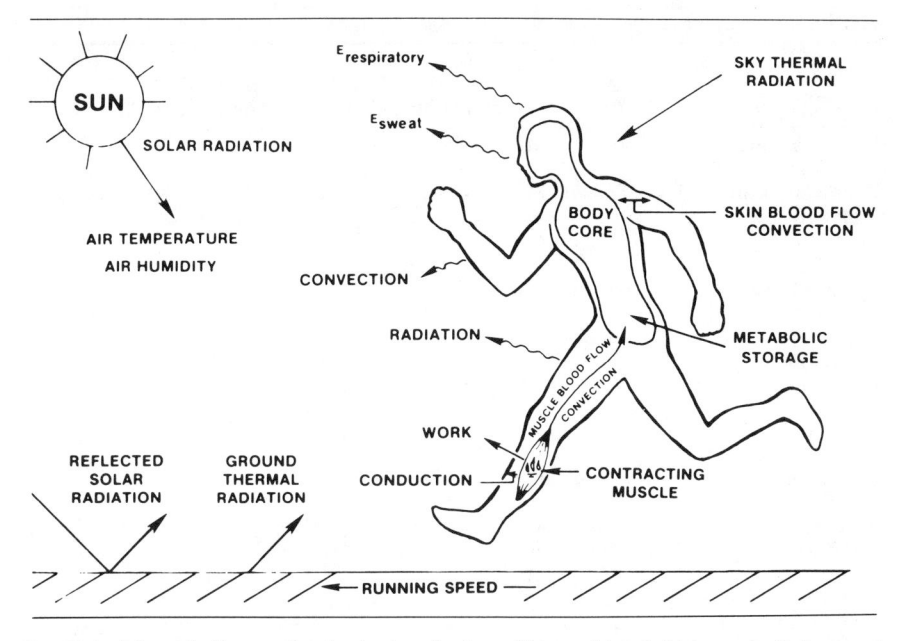

Fig. 12-1. Schematic diagram showing heat production within working skeletal muscle, its transport to the body core and to the skin, and its subsequent exchange with the environment. (29)

dissipation produced by direct and indirect effects of $\bar{T}_{sk}$ on sweat rate and SkBF (29). When T_a falls, $\bar{T}_{sk}$ declines by a smaller amount so that the $\bar{T}_{sk}$-to-T_a gradient widens, and heat loss by convection and radiation increases. This decline in $\bar{T}_{sk}$ directly and reflexly reduces both SkBF (3, 5) and sweat rate (46, 64). As a result, the reduction in evaporative cooling compensates for enhanced conductive and radiant heat loss. Heat transfer to the skin is maintained because the decline in $\bar{T}_{sk}$ also widens the T_c-to-$\bar{T}_{sk}$ gradient, thus compensating for the reduction in SkBF.

Sweat Rate

Sweating is the primary effector mechanism for dissipating heat under conditions of thermal stress. Each gram that evaporates from the surface of the skin removes 0.58 kilocalorie (kcal) of heat. It results from activating sympathetic cholinergic nerve fibers innervating eccrine sweat glands distributed over the general body surface (59), and is responsive to thermal and nonthermal input impinging on the central controller (29). Recent evidence suggests that stimulation of adrenergic fibers may also contribute to sweating control (59).

Several studies have described the effects of age on the sweating response during passive heating (14, 19, 24, 25, 61) (Table 12-2). Fennell and Moore (24) exposed older (65-to-89-year-old) and younger (20-to-24-year-old) men for 120 minutes at 26-27° C while one hand was immersed in 42.5° C water for 60 minutes. They reported a significantly ($p < 0.01$) higher T_c (37.67 ± 0.25° C) at the onset of sweating in old men compared with the value (37.15 ± 0.12° C) in young men. Similarly, Crowe and Moore (14) exposed older (70-to-82-year-

TABLE 12-2. *Effect of age on the sweating response*

Investigator	Age (yrs)	Sex	T_c at Sweating Threshold	Sweating Capacity	State of Conditioning	State of Acclimation
Hellon & Lind (1956)	45–57	M	↔	↔	—	—
Robinson et al. (1965)	44–60	M	—	↓	—	Accl
Lind et al. (1970)	39–53	M	—	↓	—	—
Fennell & Moore (1973)	65–89	M	↑	—	—	—
Crowe & Moore (1973)	70–82	M	↑	—	—	—
Ellis et al. (1976)	>70	M/F	—	↓	—	—
Foster et al. (1976)	≥70	M	↑	↓	—	—
		F	↑	↓	—	—
Collins et al. (1977)	69–90	M/F	↔	—	—	—
Schoenfeld et al. (1978)	46–63	M	—	↓	—	—
	46–63	F	—	↓	—	—
Davies (1979)	60.2* ±10.4	M	—	↓	athletes	—
Drinkwater & Horvath (1979)	12–68	F	—	↓	—	—
Drinkwater et al. (1982)	57.7** ±1.9	F	↔	↔	physically active	—
Drinkwater & Horvath (1983)	60.0 ±2.6	F	↔	↔	—	—

Arrows represent an increase (↑), decrease (↓), or no change (↔) in the variable compared with younger subjects. Dashed (—) lines indicate that no data were reported.
*Mean ± SD.
**Mean ± SE.

old) and younger (16-to-20-year-old) men for 120 minutes at 30° C while immersing one hand in 42.5° C water for 60 minutes. They reported significant differences between older and younger subjects in the T_c threshold at the onset of sweating (older men, 37.36 ± 0.33° C; younger men, 36.75 ± 0.26° C), change in T_c from beginning of exposure to onset of sweating (older men 0.403 ± 0.28° C; younger men 0.169 ± 0.14° C), and experimental time elapsed until the onset of sweating (older men, 42.3 ± 21 min; younger men, 21.5 ± 11.4 min). Hellon and Lind (34) showed older men (45 to 57 years of age) had a significantly ($p < 0.01$) longer elapsed experimental time (29 minutes vs. 15 minutes) before the onset of sweating than younger (18 to 23 years of age) men exposed at 26° C. There were no significant differences between groups in T_{re} or $\bar{T}_{sk}$ at the respective times for the onset of sweating. During a 10-minute exposure to extreme heat (80 to 90° C, 3 to 4% relative humidity), Shoenfeld et al. (61) showed lower sweat production in both older men and women (46 to 63 years of age) than in young subjects (18 to 35 years of age). Young male subjects produced 320.6 ± 132.5 g·m^{-2} of sweat during the 10-minute exposure; older males produced only 267.3 ± 98.3 g·m^{-2}. Corresponding values for young and old females were 222.0 ± 91.8 and 167.6 ± 94.4 g·m^{-2}, respectively. Ellis et al. (23) reported that 14 of 19 men and women over 70 years of age showed either the absence of sweating or little sweating on the forearm following injection of methacholine into the dermis. However, no data were presented in this study. Foster et al. (25) measured sweating in old (≥70) and young men (x̄ = 35) and women (≤35) during indirect heating or after injecting methacholine intradermally at the forearm. The older men demonstrated higher T_c thresholds for the onset of sweating at 6 different sites ($p < 0.10$), lower maximal sweating on the chest and forearm ($p < 0.10$), reductions in sweat rate per gland ($p < 0.01$), and no significant reductions in the number of active sweat glands on the chest. Kuno (41) also reported that the total number of sweat glands does not decline with age. Likewise, older women had significantly ($p < 0.01$) higher T_c thresholds for the onset of sweating and lower maximal sweat rates on the chest. Older women had the lowest chest sweating rates of all subjects, averaging only 0.11 $\mu l \cdot min^{-1} \cdot cm^{-2}$; older men averaged 0.57 $\mu l \cdot min^{-1} \cdot cm^{-2}$. On the other hand, Drinkwater et al. (19) observed that in older (57.7 ± 1.9 yr) and younger (38.4 ± 2.1 yr) physically active women exposed for 2 hours at rest in 40° C heat, there were no differences in the T_c threshold for the onset of sweating, regional sweating, or total sweat loss in $g \cdot m^{-2} \cdot h^{-1}$.

A number of studies have described the effects of age on the sweating response during exercise (20, 21, 44) (Table 12-2). Lind et al. (44) reported that older (39 to 53 years of age) miners, while performing physical labor at 35° C db/28.7° C wb, produced 8% less sweat and averaged 0.16° C higher T_{re} than younger (23 to 31 years of age) miners. All subjects performed the same work, suggesting that the older miners exercised at a greater %$\dot{V}O_2$ max. The latter observation might explain the higher T_{re} in the older men, but not the diminished sweating response. Drinkwater and Horvath (20, 22) reported no significant differences in evaporative heat loss ($w \cdot m^{-2}$) or T_{re} thresholds for the onset of sweating between older and younger women exercising in the heat. In a separate study (21) in which they observed the thermal responses of females 12 to 48 years old during exercise in 35° C heat, there was a significant decline in evaporative heat loss associated with significant elevations in T_{re} and $\bar{T}_{sk}$ when the data were analyzed using polynomial regression analysis.

Skin Blood Flow

The second major physiological adjustment that humans make to thermal stress is active vasodilatation of cutaneous blood vessels (57). At a constant $\bar{T}_{sk}$, SkBF increases in proportion to increasing T_c and carries heat convectively from the core to the skin. Increasing $\bar{T}_{sk}$ potentiates the vasodilator response to increasing T_c by shifting the SkBF:T_c relationship to a lower T_c without changing the gain of the system (51). This increase in SkBF in response to thermal stimuli is due to the withdrawal of constrictor tone in superficial veins and resistance vessels in acral areas (26, 27) and to active vasodilation mediated by increased activity in vasodilator nerve fibers innervating cutaneous vessels in the limbs, head, and trunk (6, 7, 56). In the presence of sweating, increasing SkBF provides the heat necessary for evaporation. In the absence of sweating, increasing SkBF raises $\bar{T}_{sk}$ and increases heat loss by radiation and convection. The recent observation that active vasodilatation is absent during prolonged heating in patients with anhidrotic ectodermal dysplasia suggests an association between active vasodilatation and sudomotor activity (9). During exercise, initiation of vasodilatation occurs at a higher T_c (40); however, this shift in the T_c:SkBF relationship is not proportional to exercise intensity (38, 47, 70).

TABLE 12-3. *Effect of age on forearm blood flow (FBF) at rest*

Investigator	Age (yrs)	Sex	T_c	$\bar{T}_{sk}$	FBF	State of Conditioning	State of Acclimation
Hellon et al. (1956)	39–45	M	↑	↔	↑	—	—
Hellon & Lind (1958)	41–57	M	↑	↑	↑	—	—
Lind et al. (1970)	39–53	M	↑	—	↑	—	—
Wagner et al. (1972)	46–67	M	↑*	↑*	↑	—	unaccl
Drinkwater et al. (1982)	57.7** ±1.9	F	↔	↔	↔	physically active	—
Drinkwater & Horvath (1983)	60.0 ±2.6	F	↔	↔	↔	—	—

Arrows represent an increase (↑), decrease (↓), or no change (↔) in the variable compared with younger subjects. Dashed (—) lines indicate that no data were reported.
*Represent temperatures measured during exercise.
**Mean ± SE.

Differences in forearm blood flow (FBF), as a measure of SkBF (16, 39) have been observed between older and younger subjects (35, 36, 44, 68) (Table 12-3). Hellon and Lind (35) showed a significantly ($p < 0.01$) higher FBF in older (mean age 47.5 years) than younger men (mean age 20 years) 10 minutes after exercise in a warm (38° C db, 30.5° C wb) environment. Sixty-five minutes after exercise, while exposed to the same ambient conditions, FBF was still significantly ($p < 0.001$) elevated in the older subjects. $\bar{T}_{sk}$ was also significantly higher in older subjects at 10 ($p < 0.001$) and 65 ($p < 0.05$) minutes of recovery; however, T_{re} was significantly different only at 30 minutes. Prior to exercise, older men tended to have a higher FBF, but T_{re}, $\bar{T}_{sk}$, or FBF were not significantly different between groups. Wagner et al. (68) reported that FBF at rest following exercise in the heat (49.0° C db, 26.6° C wb) was 22% higher in older (46 to 67 years old) than younger (20 to 29 years old) men. Unfortunately, $\bar{T}_{sk}$ and T_{re} were not measured in recovery, but were higher in the older men during exercise. Assuming these differences were maintained during recovery, the older subjects had a greater thermal drive than the younger men, which could explain their elevated FBF. Hellon et al. (36) reported higher FBF in older (mean age 43 years) than younger (mean age 26 years) men immediately following and 30 minutes after the completion of exercise in the heat (37.8° C db, 29.4° C wb). Significant elevations in T_{re} were associated with the time periods during which the elevations in FBF were measured; however, $\bar{T}_{sk}$ was not significantly different between groups throughout the exposure. Contrary to the above studies, Drinkwater et al. (19) reported that both older and younger women had similar increases in T_{re} and FBF during heat exposure at rest. Similarly, Drinkwater and Horvath (22) reported finding no differences during cycle ergometer exercise, between FBF, T_{re}, or $\bar{T}_{sk}$ in older and younger women.

Physical Training

The effects of physical training on heat dissipation mechanisms and thermal tolerance in young adults (20 to 40 years old) are generally well accepted (4, 28, 44, 47, 49). The T_c threshold for the onset of sweating is reduced and the sweating rate for a given T_c is elevated following endurance training in a cool environment (4, 48). On the other hand, a clear improvement in SkBF at a given T_c following training is not well documented (10). Exercise-heat tolerance in male subjects under hot-dry and hot-wet heat conditions is markedly improved by physical training (30) and similar improvements are also observed in women (12). Since aerobic power and presumably sweating capacity decline with age (25, 53), a reduction in thermal tolerance would also be expected with advancing age. Indeed, Drinkwater and Horvath (21) showed a significant fall in tolerance time for work in the heat with increasing age. However, this observation was attributed to reduced aerobic capacity in the aged, and $\dot{V}O_2$ max can be improved in older subjects (31).

To our knowledge, no one has actually trained older men or women and assessed the changes in their thermoregulatory function or thermal tolerance; however, the temperature responses of older athletes and non-athletes to conditions of thermal stress have been measured. Davies (15) studied the thermoregulatory responses of 21 athletes (14 males, 7 females) and 4 non-athletes (males) aged 18 to 65 years to one hour of treadmill exercise in a moderate environment (21° C db, 15° C wb, RH < 50%, 2.5–5.0 m/s). The older subjects had a mean $\dot{V}O_2$ max of 60.4 ml·kg^{-1}·min^{-1}, clearly documenting their high level of fitness. This study showed that the relationship between $\dot{V}O_2$ max and T_c was independent of age and sex. For a given T_{re}, sweat rate was lower in females and older athletic subjects compared with male athletes, but those differences were resolved if relative sweat rate was plotted as a function of T_{re}.

Heat Acclimation

The question of how well older men can acclimatize to exercise in the heat was first addressed by Robinson et al. (55). In this investigation, 4 exercise physiologists who originally acclimated to exercise in the heat in 1942 (mean age 32 years) were brought back for restudy in 1963 (mean age 52 years). Insofar as possible, the environmental conditions were duplicated (40° C db, 23.5° C wb, 55 m/min air movement). The work consisted of walking 5.6 km/h up a 5.6% grade (4.0% for one subject) for 5 to 13 days. Exercise duration was 65 minutes for 3 men and 85 minutes for the 4th.

According to standard criteria, the older men acclimatized in about the same way and to the same extent as when they were younger. Heart rate, T_{re}, and $\bar{T}_{sk}$ followed essentially the same patterns of change in 1963 as in 1942. In the initial study, metabolism fell an average of 7.4% during acclimatization, but did not change significantly in 1963. When overall metabolic rates for the 2 studies were compared, they averaged 15% less in 1963. Evaporative heat loss increased 15% and 17% with acclimatization in the 2 studies, but averaged 18% less overall in 1963. In 1942, sweating averaged 277 g·m^{-2}·h^{-1} per °C rise in T_{re} during work in the heat before acclimatization and 518 g·m^{-2}·h^{-1} per °C after acclimatization. Corresponding values in 1963 were 326 and 402 g·m^{-2}·h^{-1} per °C, respectively. Thus, the men "exhibited about the same degree of strain exercising at the same speed and grade as they did 21 years earlier and acclimatized about as well" (55).

In a second study from Robinson's laboratory (68), the ability of older men to acclimatize to work in the heat was compared with younger subjects. Before acclimatization, FBF at rest following work in the heat was 22% higher in older than in younger men. After acclimatization, FBF was lower in both older and young subjects, but the greater evaporation of the younger men resulted in a greater reduction in T_{re} than in the older men. Unfortunately, the experimental design did not allow a direct comparison of acclimatization of older and younger subjects. However, when the relationship of evaporative heat loss to T_{re} was used to assess group heat acclimatization, prepubertal boys had the lowest evaporative rates relative to T_{re} and $\bar{T}_{sk}$ while older men had the next lowest evaporative rates. In a more recent study by Dill et al. (17), subjects aged 58 to 85 years walked 10 times in 2 weeks at 100 m/min for one hour in the desert. Based on final T_{re}, there was no evidence of heat acclimation at the end of the 2-week period, but sweat chloride concentration did fall in some subjects, suggesting partial acclimation. Sixty-minute exposures may not have been sufficient to produce acclimation in these subjects (43), although 65 minutes seemed to be sufficient in the study by Robinson et al. (55).

SUMMARY

There is considerable evidence that during heat waves older people are more susceptible to fatal thermal injuries than younger individuals (1, 37, 42, 62, 66, 67); however, it is often difficult to separate the effects of existing disease processes from temperature regulatory dysfunction in such instances. Moreover, many of these victims are probably unacclimated, unfit, and relatively obese.

What is the evidence for an age-related dysfunction of temperature regulation? If the thermoregulatory system is analyzed by evaluating how sweating and SkBF relate to T_c and $\bar{T}_{sk}$ as described by Robinson (54) and more recently adopted by other researchers (10, 29, 45), the evidence is meager. The T_c threshold for the onset of sweating is elevated in older people (14, 24, 25); however, it is also well known that untrained and unacclimated persons have T_c:sweating relationships that are shifted to the right (48). In most of the studies reviewed, the effects of fitness and acclimation state were not considered (Table 12-2). Thus all, or at least part, of the observed shift in this relation could be attributed to reductions in aerobic power and/or a lack of heat acclimation. Many of the subjects showing marked reductions in sweating sensitivity were above 70 years of age. There may be an effect of age on the sweating mechanism in this population, but a carefully controlled study which screens for the effects of disease on central and peripheral control mechanisms must be performed before such a conclusion can be drawn. With regard to alterations in SkBF with age, the data are even less clear. None of the studies reviewed above showed changes in SkBF independent of T_c and $\bar{T}_{sk}$ (Table 12-3). Moreover, none considered the effects of acclimation state. Thus, in terms of these criteria, there is no conclusive evidence to support the notion that advancing age per se is causally related to a dysfunction of the temperature regulatory system.

A second issue is whether or not heat intolerance is a function of age. Once again, there is considerable evidence indicating that older people do not perform well in the heat (14, 17, 21, 24), but this lack of tolerance could be attributed to loss of acclimation (69), heat intolerance per se (60, 71), or to a low aerobic power (15, 21). Moreover, there is some evidence that thermal tolerance is unaffected by decreased sweating in older men up to 60 years of age (55). In general, men are prolific sweaters and a 10 to 20% reduction in sweating capacity may not affect thermal tolerance.

In conclusion, when rigid criteria are applied to the relatively few studies which have addressed the issue of how age affects temperature regulation, the concept that heat tolerance and thermoregulatory function are compromised with advancing age is not supported. A comprehensive well-controlled study which screens for disease and normalizes for differences in aerobic power, body composition, body weight/surface area ratio, and state of acclimation is required to answer the questions posed at the beginning of this review.

REFERENCES

1. Applegate, W. B., J. W. Runyan, L. Brasfield, M. L. Williams, C. Konigsberg, and C. Fauche. Analysis of the 1980 heat wave in Memphis. *J. Am. Geriatrics Soc.* 29:337–342, 1981.
2. Astrand, I. Aerobic work capacity in men and women with special reference to age. *Acta Physiol. Scand.* 49 (Suppl. 169): 7–92, 1960.
3. Barcroft, H., and O. G. Edholm. Temperature and blood flow in the human forearm. *J. Physiol.* (Lond.) 104:366–376, 1946.
4. Baum, K., K. Bruck, and J. P. Schwennicke. Adaptive modifications in the thermoregulatory system of long-distance runners. *J. Appl. Physiol.* 40:404–410, 1976.
5. Bevegard, B. S., and J. T. Shepherd. Regulation of the circulation during exercise in man. *Physiol. Rev.* 47:178–213, 1967.
6. Blair, D. A., W. E. Glover, and I. C. Roddie. Vasomotor fibers to skin in the upper arm, calf, and thigh. *J. Physiol.* (Lond.) 153:232–238, 1960.
7. Blair, D. A., W. E. Glover, and I. C. Roddie. Cutaneous vasomotor nerves to the head and trunk. *J. Appl. Physiol.* 16:119–122, 1961.
8. Boulant, J. A. Hypothalamic control of thermoregulation. In: *Handbook of the Hypothalamus*, Vol. 3, Part A. *Behavioral Studies of the Hypothalamus.* 1–82. P. J. Morgane, and J. Panskepp (eds.) New York: Marcel Dekker, 1980.
9. Brengelmann, G. L., P. R. Frenno, L. B. Rowell, J. E. Olerod, and K. K. Kraning. Absence of active cutaneous vasodilation associated with congenital absence of sweat glands in man. *Am. J. Physiol.* 240:H571–H575, 1981.
10. Brengelmann, G. L. Circulatory adjustments to exercise and heat stress. *Annu. Rev. Physiol.* 45:191–212, 1983.
11. Burton, A. C. The operating characteristics of the human thermoregulatory mechanisms. In: *Temperature, Its Measurement and Control in Science and Industry.* 522–528. New York: Reinhold, 1941.
12. Cohen, J., and C. V. Gisolfi. Effects of interval training on heat tolerance of young women. *Med. Sci. Sports Exerc.* 14:46–52, 1982.
13. Collins, K. J., C. Dore, A. N. Exton-Smith, R. H. Fox, I. C. MacDonald, and P. M. Woodward. Accidental hypothermia and impaired temperature homeostasis in the elderly. *Br. Med. J.* 1:353–356, 1977.
14. Crowe, J. P., and R. E. Moore. Physiological and behavioural responses of aged men to passive heating. *J. Physiol.* (Lond.). 236:43P–44P, 1973.
15. Davies, C. T. M. Thermoregulation during exercise in relation to sex and age. *Eur. J. Appl. Physiol.* 42:71–79, 1979.
16. Detry, J.-M. R., G. L. Brengelmann, L. B. Rowell, and C. Wyss. Skin and muscle components of forearm blood flow in directly heated resting man. *J. Appl. Physiol.* 32:506–511, 1972.
17. Dill, D. B., F. W. Kasch, M. K. Yousef, L. F. Soholt, and D. L. Wolfenbarger. Cardiovascular responses and temperature regulation in relation to age. *Aust. J. Sports Med.* 7:99–106, 1975.
18. Dillman, V. M. In: *The Law of Deviation of Homeostasis and Diseases of Aging.* H. T. Blumenthal (ed.) 155–272, Boston: Jon Wright PSG, Inc., 1981.
19. Drinkwater, B. L., J. F. Bedi, A. B. Loucks, S. Roche, and S. M. Horvath. Sweating sensitivity and capacity of women in relation to age. *J. Appl. Physiol.: REEP* 53:671–676, 1982.
20. Drinkwater, B. L., and S. M. Horvath. Thermoregulatory response of postmenopausal women to exercise in the heat. In: *Proceedings, NIA Conference on Exercise in the Elderly* (Washington, D.C.) as reported in reference 19, p. 675, 1977.
21. Drinkwater, B. L., and S. M. Horvath. Heat tolerance and aging. *Med. Sci. Sports Exerc.* 11:49–55, 1979.
22. Drinkwater, B. L., and S. M. Horvath. Physiological adaptation of women to heat stress. In: *Terminal Progress Report on National Institute for Occupational Safety and Health*, 1–74, February 1983.
23. Ellis, F. P., A. N. Exton-Smith, K. G. Foster, and J. S. Weiner. Eccrine sweating and mortality during heat waves in very young and very old persons. *Isr. J. Med. Sci.* 12:815–817, 1976.
24. Fennell, W. H., and R. E. Moore. Responses of aged men to passive heating. *J. Physiol.* (Lond.) 231:118P–119P, 1973.

25. Foster, K. G., F. P. Ellis, C. Dore, A. N. Exton-Smith, and J. S. Weiner. Sweat responses in the aged. *Age and Ageing* 5:91–101, 1976.
26. Fox, R. H., R. Goldsmith, D. J. Kidd, and H. E. Lewis. Blood flow and other thermoregulatory changes with acclimatization to heat. *J. Physiol.* (Lond.) 166:548–562, 1963.
27. Gaskell, P. Are there sympathetic vasodilator nerves to the vessels of the hands? *J. Physiol.* (Lond.) 131:647–656, 1956.
28. Gisolfi, C. V. Temperature regulation during exercise: Directions—1983. *Med. Sci. Sports Exerc.* 15:15–20, 1983.
29. Gisolfi, C. V., and C. B. Wenger. *Temperature Regulation During Exercise.* Exercise and Sports Sciences Reviews, 12:339–372, Collamore Press, 1984.
30. Gisolfi, C., N. Wilson, and B. Claxton. Work-heat tolerance of distance runners. *Ann. N.Y. Acad. Sci.* 301:139–150, 1977.
31. Hagberg, J. M., W. K. Allen, D. R. Seals, B. F. Hurley, A. A. Ehsani, and J. O. Holloszy. A hemodynamic comparison of young and older endurance athletes during exercise. *J. Appl. Physiol.* 58:2041–2046, 1985.
32. Hardy, J. D. Physiology of temperature regulation. *Physiol. Rev.* 41:521–606, 1961.
33. Hardy, J. D. The "set-point" concept in physiological temperature regulation. In: *Physiological Controls of Regulations,* W. S. Yamamoto and J. R. Brobeck (eds.) 98–116. Philadelphia: W. B. Saunders, 1965.
34. Hellon, R. F., and A. R. Lind. Observations on the activity of sweat glands with special references to the influence of aging. *J. Physiol.* (Lond.) 133:132–144, 1956.
35. Hellon, R. F., and A. R. Lind. The influence of age on peripheral vasodilation in a hot environment. *J. Physiol.* (Lond.) 141:262–272, 1958.
36. Hellon, R. F., A. R. Lind, and J. S. Weiner. The physiological reactions of men of two age groups to a hot environment. *J. Physiol.* (Lond.) 133:118–131, 1956.
37. Henschel, A., L. Burton, and L. Morgalies. An analysis of the deaths in St. Louis during July 1966. *Am. J. Public Health* 59:2232–2240, 1969.
38. Johnson, J. M. Responses of forearm blood flow to graded leg exercise in man. *J. Appl. Physiol.: REEP.* 46:457–462, 1979.
39. Johnson, J. M., and L. B. Rowell. Forearm skin and muscle vascular responses to prolonged leg exercise in man. *J. Appl. Physiol.* 39:920–924, 1975.
40. Johnson, J. M., L. B. Rowell, and G. L. Brengelmann. Modification of the skin blood flow—body temperature relationship by upright exercise. *J. Appl. Physiol.* 37:880–886, 1974.
41. Kuno, Y. *Human Perspiration,* 329–333. Springfield, 1956.
42. Levine, J. A. Heat stroke in the aged. *Am. J. Med.* 47:251–255, 1969.
43. Lind, A. R., and D. E. Bass. Optimal exposure time for development of acclimatization to heat. *Fed. Proc.* 22:704–708, 1963.
44. Lind, A. R., P. W. Humphreys, K. J. Collins, K. J. Foster, and K. F. Sweetland. Influence of age and daily duration of exposure on responses of men to work in heat. *J. Appl. Physiol.* 28:50–56, 1970.
45. Nadel, E. R. A Brief Overview. In: *Problems with Temperature Regulation During Exercise,* E. R. Nadel (ed.) 1–10. New York: Academic Press, 1977.
46. Nadel, E. R., R. W. Bullard, and J. A. J. Stolwijk. Importance of skin temperature in the regulation of sweating. *J. Appl. Physiol.* 31:80–87, 1971.
47. Nadel, E. R., E. Cafarelli, M. F. Roberts, and C. B. Wenger. Circulatory regulation during exercise in different ambient temperatures. *J. Appl. Physiol.: REEP.* 46:430–437, 1979.
48. Nadel, E. R., K. B. Pandolf, M. F. Roberts, and J. A. J. Stolwijk. Mechanisms of thermal acclimation to exercise and heat. *J. Appl. Physiol.* 37:515–520, 1974.
49. Pandolf, K. B. Effects of physical training and cardiorespiratory physical fitness on exercise-heat tolerance: Recent observations. *Med. Sci. Sports* 11:60–65, 1979.
50. Piwoka, R. W., and S. Robinson. Acclimatization of highly trained men to work in severe heat. *J. Appl. Physiol.* 22:9–12, 1967.
51. Roberts, M. F., and C. B. Wenger. Control of skin circulation during exercise and heat stress. *Med. Sci. Sports* 11:36–41, 1979.
52. Roberts, M. F., C. B. Wenger, J. A. J. Stolwijk, and E. R. Nagel. Skin blood flow and sweating changes following exercise training and heat acclimation. *J. Appl. Physiol.: REEP.* 43:133–137, 1977.
53. Robinson, R. Experimental studies of physical fitness in relation to age. *Arbeitphysiologie* 10:255–323, 1938.
54. Robinson, S. Physiological adjustments to heat. In: *Physiology of Heat Regulation and the Science of Clothing,* L. H. Newburgh (ed.) 193–231. Philadelphia: W. B. Saunders, 1949.
55. Robinson, S., H. S. Belding, F. C. Consolazio, S. M. Horvath, and E. S. Turrell. Acclimatization of older men to work in heat. *J. Appl. Physiol.* 20:583–586, 1965.
56. Roddie, I. C., J. T. Shepherd, and R. F. Whelan. The contribution of constrictor and dilator nerves to the skin vasodilatation during body heating. *J. Physiol.* (Lond.) 136:489–497, 1957.
57. Rowell, L. B. Active neurogenic vasodilation in man. In: *Vasodilatation,* P. M. Vanhoutte and I. Leusen (eds.) 1–17. New York: Raven Press, 1981.

58. Saltin, B., and L. Hermansen. Esophageal, rectal, and muscle temperature during exercise. *J. Appl. Physiol.* 21:1757–1762, 1966.
59. Sato, K., and F. Sato. Pharmacologic responsiveness of isolated single eccrine sweat glands. *Am. J. Physiol.* 240:R44–R51, 1981.
60. Senay, L. C. Jr., and R. Kak. Body fluid responses of heat tolerant and intolerant men to work in a hot wet environment. *J. Appl. Physiol.* 49:55–59, 1976.
61. Shoenfeld, Y., R. Udassin, Y. Shapiro, A. Ohri, and E. Sohar. Age and sex difference in response to short exposure to extreme dry heat. *J. Appl. Physiol.: REEP.* 44:1–4, 1978.
62. Schuman, S. H. Patterns of urban heat wave deaths and implications for prevention: Data from New York and St. Louis during July 1966. *Environ. Res.* 5:59–75, 1972.
63. Stitt, J. T. Fever versus hyperthermia. *Fed. Proc.* 38:39–43, 1979.
64. Stolwijk, J. A. J., and E. R. Nadel. Thermoregulation during positive and negative work exercise. *Fed. Proc.* 32:1607–1613, 1973.
65. Thauer, R. Thermosensitivity of the spinal cord. In: *Physiological and Behavioral Temperature Regulation,* J. D. Hardy et al. (eds.) 472–492. Springfield, IL: Charles C. Thomas, 1970.
66. U.S. Department of Health and Human Services. Heatstroke—United States 1980. *Morbility and Mortality Weekly Rep.* 30:277–279, 1981.
67. U.S. Department of Health and Human Services. Illness and death due to environmental heat—Georgia and St. Louis, Missouri, 1983. *Morbidity and Mortality Weekly Rep.* 33:325–326, 1984.
68. Wagner, J. A., S. Robinson, S. P. Tzankoff, and R. P. Marino. Heat tolerance and acclimatization to work in the heat in relation to age. *J. Appl. Physiol.* 33:616–622, 1972.
69. Williams, C. G., C. H. Wyndham, and J. F. Morrison. Rate of loss of acclimatization in summer and winter. *J. Appl. Physiol.* 22:21–26, 1967.
70. Wenger, C. B., M. F. Roberts, J. A. J. Stolwijk, and E. R. Nadel. Forearm blood flow during body temperature transients produced by leg exercise. *J. Appl. Physiol.* 38:58–63, 1975.
71. Wyndham, C. H., N. B. Strydom, C. G. Williams, and A. Heyns. An examination of certain individual factors affecting the heat tolerance of mine workers. *S. Afr. J. Inst. Min. Metall.* September, 1967, 79–91.

13

Heat Stroke in Northern Climates

RICHARD L. HUGHSON, PH.D.

University of Waterloo

The northern temperate climate typically fluctuates markedly with the seasons. In Canada and the northern United States, winter maximum temperatures are frequently below 0° C, while summer maximum temperatures often rise to 30° C or above. For athletes who compete in year-round or summer season sports, the loss of heat acclimatization during the cold winter months presents a major problem.

Lack of early season heat acclimatization has been associated with heat injury in mass participation road running. In the June 11, 1978, Waterloo 10-kilometer (km) road race, 11 people were hospitalized for exertional heat injury (6). By examination of the conditions under which these runners participated, it is possible to highlight some of the major risk factors. First, the runners all lacked heat acclimatization. As seen in Fig. 13-1, the daily mean temperature for the days preceding June 11, 1978, was in the range of 19.7° C. Further, the temperature when the race started at 1 P.M. was 25.1° C (Fig. 13-2), with a relative humidity of 46%. The wind velocity was 16 knots. These conditions taken in isolation did not seem to be extreme. Taken with the lack of acclimatization, they proved to be quite stressful. Of the 11 injured runners, 3 were young females (ages 14 to 18 years) and 8 were males (ages 17 to 38 years). It is significant that all 11 of these injured runners were novices to the sport of competitive road running.

The finding of inexperience as a significant risk factor predisposing to heat injury was not unique to the Waterloo 1978 run. A women's road run in Toronto, Ontario, on August 13, 1978, had 11 heat-injured participants admitted to hospital (6). These women (ages 13 to 30 years) were all novices to 10-km road running. On this day, the environmental temperature was 31.8° C, with 61% humidity. While most of the participants could be expected to be heat acclimatized at this time of the summer season, the extreme environmental heat stress placed an excessive burden on the thermoregulatory system in exercise. Other mass participation types of road runs have had similar experiences with novice runners. Hanson and Zimmerman (2) reported cases of exertional heat stroke in inexperienced male runners (ages 24 to 37 years).

Heat stroke can also occur in athletes who are relatively experienced with competition. Hart et al. (3) reported a 41-year-old man who collapsed after 9 km of a 10-km run in Hamilton, Ontario, June 10, 1979. The environmental

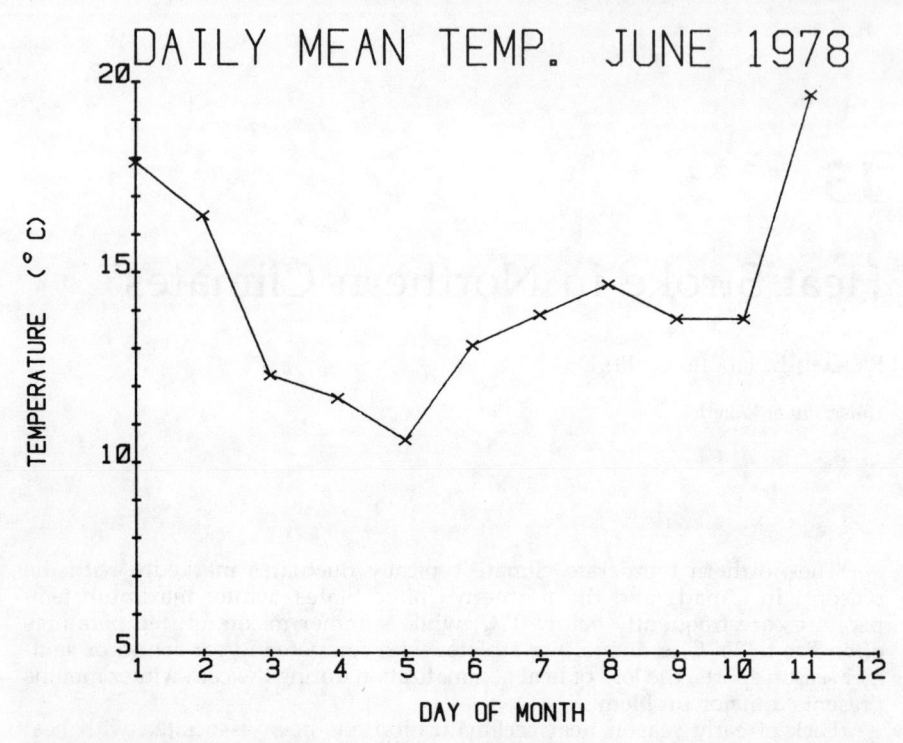

Fig. 13-1. *The mean temperature recorded during the month of June 1978 in Waterloo, Ontario. The Waterloo 10-km race was held on June 11.*

heat load was quite severe, with a temperature of 31.6° C and humidity of 80% at the 1:45 P.M. start time. This runner suffered heat-induced renal failure and was hospitalized for 4 weeks. The significant observation on this runner was that he had been actively training for 9 years prior to the injury and had completed 3 42.2-km marathons. In spite of this, he suffered a severe injury. A fatal heat stroke was reported in a 29-year-old man who was experienced in marathon running (15). This man was competing in England when the temperature was 19° C with a relative humidity of 30%. Relatively low environmental temperatures were noted in other cases of exertional heat stroke. One case reported by Hanson and Zimmerman occurred at 15° C (2), whereas Sutton et al. reported 29 cases of heat injury at 16° C (14). In New Zealand, 16 injured runners were hospitalized due to exertional heat injury suffered in an 11-km run with an environmental temperature of 21.3° C (13). The observations in Australia indicate that even with effective temperatures of 5 to 15° C, a small percentage (typically less than 0.6%) of runners is expected to collapse (12). Some of these will require hospitalization.

Absence of sweating is a primary defect of the thermoregulatory system of the nonathletic heat stroke patient. However, in most cases of exertional heat stroke, the sweating is still profuse at the time of collapse (2, 6, 12). The ability of the thermoregulatory system must be considered in light of the metabolic heat load, environmental conditions, and the efficiency of evaporative heat loss.

During even relatively short distance competitive pace runs, the rectal

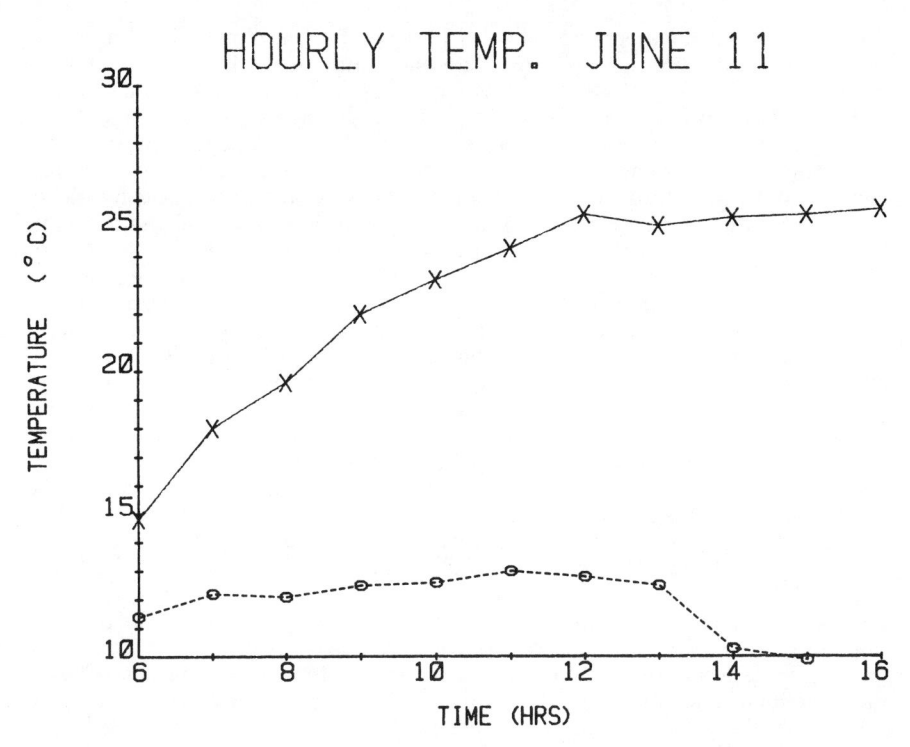

Fig. 13-2. *The dry bulb (X, solid line) and web bulb (O, dotted line) temperatures recorded hourly on the day of the Waterloo 10 km race. The race started at 1 P.M. (1300 hours).*

temperature can be expected to rise to 40° C or above (7, 11) if the environmental conditions are not severe. We recently reported on the effect of environmental heat load during 8-km road running (7). The environmental heat load was measured by the wet bulb-globe temperature (WBGT) index. In relatively cool conditions, WBGT = 18 to 20° C, the 2 male and 2 female subjects had run times of 25:11 to 43:45 for 8 km. The rectal temperatures observed ranged from 39.6 to 40.1° C at the completion of the run. Two subjects were also studied under hot conditions (WBGT = 28° C). A novice female runner slowed her run time from 43:45 to 47:00, yet had a rectal temperature of 40.4° C as opposed to 39.6° C under the cooler condition. An elite male runner slowed his time from 25:11 to 26:42. In spite of this, his rectal temperature increased to 40.2° C from 40.0° C at the end of the run. It is clear from these observations that environmental heat stress can place a major burden on thermoregulation in exercise.

The contribution of metabolic heat production, solar heat load, and evaporative cooling can be considered in a theoretical discussion. A typically fit masters athlete might cover 10 km in 48 minutes. If he weighs 65 kilograms (kg), the predicted oxygen cost would be 38 ml $O_2 \cdot kg^{-1} \cdot min^{-1}$. This amounts to 12.35 kilocalories (kcal) $\cdot min^{-1}$ (862 W), for a caloric equivalent of 5 kcal per liter O_2^{-1}. Allowing for 10% external work and 7% respiratory heat loss (11), the total heat load to the body is approximately 725 W. Solar radiation could contribute 175 W to the total rate of heat gain (8). The body must balance this 1,000 W heat load. Sweating releases 2,500 J $\cdot ml^{-1}$ (8). For unacclimatized individuals, sweat rates are typically 1.0 liter per hr^{-1}; acclimated runners can sweat 2.0 or more liters per hr^{-1} (8). The maximum rate of heat loss by evaporation would be 700 to 1,400 W. However, Gisolfi and Copping (1) and Pugh et al. (11) have indicated that sweating is normally 50% efficient. The net rate of heat loss by evaporation is then 250 to 700 W. Even at maximum sweat rates, the thermoregulatory system depends on convective heat loss to maintain thermal equilibrium. Elevated environmental temperatures and humidity combined with solar radiation can impose severe stress on the thermoregulatory capacity of the unacclimatized athlete. It is possible for even a maximally activated sweating mechanism to be inadequate for thermoregulation.

It appears that the major mechanism which can prevent heat injury is self-awareness of athletic potential for a given set of environmental circumstances. Most heat stroke victims in mass participation runs are novices. Typically, the elite distance runner carefully monitors his physical status during a run (9). On the other hand, novice runners attempt to dissociate from the uncomfortable sensations of the effort (9). In agreement with this latter statement, most of the injured runners in the Waterloo 10-km had completed distances up to 2 km without any reflection of having run that section of the course (6). Education of the runners to the dangers of exertional heat stroke can provide valuable protection. The 1979 Waterloo 10-km run was held under conditions similar to the 1978 run (dry bulb = 24.4° C, WBGT = 18.6° C), again with little opportunity for heat acclimatization (5). Unlike the 1978 run, only 5 people were treated at the race site for minor heat injury. No hospitalizations took place. Prior to the run, a red warning (4) was given to the runners.

A population of older male exercisers (ages 60 to 67 years) has also shown the benefits of education (10). These men self-regulated their exercise pace to achieve aerobic training. The men were studied in the heat acclimatized state under cool (WBGT = 14.8° C) and hot (WBGT = 25.6° C) conditions. There was no significant difference in exercise heart rate (cool = 136, hot = 135), mean skin temperature change (cool = -0.08, hot = -0.90) or mean rectal temperature change (cool = 1.29, hot = 1.30° C). However, to achieve these similar responses in the hot conditions, the men self-selected a pace which was slower (cool = 122 m · min^{-1}, hot = 110.8 m · min^{-1}, $P < 0.05$). From these observations, it is clear that problems with thermal balance during exercise in the heat are a consequence of failure to observe the warning signs of impending heat injury.

REFERENCES

1. Gisolfi, C. V., and J. R. Copping. Thermal effects of prolonged treadmill exercise in the heat. *Med. Sci. Sport* 6:108–113, 1974.
2. Hanson, P. G., and S. W. Zimmerman. Exertional heatstroke in novice runners. *J.A.M.A.* 242:154–157, 1979.
3. Hart, L. E., B. P. Egier, A. G. Shimizu, P. J. Tandan, and J. R. Sutton. Exertional heat stroke: the runner's nemesis. *Can. Med. Assoc. J.* 122:1144–1150, 1980.
4. Hughson, R. L. Primary prevention of heat stroke in Canadian long-distance runs. *Can. Med. Assoc. J.* 122:1115–1116, 1980.
5. Hughson, R. L. Long-distance running in the heat. (letter). *Can. Med. Assoc. J.* 123:607, 1980.
6. Hughson, R. L., H. J. Green, M. E. Houston, J. A. Thomson, D. R. MacLean and J. R. Sutton. Heat injuries in Canadian mass participation runs. *Can. Med. Assoc. J.* 122:1141–1144, 1980.
7. Hughson, R. L., L. A. Staudt and J. M. Mackie. Monitoring road racing in the heat. *Phys. Sportsmed.* 11:94–103, 1983.
8. Knochel, J. P. Environmental heat illness. An eclectic review. *Arch. Intern. Med.* 133:841–864, 1974.
9. Morgan, W. P., and M. L. Pollock. Psychologic characterization of the elite distance runner. *Ann. N.Y. Acad. Sci.* 301:382–396, 1972.

10. Morrison, D. G., R. L. Hughson, D. A. Cunningham, and P. A. Rechnitzer. Environment temperature influences on the performance of older men in a self-regulated exercise program. Unpublished manuscript.
11. Pugh, L. G. C. E., J. L. Corbett, and R. H. Johnson. Rectal temperatures, weight losses, and sweat rates in marathon running. *J. Appl. Physiol.* 23:347–352, 1967.
12. Richards, R., D. Richards, P. J. Schofield, and J. R. Sutton. Reducing the hazards in Sydney's 'The Sun City-to-Surf' runs, 1971 to 1979. *Med. J. Aust.* 2:452–457, 1979.
13. Roydhouse, N., H. Karn, and L. Johnson. 'Round the Bays' 11.92 km fun run for 25,000 entrants. *N. Zealand J. Sports Med.* 6:4–10, 1978.
14. Sutton, J., M. J. Coleman, A. P. Millar, L. Lazarus, and P. Russo. The medical problems of mass participation in athletic competition. The "City-to-Surf" Race. *Med. J. Aust.* 2:127–133, 1972.
15. Whitworth, J. A. G., and M. J. Wolfman. Fatal heat stroke in a long distance runner. *Br. Med. J.* 287:948, 1983.

14

Prevention of Exercise-Induced Heat Stroke

ROWLAND RICHARDS, M.B.

Medical Director, Sydney Sun "City-to-Surf" Run

DAVID RICHARDS, M.D.

Deputy Medical Director, Sydney Sun "City-to-Surf" Run

ABSTRACT

In the first 14-kilometer (km) Sydney *Sun* "City-to-Surf" Run in 1971, 29 runners (1.8% of 1,600 starters) collapsed with exercise-induced heat exhaustion, and 7 (24.1% of casualties) required hospital treatment. From 1972 to 1977 the incidence of heat exhaustion was reduced to 0.27% of 38,500 starters, but 23.3% of casualties still required hospital treatment. From 1978 to 1984, after a strategy was developed to reduce the incidence and severity of heat exhaustion, only 197 runners (0.14% of 144,950 starters) collapsed from heat exhaustion, and, of these, only 2 (1.0% of casualties) who had been treated in the on-site medical centers according to an established protocol required overnight observation in hospital. One patient who was not treated according to the protocol suffered severe complications of heat exhaustion.

Volunteer medical teams experienced in intensive care but inexperienced in the simultaneous care of scores of collapsed, comatose, or combative heat casualties used the protocol effectively. Heat stroke was prevented by effec-

---

Acknowledgements

We thank all volunteers who participated in the medical support teams for their support, encouragement and advice, particularly Dr. H. Roydhouse, Auckland; Dr. R. L. Pearce, Perth; the Perth *Daily News*; Mr. T. Phillips, St. John Ambulance NSW; and Dr. J. R. S. Hales, the Makkah Cooling Unit, for data relating to their events; New South Wales Police; Dr. J. Harley, New South Wales Medical Disaster Planning Committee; Superintendent I. McGuffog, Superintendent J. O'Leary, Station Officer J. Yates, Central District Ambulance for their cooperation; John Fairfax & Sons, publishers of the *Sun* and their staff and all members of the *Sun* "City-to-Surf" Organizing Committee for their sympathetic cooperation; and Professor J. R. Sutton, J. Burke and Dr. J. Harley for their technical and editorial advice. Our thanks also go to Mrs. V. Coleman and Mrs. B. Richards for their secretarial assistance.

tive treatment of heat exhaustion in fully staffed and equipped on-site intensive care facilities.

INTRODUCTION

Since the early 1970's, Sutton (31, 32), Hanson (12, 15), and many other individuals (4, 6, 7, 15, 16, 21, 22, 30) and organizations (1, 9) have emphasized the potentially fatal nature of exercise-induced heat exhaustion (EIHE) in fun running and have recommended measures of organization, education, and medical support to prevent its occurrence. However, only a few fatalities due to heat exhaustion have been reported in runners after competing in "fun runs" and marathons (2, 33).

Despite the growing volume of published papers and reports on heat exhaustion and heat stroke, it is still appropriate to re-emphasize some of the points which have been made relating to organization, education, and medical support and to add the need for research to evaluate the effectiveness of measures to prevent and treat heat exhaustion.

First, there is a need to clarify concepts of EIHE and exertion-induced heat stroke (EIHS) which differ from "classical heat stroke." Whereas classical heat stroke is the well-recognized condition associated with soldiers in the desert, children in closed motor vehicles, and pilgrims to Mecca, EIHE is characteristically seen in healthy young adults who participate in endurance events such as running and cycling.

EIHE may be diagnosed in the presence of the clinical triad: (1) physical exertion, (2) exhaustion and collapse, and (3) rectal temperature $\geq 38°$ C. EIHE comprises a continuum with exhaustion due to exertion at one end and heat stroke at the other end.

The purpose of this chapter is to review the methods used to prevent EIHE and EIHS in fun runs in Australia. Many of the principles used in fun runs in particular may be applied to mass participation endurance events in general.

In this paper the following definitions are used:

"Effective temperature (ET)," according to Landsberg (19), is a measure of sensation of temperature "in which, for a given air temperature and humidity, the state of comfort is equal to that experienced from an environment at a lower temperature with saturated water (100% relative humidity)." Thus, when the relative humidity is 100%, ET is the same as the air temperature and when the relative humidity is below 100%, ET is equivalent, in sensation of temperature, to a lower air temperature with 100% relative humidity.

"Corrected effective temperature (CET)," according to Gregorczuk (11), is ET corrected for the influence of global radiation (intensity of sunlight which varies in different seasons and latitude) and wind velocity.

METHODS

Data were derived from our experience in the Sydney *Sun* "City-to-Surf" (23–28), published reports of experience in other events (3, 10, 18, 29, 30) and personal communications with medical directors of fun runs and marathons and others interested in heat exhaustion.

1. Background

When appointed as Medical Director (RR) in 1976 and Deputy Medical Director (DR) in 1977, we reviewed the background information from 1971 to 1977 to identify medical and other problems and develop strategies principally designed to reduce the incidence and severity of heat exhaustion (Fig. 14-1).

SYDNEY "SUN" CITY-TO-SURF
APPROACH TO
PREVENTION OF EXERTION – INDUCED
HEAT STROKE

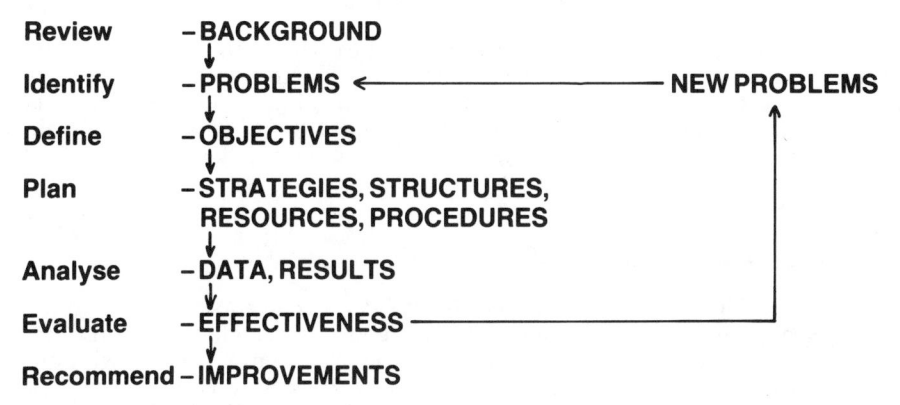

Review   – BACKGROUND
                  ↓
Identify   – PROBLEMS ←────────────────── NEW PROBLEMS
                  ↓   ↑
Define   – OBJECTIVES   │
                  ↓   │
Plan   – STRATEGIES, STRUCTURES,   │
                  RESOURCES, PROCEDURES   │
                  ↓   │
Analyse   – DATA, RESULTS   │
                  ↓   │
Evaluate   – EFFECTIVENESS ───────────────────────────────┘
                  ↓
Recommend – IMPROVEMENTS

Fig. 14-1. *Approach to prevention of exercise-induced heat exhaustion in the Sydney* Sun *"City-to-Surf."*

2. Identifying the Problems

In the first event in 1971, 29 of 1,600 starters (1.8%) collapsed with heat exhaustion and 7 (24.1% of casualties) required further hospital attention. Medical care was provided by Sutton and other doctors who had competed in the event themselves (32).

Following Sutton's (32) recommendations for preventing a recurrence of this potentially fatal situation, significant changes were made to the organization of the event. The run was conducted in August (late winter) rather than in September (early spring). Pre-run seminars were introduced to educate runners on training programs, diet, clothing, and how to avoid developing heat exhaustion. A structured medical support system was also developed.

Of the 38,500 starters from 1972 to 1977, there were 103 heat casualties (0.27% of starters) of whom 24 (23.3% of casualties) were transferred to hospital, some for several days (27). Analysis of data derived from observations relating mainly to the weather conditions on the day and the incidence of casualties revealed that the main problem was heat exhaustion, particularly on hot days. The major factors which predisposed to heat exhaustion were high ET and the individual motivation of enthusiastic amateur runners (27).

Other problems included the risk of a runner falling and being trampled at the start, medical volunteers inexperienced in thermal resuscitation, and delay in commencing effective treatment as a result of the "sick" casualties being transferred to hospital directly from the course or from the medical center.

Methods of treatment, which included covering the body with towels or sheets soaked in ice water, resulted in counter-productive peripheral vasoconstriction and a danger of electrocution if electrical equipment such as a defibrillator was used.

On the basis of this background information, we introduced changes to the overall medical management of the Sydney *Sun* "City-to-Surf" (25–28). By a process of continuing analysis and evaluation of data, progressive improvements were made during the years 1978 to 1984 (23, 24).

3. Strategies to Minimize Medical Problems

The primary objectives were to prevent heat stroke by reducing the incidence and severity of heat exhaustion, to increase the safety and effectiveness of treatment, to establish clinical and biochemical data bases specific to fun runners, and to analyze the data to evaluate the effectiveness of management. Our approach to the strategy of preventing heat stroke was evolved during the years 1978 to 1985 as follows.

4. Pre-Run Organization

All facilities were expanded and the event was moved still earlier, to the first week in August (late winter). Fifty invited runners and 500 proven faster runners were placed in the front rows at the start; the remainder were requested to start from time zones (50', 60', 70', 80' and over) related to their expected finishing times, in order to reduce the risk of a fall at the start.

5. Pre-Run Education

Two pre-run seminars were held, 3 months and 3 weeks prior to the event respectively; 10 weekly newspaper articles were published; radio phone-in and television interviews were arranged; medical information was included on the entry forms and the booklet "Information for Runners" (received on registration); and the entry form was modified to include a waiver of liability and permission to use information for medical research. The emphasis was on safety and prevention of heat exhaustion and included advice on training, diet, clothing, fluid intake sufficient to ensure plentiful pale urine, and when to slow down or stop running.

Medical identity cards for those who had medical problems were available to be pinned to the chest number when registering at the start. The runner was requested to provide information as to diagnosis of medical problem(s) and medication(s) in order to provide prompt treatment in the event of collapse.

6. Pre-Run Briefing

Comprehensive administrative instructions, a protocol of management for collapsed casualties, and a form for documentation of casualties were circulated at briefing sessions with key members of the medical team prior to the run, and again with all members in the medical center on run day.

7. Run Day Medical Support

From 1978 to 1982 volunteers from an inner-city teaching hospital (Sydney Hospital) provided most of the personnel and equipment for the medical center and laboratory facilities for biochemical analysis of blood samples taken from casualties prior to the commencement of treatment. In 1983, after the partial closure of this hospital, the medical support consisted of 1 doctor with previous experience, comprehensive administrative instructions (refined over the years), a protocol of management for collapsed casualties, and volunteer hospital disaster teams consisting of 1 doctor and 2 nurses from 12 inner-city and other metropolitan hospitals. All were experienced in intensive care but inexperienced in the simultaneous management of scores (65 in 1983) of collapsed casualties, most of whom were (46 in 1983) combative, confused or comatose, and suffering from heat exhaustion. Approximately 80% were admitted to the medical center (see below) within 20 minutes of the first arrival. Another inner-city hospital provided laboratory facilities for the biochemical analysis of blood samples.

8. Medical and First Aid Centers

Two separate fully staffed and equipped medical centers were established, one in the Bondi Beach pavilion adjacent to the finish line and one in a Scout Hall some 300 meters from the finish, on the opposite side of the road taken by the runners. In the 2 medical centers a total of 45 beds plus 45 emergency "beds" (a mattress under each bed) enabled intensive care to be provided, simultaneously if necessary, for 90 casualties. First aid was provided by St. John Ambulance (StJ) members in 16 first aid posts located in minibuses at approximately 1-km intervals along the course and in 4 first aid centers in the finish area on both sides of the road.

Transport and communications were provided by the Central District Ambulance (CDA) and the New South Wales Disaster Organization, which used the occasion as the principal annual practice for disaster procedures, equipment, and personnel. A further network of communication was provided by the Wireless Institute Citizen Emergency Network (WICEN).

9. Treatment and Documentation

On admission after triage, vital signs were recorded together with the rectal temperature. Heat casualties were rapidly rehydrated with intravenous isotonic saline or glucose/saline infusions after blood was taken for biochemical analysis. Local active cooling was achieved with cold packs (ice, gel, and now instant cold packs) placed over the major vessels in the neck, axillae, and groin. Intravenous dextrose 50% was administered if hypoglycemia was suspected, along with oxygen by mask. Sedative medications were specifically avoided to prevent prolonged confusion. Cardiopulmonary resuscitation took precedence over all other treatment.

All observations and treatment were fully documented together with full name, race number, previous, recent and present medical conditions, and other relevant history.

10. Post-Run After-Care

On discharge, all who had suffered from heat exhaustion were given printed details of their illnesses, what action to take should specified complications arise, and an invitation to attend the hospital (which provided laboratory facilities) 2 and 9 days later to report progress and have blood taken for further analysis.

11. Post-Run Debriefing

A post-run debriefing seminar was attended by all available members of the medical teams. All aspects of the race were discussed, and recommendations were made to the organizing committee for future implementation.

12. Post-Run Research

In 1978 and 1980 biochemical studies were conducted on volunteer "controls" (who did not collapse) 2 weeks pre-run, on run day, and 2, 9, and 30 days post-run. Similar biochemical studies were conducted on the collapsed heat casualties in groups according to initial rectal temperature (38.0–39.9° C, 40.0–41.9° C, and ≥42° C) on run day (prior to intravenous therapy), and 2, 9, and 30 days post-run. Initial results were reported in 1979 (25).

RESULTS

Weather Conditions, Incidence and Severity of Heat Exhaustion

The correlations between weather conditions (expressed as CET) and the reduced incidence of heat casualties in 1978 to 1984 compared with 1972 to 1977 are shown in Fig. 14-2. This relationship enabled us to predict in 1983 and 1984 the total number of casualties and heat casualties, given the expected environmental conditions and expected number of starters (24) (Fig. 14-3). The CET is positively correlated to atmospheric temperature, relative humidity, and global radiation and negatively correlated to wind velocity (11). Although the severity of heat exhaustion was reduced from 1972 to 1977, 24 cases still required hospital treatment, some for several days. This represented a reduction from 1.8% of starters and 24.1% of casualties in 1971 to 0.27% of 38,500 starters and 23.3% of casualties during 1972 to 1977 (27). The main causes of collapse in 275 casualties from 1978 to 1984 (see Table 14-1) were heat exhaustion (71.6%) and physical exhaustion without hyperthermia (21.8%) (23).

From 1978 to 1984 there was a further reduction in the incidence of heat casualties (0.14% of 144,950 starters) and the severity of heat exhaustion. Only 2 (1.0% of 196 casualties), who had been treated in the medical centers according to our protocol but remained confused, required overnight observation in hospital (23, 27).

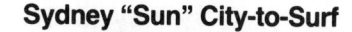

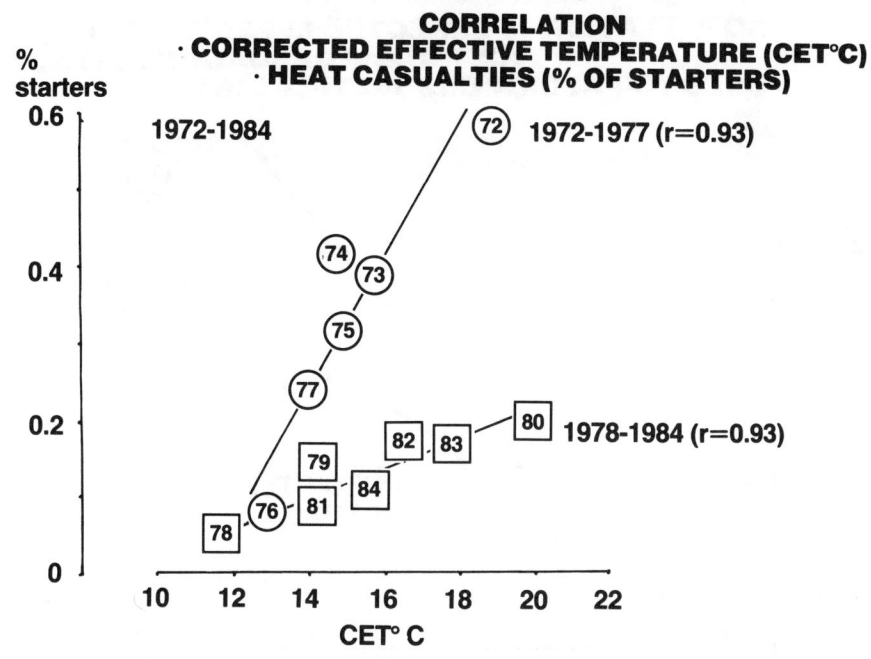

Fig. 14-2. *Relationship of corrected effective temperature to incidence of collapse in the Sydney Sun "City-to-Surf."*

Failure to provide prompt on-site therapy for EIHE probably facilitated the development of complications in 1 case from the Sydney *Sun* "City-to-Surf," and death in 1 case in another run (33). These 2 cases serve to reinforce the importance of prompt on-site therapy for EIHE.

Two Illustrative Cases of Heat Injury

A 29-year-old insulin-dependent diabetic male collapsed in coma 1 hour after the start and 1 km from the finish of the 1984 Sydney *Sun* "City-to-Surf." In the ambulance 40 minutes after collapse, his systolic blood pressure was 70 mmHg. He was given 2,500 ml intravenous fluids prior to admission to a hospital emergency department 70 minutes after collapse. On admission he was obtunded, rectal temperature was 39.5° C, and blood pressure 160/60 mmHg. He was given 100 ml of dextrose 50% intravenously and transferred to the intensive care ward where 60 minutes later the rectal temperature was 40° C, blood pressure 160/60 mmHg, and pulse rate 100/minute. Active cooling was commenced (170 minutes after collapse) by immersion in an ice bath. Rectal temperature, which was reduced to 38° C after a further 110 minutes (5 hours after collapse), fell to 35.8° C after removal from the ice bath, but rose again to 38.9° C 4 hours later. The subsequent course was complicated by coma, hypotension, hypoglycemia, prolonged hyperthermia, dehydration, disseminated intravascular coagulation (DIC), and lactic acidosis, as well as

Sydney "SUN" City-to-Surf
CORRELATION - CORRECTED EFFECTIVE TEMP. (CET°C) and CASUALTIES 1978-82 USED TO PREDICT CASUALTIES 1983

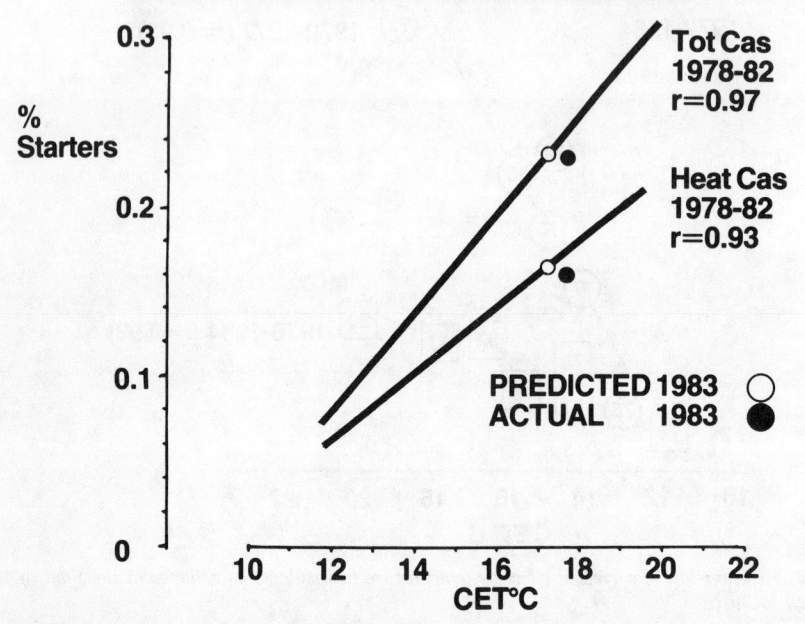

Fig. 14-3. *Prediction of number of cases of exercise-induced heat exhaustion in the Sydney Sun "City-to-Surf."*

liver, pancreatic, and renal damage. He was ultimately discharged well 13 days after admission.

A previously fit 32-year-old male collapsed 0.5 km from the finish of an 11 km fun run held in South Australia in November (early summer) when the midday temperature was 38° C. One hour after collapse when admitted to the local hospital, he was disoriented, suffered peripheral circulatory failure, and had a recorded temperature of 42° C. After 3 hours of intravenous therapy, his temperature was reduced to 38° C. Some hours later he became comatose, assumed a decerebrate posture, and developed disseminated intravascular coagulation and hepatocellular failure. Despite energetic treatment in the intensive care unit of a large public hospital, he did not regain consciousness and died 84 hours after collapse. At autopsy, findings included multiple intracranial hemorrhages, marked cerebral edema, pulmonary edema, and acute renal tubular necrosis.

Prompt on-site therapy for heat exhaustion might have prevented the serious complications suffered by these 2 men.

Age and Sex Profile

The age and sex distribution of 33,700 entrants and 46 heat casualties in 1983 Sydney *Sun* "City-to-Surf" showed a disproportionate incidence of heat exhaustion in males aged 19 to 39 years and in females aged 19 to 29 years. Females represented 4% of runners in 1971–1974, from 6 to 15% in 1975 to 1979, and approximately 21% in 1980 to 1984. Females represented 15% of casualties from 1980 to 1984. There were no heat casualties among those aged below 12 years or over 50 years in 1983 (23).

History Profile

Of the 179 male heat casualties (Table 14-1), 23% had suffered some recent illness (respiratory or gastrointestinal) which predisposed them to dehydration before and during the event; in 56% the intake of fluids before or during the event was inadequate (most had taken no fluid and some had not eaten breakfast). At least 81%, including 6% who were registered athletes, had trained for 3 months or longer before the event, and at least 15% had trained for less than 3 months. Records were incomplete for the remaining 4%. Of the 18 female heat casualties, at least 46% had suffered a recent illness and at least 15% were registered athletes (23).

TABLE 14-1. *Casualties Treated in the Medical Centers 1978–1984*
(275 casualties = 0.19% of 144,950 starters)

Conditions treated	n	% of total casualties
Heat exhaustion (initial rectal temperature ≥38° C)	197	71.6
Other exhaustion (initial rectal temperature ≤38° C)	60	21.8
Cardiac arrest	3	1.1
Asthma	4	1.5
Other, including injuries	11	4.0
Total	275	100.0

Clinical Profile

Some male casualties who had initial rectal temperatures (IRTs) ≥42° C did not appear "ill" (22% were lucid and 89% had moist or sweating skin), while others with lower IRTs (38.0 to 39.9° C) did appear "ill" (2% were unconscious or had seizures and 5% had dry skin). None of the female casualties had a recorded IRT ≥42° C (23). Biochemical studies have been performed and are unhelpful in quantifying thermal illness (25).

Effectiveness of Treatment

Treatment in the medical centers was commenced in most cases within 15 minutes of collapse. The mean time taken for the rectal temperature to fall to below 38° C was 31 ± 12 (SD) minutes for all 196 (male and female) victims of heat exhaustion treated in the medical centers. In 41 male casualties who had IRTs ≥42° C, it took 49 ± 14 minutes to reduce the temperatures to <38° C (Fig. 14-4) (23).

During the period 1971 to 1977, in which 132 of 40,082 starters (0.33%)

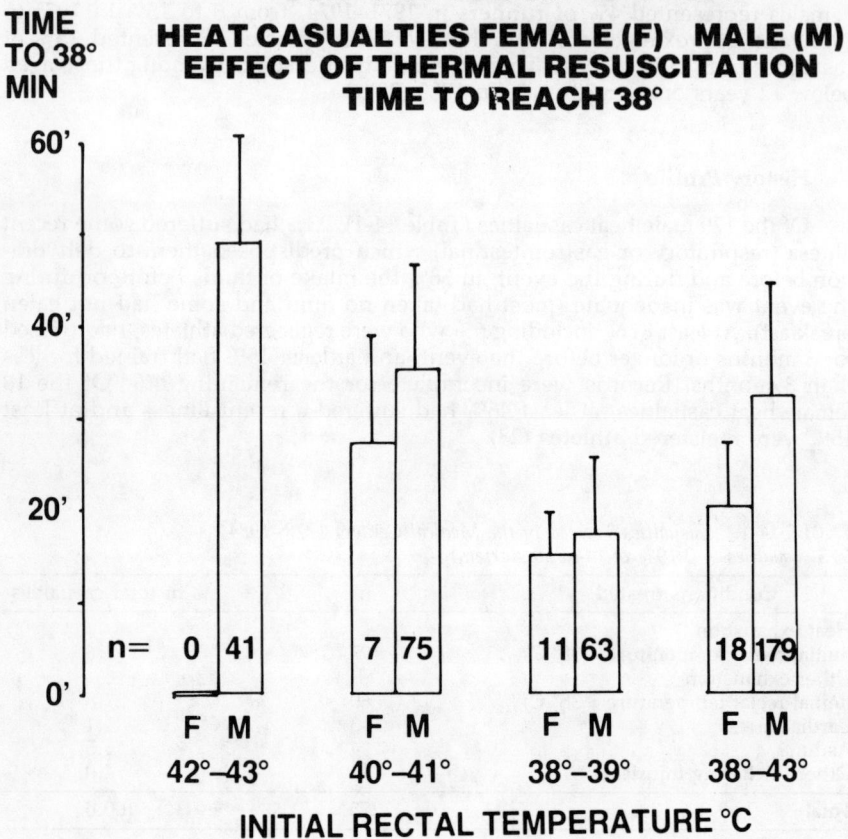

"SUN" CITY-TO-SURF 1978–1984
**HEAT CASUALTIES FEMALE (F)   MALE (M)
EFFECT OF THERMAL RESUSCITATION
TIME TO REACH 38°**

Fig. 14-4. *Times taken to restore normothermia.*

suffered from heat exhaustion, 31 (23.5% of heat casualties) were admitted to hospital for further management (see Fig. 14-5). By contrast, during the period 1978 to 1984, in which 197 of 144,950 starters (0.14%) suffered from heat exhaustion, only 2 (1.0% of heat casualties) treated according to the protocol of management were admitted to hospital for further management of heat exhaustion. One was treated in the medical center and taken directly to hospital suffering complications probably due to delay in treatment (23).

DISCUSSION

Rectal temperatures of 42 to 43° C were recorded in 41 males with heat exhaustion among 144,950 runners in the Sydney *Sun* "City-to-Surf" from 1978 to 1984. There have been no deaths and no long-term morbid sequelae from heat exhaustion. These results may be attributed to the methods employed to reduce the incidence and severity of heat exhaustion and prevent heat stroke.

Sydney "Sun" City-to-Surf

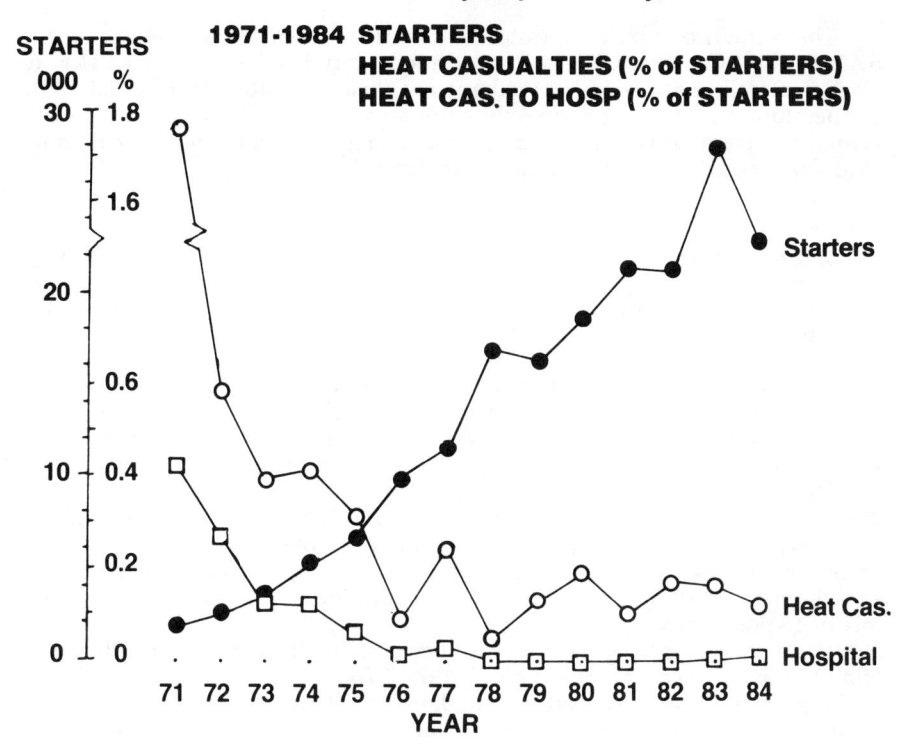

1971-1984 STARTERS
HEAT CASUALTIES (% of STARTERS)
HEAT CAS. TO HOSP (% of STARTERS)

Fig. 14-5. *Distribution of numbers of starters, numbers of casualties and incidence of hospitalization in the Sydney Sun "City-to-Surf" over several years.*

1. Concepts and Definitions of Heat Exhaustion and Heat Stroke

Both Harts and their coworkers (14, 15) noted that "classical heat stroke" is commonly a disorder of the elderly and is associated with coma, hyperpyrexia (up to 47° C), predisposing illness, dry skin, respiratory alkalosis, and a high mortality rate (10 to 80%).

EIHE is typically a disorder of young athletes and is associated with central nervous system disturbance, pyrexia (up to 43° C), sweating skin, lactic acidosis, marked hyperuricemia, and marked elevation of enzyme levels. Complications include rhabdomyolysis, disseminated intravascular coagulation (DIC), and acute renal failure.

It is clear that the picture of heat exhaustion we have seen is consistent with the criteria for exertion-induced heat exhaustion and with the statement by Lind (20) and others that "heat exhaustion and heat stroke represent different degrees of severity on a continuum."

Many writers regard central nervous system (CNS) disturbance as essential to a diagnosis of heat stroke (6, 13, 15, 31). This is potentially dangerous, as delays in treatment may occur while the casualty remains lucid. Many agree that sweating is often present but disagree as to the temperature levels which differentiate heat exhaustion from heat stroke: 39 to 41° C (6), 41° C (13), 42° C (7, 15).

2. Effects of Weather Conditions (23)

The incidence of collapse (total casualties) experienced by runners in the Sydney *Sun* "City-to-Surf" has been directly correlated to the CET. The incidence of collapse due to heat exhaustion (heat casualties with initial rectal temperature $\geq 38°$ C) is also directly correlated to the CET. The grave risk of running in conditions of high atmospheric temperature (38° C) was demonstrated in the case reported from South Australia (33).

3. Comparison of Wet Bulb Globe Temperature (WBGT) and CET (24)

It is generally recommended that a run should be stopped when the WBGT exceeds 28° C (1). However, the estimation of WBGT immediately before the run has limitations. The effect of wind (or, particularly, the absence of it) is not taken into account in the measurement of WBGT. Although wind may vary in direction and velocity (in relation to the runners) in different parts of the course and from time to time, the presence of it is an important environmental factor and is included in the calculation of CET.

The CET includes the effect of global radiation and wind and correlates closely with both total casualties ($r = 0.97$) and heat casualties ($r = 0.93$). It is the preferred estimation in predicting the percentage of starters who may become casualties. It may also be used to determine if the run should be stopped or if the runners should be warned to take additional care to avoid hyperthermia or hypothermia.

The accuracy of the predicted number of casualties depends on the reliability of the weather forecasts to predict the CET, the accuracy of the estimate of the number of starters, and the similarity of the runner population to that of previous years. Obviously, Sydney *Sun* "City-to-Surf" statistics should not be used to predict thermal injury in other events. Organizers of other events must establish their own methods.

4. Clinical Features of Heat Exhaustion (23)

The characteristic clinical features are feeling hot, ill, confused, and nauseated; looking pale (sometimes flushed) with moist (sometimes dry) skin; and behaving in an abnormal way (clumsy movements, confused, combative, fitting, or unconscious). However, some victims with high temperatures ($\geq 42°$ C) remain lucid and have pale sweaty skin and do not appear to be ill, while others with lower temperatures (38.0–39.9° C) may be unconscious, have dry flushed skin and appear to be more seriously ill.

Wide variations were noted in heart rate (100 to 160 beats/minute), blood pressure (80/20 to 180/100 mmHg), and respiratory rate (15–60/minute). These variations probably reflected the result of competition for blood in the exercising muscles to enable increased metabolism, in the circulation to prevent hypovolemic shock, and in the skin to increase evaporation of sweat.

5. Treatment

All runners with heat exhaustion (collapsed with an IRT $\geq 38°$ C) were resuscitated by rapid intravenous rehydration and the application of instant cold packs (for example, "Kwik Kold") over the neck, axillary, and femoral vessels in more severe cases. If hypoglycemia was suspected in patients with persistent CNS disturbance, a 50% solution of glucose (50 ml) was administered intravenously.

Runners with medical problems such as diabetes or asthma should complete and carry medical identity cards, and their organizations should advise on the risks of, and how to avoid, heat exhaustion. The 2 illustrative cases exhibited delays after collapse before the commencement of rehydration of 40 and 60 minutes. The times taken after collapse to reduce the maximum recorded rectal temperature from 40 and 42 to 38° C were 5 and 4 hours, respectively. These data suggest that delay in commencing treatment and reducing the temperature resulted in severe complications (17) and death (33).

In managing 41 cases of heat exhaustion in patients with initial rectal temperatures of ≥42° C, we have reduced the temperature by at least 4° C to 38° C in a mean time of 49 minutes ± 14 minutes without reported complications when treatment was commenced within 15 minutes of collapse.

Hanson and Zimmerman (13) reported 4 cases who were treated within 15 minutes of collapse. The time taken for rectal temperatures of 40.5 to 42.5° C to be reduced to 39.5° C was 30 to 120 minutes. All suffered some complications and remained in hospital for 28 to 96 hours.

Hart et al. (15) reported one case admitted to hospital 20 minutes after collapse, but the time taken for rectal temperature to be reduced to 38° C was 5 hours. Despite a maximum reported rectal temperature of only 40.3° C, he remained unconscious for 6 hours, and suffered DIC and acute renal failure requiring dialysis. It would appear that the critical time spent at temperatures ≥40° C, rather than the limit of 42° C suggested by Bynum et al. (7), between collapse and commencement of treatment is greater than 15 minutes and less than 40 minutes and that the critical time after collapse to reduce the temperature to 38° C is 1 to 4 hours.

6. Motivation of Enthusiastic Amateur Fun Runners and Heat Exhaustion

It is generally acknowledged that those most likely to suffer heat exhaustion in fun runs are the highly motivated enthusiastic amateur fun runners (5, 13, 16) rather than elite athletes who are adequately conditioned for competition and who have learned to "listen to their bodies" (16), or the unfit who do not run fast enough to generate more heat than they can dissipate. When one considers the large numbers at risk and the emphasis placed on the dangers of heat exhaustion, the mortality rate is low if the few reported cases (2, 33) reflect the true picture.

It could be that many cases of serious heat exhaustion occurred in other events and were not recorded, as was the case in the "Great North Marathon" (4) or that deaths from heat exhaustion have been incorrectly recorded as myocardial infarction (2).

Heat exhaustion in the Sydney *Sun* "City-to-Surf" appears to be more likely to occur in highly motivated individuals who do not heed advice after recent illness and who do not maintain adequate hydration (17).

7. Reduced Incidence and Severity of Heat Exhaustion

The results of our study indicate a significant reduction in the incidence of casualties during the period 1978 to 1984, compared with that in the period

1971 to 1977. This is probably due to the combination of improved fitness of the runners and continuing education of runners in the prevention of heat exhaustion.

The reduced incidence of admissions to hospital, a measure of severity, may be explained in part by increased education and the improved fitness of runners, but is more probably due to the efficient deployment of the medical team and the effective use of a protocol of management introduced in 1978 which was based on rapid intravenous rehydration and the local application of cold packs over large vessels.

In the Makkah Body Cooling Unit (17) which was established to treat classical heat stroke in pilgrims to Mecca, a cooling rate of 0.3° C every 5 minutes (that is, a fall of 3° C in 50 minutes) was achieved in 69 patients by blowing warm moist air over the patient suspended on a net in a cooling chamber. The emphasis was on body cooling. Rehydration was not discussed.

The traditional cooling methods of immersion in an ice bath, the use of ice water in towel packs, and spraying the body with cold water have been abandoned by the Makkah Body Cooling Unit because of the counterproductive effect of peripheral vasoconstriction, shivering, discomfort to the patient and medical staff (when the skin is rubbed with ice), slow cooling, the danger of using electrical equipment, the difficulty of monitoring vital functions, and the problems associated with patients suffering from uncontrolled diarrhea and vomiting, especially when they are immersed in a bath. For similar reasons, we have concentrated on local cooling (the application of cold packs over the major neck, axillary, and femoral vessels) as the preferred method of active body cooling.

It is of interest that Cabanac (8) has shown that face-fanning ("a spontaneous behavioral self defence against hyperthermia"), can reduce the tympanic temperature by approximately 1.4° C. Face-fanning, combined with cooling the forehead and face by moist cold towels, may reduce the brain temperature from a critical level in the presence of a high rectal temperature, especially when other measures are not available.

While late complications after discharge have not been reported to us, it was considered prudent to provide all discharged casualties with printed statements of the nature of their illness, the complications which should be reported if they occurred, and an invitation to attend for further observation and blood tests 2 and 9 days later. There have been no observed or reported complications resulting from rapid rehydration, most probably due to the fact that most casualties were healthy young adults.

8. Provision of Medical Resources

We have shown that by using the data obtained from previous runs, weather forecasts (CET), and number of entries, the total number of casualties and the number of heat casualties can be predicted with sufficient accuracy to enable the optimum use of human and material resources (Fig. 14-3). In addition, the CET forecast can be used to determine whether the event should be stopped or the runners advised of the increased risk of developing hyperthermia or hypothermia.

9. Disaster Teams

Since 1983, volunteer disaster teams from 12 inner-city and metropolitan hospitals, with equipment and medical supplies, have assisted a small team with experience of previous years' runs in providing adequate medical cover for the medical centers. The experience of participating in a real disaster situation provided excellent and realistic training for the disaster teams. It is of interest that the members of the disaster teams, some of whom were experienced in intensive care, but were unfamiliar with the venue and problems associated with the resuscitation of combative casualties suffering from heat exhaustion, were generally able to use the protocol of management effectively (23).

In addition, the disaster teams with their equipment, together with the ambulance "disaster vans" containing emergency medical supplies and equipment, were on site and readily available in the event of a major disaster not related to running.

10. Effectiveness of Strategy

The incidence and severity of heat exhaustion have been reduced and heat stroke has been prevented in the Sydney *Sun* "City-to-Surf." The effectiveness of comprehensive administrative instructions, a protocol of management of collapsed casualties, and complete documentation of history and all observations has been demonstrated. The value of data based on post-run debriefing and research to identify new problems and redefine objectives and strategies with changing circumstances from year to year has also been demonstrated. It may be argued that the elaborate medical support provided in the Sydney *Sun* "City-to-Surf" is unnecessary as many would recover without treatment. However, our experience suggests that prompt thermal resuscitation may prevent complications of thermal injury.

REFERENCES

1. American College of Sports Medicine. Prevention of thermal injuries during distance running. Position stand. *Med. Sci. Sports Exerc.* 16:ix–xiv, 1984.
2. Bassler, T. J. Heat stroke in a "run for fun." *Br. Med. J.* 1:197, 1979.
3. Bloomfield, J. The Perth "City-to-Surf" Fun Run 1980. *Sports Coach* 5:9–13, 1981.
4. Bryson, L. G. and A. Seymour. Popular marathons. *Br. Med. J.* 288, 1613, 1984.
5. Budd, G. M. Effects of heat on health, comfort and performance. *Occupational Health*, May, 1979, 16–22.
6. Burke, L. M., L. Piterman, and R. S. D. Read. Safety and supervision in fun runs. *Aust. J. Sports Med. Ex. Sci. J.* 14:125–128, 1982.
7. Bynum, G. D., K. B. Pandoff, W. H. Schuette, R. F. Goldman, D. E. Lees, J. Whang-Peng, E. R. Atkinson and J. M. Bull. Induced hyperthermia in sedated humans and the concept of critical thermal maximum. *Am. J. Physiol.* 235:R228–R236, 1978.
8. Cabanac, M. Face fanning: a possible way to prevent or cure brain hyperthermia. In: *Heat Stroke and Temperature Regulation*, M. Khogali and J. R. S. Hales (eds.) 213–221. Sydney: Academic Press, 1983.
9. Consensus Conference—Popular marathons, half-marathons, and other long distance runs: recommendations for medical support. *Br. Med. J.* 288:1355–1359, 1984.
10. Duras, P. I., J. W. Russell, and A. Kretsch. Illness and injury during the 1980 Big M Melbourne Marathon. *Aust. Sports Med. Ex. Sci. J.* 15:35–39, 1983.
11. Gregorczuk, M. Diagram biocyclometryczny. *Przeglgeofig* 11:57–60, 1966.
12. Hanson, P. G. Heat injury in runners. *Phys. Sports Med.* 7:191–196, 1979.
13. Hanson, P. G. and S. W. Zimmerman. Exertional heat stroke in novice runners. *J.A.M.A.* 242:154–157, 1979.
14. Hart, G. R., R. J. Anderson, C. P. Crumpler, A. Shulkin, G. Reed, and J. P. Knochel. Epidemic classical heat stroke: clinical characteristics and course of 28 patients. *Medicine* (Baltimore) 61:189–197, 1982.
15. Hart, L. E., B. R. Eiger, A. G. Shimizu, P. J. Tandan, and J. R. Sutton. Exertional heat stroke: The runner's nemesis. A case report. *Can. Med. Assoc. J.* 122:1144–1150, 1980.

16. Hughson, R. L., H. J. Green, M. E. Houston, J. A. Thomson, D. R. MacLean, and J. R. Sutton. Canadian mass participation runs. *Can. Med. Assoc. J.* 122:1141–1144, 1980.
17. Khogali, M. The Makkah body cooling unit. In: *Heat Stroke and Temperature Regulation*, M. Khogali and J. R. S. Hales (eds.) 139–148. Sydney: Academic Press, 1983.
18. Kretsch, A., R. Grogan, P. Duras, F. Allen, J. Sumner and I. Gillam. 1980 Marathon study. *Med. J. Aust.* 141:809–814, 1984.
19. Landsberg, H. E. A. Limited review of physical parameters: The assessment of human bioclimate. Technical notes No. 123 in *World Meteorological Organization*, 10–20, 1972.
20. Lind, A. R. Pathophysiology of heat exhaustion and heat stroke. In: *Heat Stroke and Temperature Regulation*, M. Khogali and J. R. S. Hales (eds.) 179–188. Sydney: Academic Press, 1983.
21. Nicholson, R. and K. W. Somerville. Heat stroke in a "run for fun." *Br. Med. J.* 1:1525–1526, 1979.
22. Noble, H. B. and D. Bachman. Medical aspects of distance race planning. *Phys. Sports Med.* 7:78–84, 1979.
23. Richards, R. and D. Richards. Exertion-induced heat exhaustion and other medical aspects of "City-to-Surf" fun runs. *Med. J. Aust.* 141:799–805, 1984.
24. Richards, R., D. Richards, and R. Whittaker. Method of predicting the number of casualties in the City-to-Surf fun runs. *Med. J. Aust.* 141:805–808, 1984.
25. Richards, D., R. Richards, P. Schofield, V. Ross. Biochemical and haematological changes in Sydney's *The Sun* "City-to-Surf" fun runners. *Med. J. Aust.* 2:449–453, 1979.
26. Richards, R., D. Richards, P. Schofield, V. Ross, and J. R. Sutton. Reducing the hazards in Sydney's *The Sun* "City-to-Surf" runs, 1971 to 1979. *Med. J. Aust.* 2:453–457, 1979.
27. Richards, D., R. Richards, P. Schofield, V. Ross, and J. R. Sutton. Management of heat exhaustion in Sydney's *The Sun* "City-to-Surf" fun runners. *Med. J. Aust.* 2:457–461, 1979.
28. Richards, R., D. Richards, P. Schofield, V. Ross, and J. R. Sutton. Organization of *The Sun* "City-to-Surf" fun run, Sydney. *Med. J. Aust.* 2:470–474, 1979.
29. Roydhouse, N. "Round-the-Bays" 1980 medical report. *N. Zealand J. Sports Med.* 8:14–16, 1980.
30. Roydhouse, N., H. Karn and L. Johnson. "Round-the-Bays" 11.92 km fun run for 25,000 entrants. N. Zealand J. Sports Med. 6:4–10, 1978.
31. Sutton, J. R. Heat illness. In: *Sports Medicine*. R. H. Strauss (ed.) 307–322. Philadelphia: W. B. Saunders, 1984.
32. Sutton, J. R., M. J. Coleman, A. P. Millar, L. Lazarus, and P. Russo. The medical problems of mass participation in athletic competition. The "City-to-Surf" race. *Med. J. Aust.* 2:127–133, 1972.
33. To, L. B. Fatal heat stroke in a "fun run." *Med. J. Aust.* 2:104–105, 1980.

15

Providing Medical Care In Fun Runs and Marathons In Australasia

ROWLAND RICHARDS, M.B.

Medical Director, Sydney Sun *"City-to-Surf" Run*

DAVID RICHARDS, M.D.

Deputy Medical Director, Sydney Sun *"City-to-Surf" Run*

ABSTRACT

First aid and treatment of minor injuries in fun runs and marathons in Australia and New Zealand are generally provided by St. John Ambulance members and in a few events by Red Cross members. Intensive care based on previous experience is provided in on-site facilities in both the Sydney *Sun* "City-to-Surf" (35,000 entries) and the Auckland *Star* "Round-the-Bays" (70,000 entries) runs. Volunteer medical team members drawn from several sources (hospitals, military medical establishments, sports medicine groups, and private practitioners) perform effectively when provided with comprehensive administrative instructions, a protocol of management, and a form for documentation. In other small events, less comprehensive on-site facilities are provided, and most casualties are transported by ambulance directly from the

---

Acknowledgements

We thank all volunteer members of the medical support teams for their support, encouragement and cooperation, including Dr. J. Robinson and staff, Sydney Hospital; Dr. K. Abraham and staff, Royal Prince Alfred Hospital; Professor L. Lazarus, and staff, St. Vincent's Hospital; New South Wales Police; New South Wales Disaster Organisation; Central District Ambulance; sports medics and private medical practitioners; specialist doctors, nurses, physiotherapists and students; disaster teams from metropolitan hospitals; and Lewisham Sports Medicine Research Institute. We pay tribute to John Fairfax & Sons, publishers of the *Sun*; Mr. A. Forsyth, Run Organiser, and staff; Mr. G. Carruthers, Run Director; and members of the *Sun* City-to-Surf Organising Committee for their sympathetic cooperation and for their constant courses for the safety of runners. Equipment and medical and other supplies were generously donated by Terumo Corporation, Honeywell Pty Ltd and Abbott Australasia Pty Ltd., and by the distributors of "Staminade," "Kwik Kold," & "Kwik Wrap." Our particular thanks go to Mrs. V. Coleman and Mrs. B. Richards for their secretarial assistance; to the staff of the *Sun* for the art work, and to Professor J. R. Sutton and J. Burke for their technical and editorial advice.

course to the local hospital. Delay in commencing definitive treatment in 1 case resulted in death from heat exhaustion, and in another in severe complications. It is concluded that first aid and intensive care should be provided in on-site facilities and the extent determined by critical evaluation of previous experience.

INTRODUCTION

Adventurous individuals who choose risk-taking pursuits such as mountain climbing, walking across deserts, and exploring other hostile environments make personal choices to participate and accept responsibility for their own safety. Despite taking precautions when challenging nature, there are many obituaries and monuments to recognize those who failed.

Elite athletes and others who are induced by promoters to participate in punishing events, almost to the point of self-destruction, are protected to some extent by the safety precautions observed by the promoters. The safety rules are generally more stringent than those which apply in the case of less strenuous mass participation "fun run" events.

Enthusiastic amateur fun runners are usually enticed by friends or induced by promoters to participate and may suffer a fate similar to others who fail to observe accepted safety precautions. Responsible bodies such as the American College of Sports Medicine (1), Consensus Conference in the United Kingdom (5), and Road Runners of America have published guidelines for the organization and medical support of endurance events to avoid thermal injury, particularly heat exhaustion.

All emphasize the need for adequate organization of the event, education of competitors and organizers, and medical care for those who disregard the advice given or are injured despite following the guidelines. Few, however, emphasize the need for scientific research and coordinated collection and analysis of data to evaluate the effectiveness of such organization, education, and medical support. Over the past 8 years, the organizers of the Sydney *Sun* "City-to-Surf" run have developed a comprehensive program of safety measures to protect runners from injury and illness and to evaluate the results of such a program. The purpose of this chapter is to review this program and others used in Australasia to protect runners from injury and illness.

METHODS

Data were derived from experience in the Sydney *Sun* "City-to-Surf" runs (9, 11–15, 18), published reports from other events (2–4, 6, 7, 16, 17), and personal communications with members of St. John Ambulance (StJ), Australian Sports Medicine Federation, and medical directors of endurance running events.

RESULTS

Of the 22 events reviewed, the Sydney *Sun* "City-to-Surf" 14-kilometer (km) run (≤35,000 entries per year) experience is given in some detail as it includes most of the items covered in the other 21 events for which we have some (mostly incomplete) information. The most complete data from other events relate to the Auckland *Star* "Round-the-Bays" 12-km run (≤80,000 entries per year) which also has a highly organized medical support team of a size (approximately 250–350 members) similar to the Sydney run. This represents approximately one medical support team member per 100 runners in the "City-to-Surf" and one per 300 runners in the "Round-the-Bays."

Significant numbers of heat casualties have been reported in both events. In the other events in 1984 and 1985 for which we have information, organized medical support teams were provided in 6 events of 10 km or more with 1,000 to 5,000 runners, and in 2 42-km marathons (one of 5,000 runners (Sydney *Wang*) and one of 600 runners (Sydney *Xerox*). In the remaining 15 events of less than 10 km, only first aid cover was provided. Details of numbers involved were not available. In addition to the *Sun* "City-to-Surf" and the *Star* "Round-the-Bays" runs, heat casualties were reported in one 42-km marathon (Melbourne "Big M") and 2 other events, the Perth *Daily News* "City-to-Surf" 12-km run, and the Sydney "Yellow Pages" 14-km run. A summary of selected events is shown in Table 15-1.

No heat casualties were reported in events of 10 km or less. With a few notable exceptions, the medical support was adequate in the circumstances. Details of events with organized medical support follow.

Sydney *Sun* "City-to-Surf" 14-km run
1978 to 1985; 20,000 to 35,000 entrants

The events began at 10 a.m. on the first Sunday in August (late winter) and covered a distance of 14 km, commencing at the Sydney Town Hall, on roads winding through the eastern suburbs of Sydney to Bondi Beach. Entry was unconditional, and entrants were recorded in the computer by age, sex, division, class, and team name. Starters represented approximately 80% of entrants plus late entrants. Those who registered a finishing time represented approximately 95% to 97% of starters. The names and finishing times of all entrants (excluding late entries) who completed within 150 minutes were published in *The Sun*.

From 1978 to 1984, 1.3% of 144,950 starters required first aid for minor injuries; 0.19% of starters required intensive care for medical emergencies including 0.14% (range 0.05 to 0.19%) of starters who suffered from heat ex-

TABLE 15-1. *Summary of selected events in Australasia 1971 to 1985*

Event	Distance (Km)	Years	Entrants (estimated, if no published data)	Reported Heat Casualties (% of entrants)*
Sun "City-to-Surf"	14	1971–84	2,000–33,700	0.04–1.50
Star "Round-the-Bays"	12	1972–85	1,200–80,000	0–0.30
Melbourne "Big M"	42	1977–80	5,000	0–12.00
Daily News "City-to-Surf"	12	1975–84	500–4,000	0.05–0.13
Wang Marathon	42	1984–85	4,000	0
Xerox Marathon	42	1984	600	0
Yellow Pages	14	1984	1,000	0.30
Others (15)	<10	1984	200–5,000	0

*Heat casualties as percentage of actual starters (approximately 80% of entrants) are underestimated by approximately 25%.

haustion. Chafing, sprains, strains, cramps, and blisters were the common minor injuries, and heat exhaustion was the most common medical emergency (9).

An outline of the organization of the event and of the medical support which has evolved during the years 1978–1985 follows.

1. ORGANIZATION OF THE EVENT: The organizing committee was composed of the run organizer from the *Sun* newspaper, run director, medical director, and representatives from the police, amateur athletic associations, and the *Sun*. The committee was responsible for deploying over 2,000 officials, including over 350 members of the medical support team (Fig. 15-1).

The emphasis was on safety for the runners and spectators. This was achieved by organizing the event in expected cool weather conditions; providing adequate crowd and traffic control, communications, drinks, and toilet facilities; educating runners, medical team, and organizers; providing sufficient medical support for first aid and intensive care for runners and for casualties in disasters not related to running; and researching the effectiveness of overall organization and management of casualties.

2. EDUCATION: Runners received advice upon registration on how to train, what to eat and drink, what to wear, and how to avoid injury, heat exhaustion, and other medical problems (9). The organizers, StJ, and medical team members received advice on the medical arrangements by comprehensive administrative instructions, pre-run briefings, and several monthly and other ad hoc meetings. At a post-run debriefing seminar attended by all avail-

SYDNEY "SUN" CITY-TO-SURF

ORGANIZATION
1985

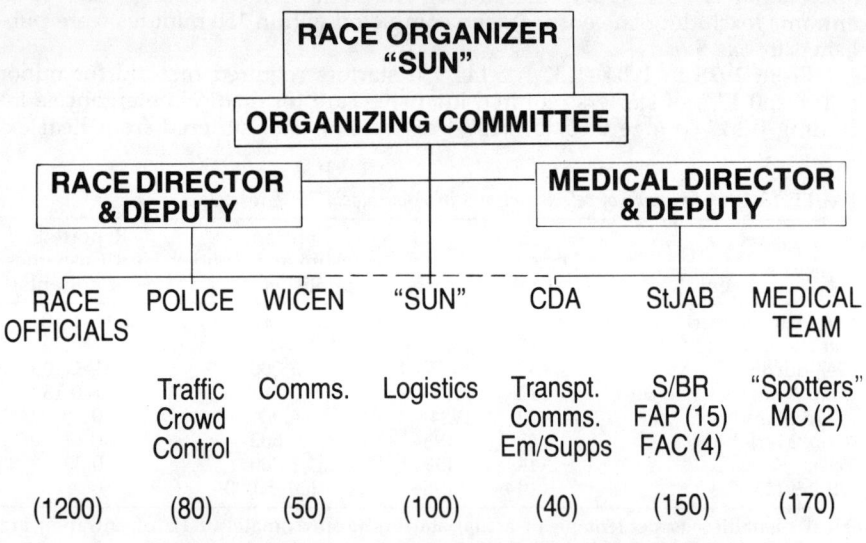

Fig. 15-1. *Organization of the Sydney* Sun *"City-to-Surf."*

able personnel, recommendations were made to the organizing committee for improvements in future events.

3. ORGANIZATION OF MEDICAL SUPPORT IN 1985: The organizational structure was developed to achieve the primary objectives of providing (a) prompt identification of injured, exhausted, and collapsed casualties; (b) rapid transport of casualties to first aid and medical centers on site; (c) immediate triage, diagnosis, and effective treatment of casualties; and (d) facilities and resources capable of coping with a major disaster not related to running.

StJ members provided first aid and treatment of minor injuries; medical team (MT) members provided prompt identification ("spotters") and intensive care for medical emergencies; Central District Ambulance (CDA) Disaster Organization provided emergency supplies and equipment, transport, and medical communications; Wireless Institute Citizen Emergency Network (WICEN) provided an additional medical communication network combined with a network covering the whole event; New South Wales Police provided crowd and traffic control and a further communication network linked with the CDA Disaster Organization (Fig. 15-2).

4. DEPLOYMENT OF MEDICAL SUPPORT IN 1985: The first aid and medical teams were deployed in the registration area (Sydney Town Hall on two levels), at the start, along the course, and at the finish. The CDA was also deployed at the start, along the course, and at the finish. The final deployment of the medical team members and equipment was based on the prediction of the number of casualties to be expected (11). This number was calculated from previous experience, estimated number of runners, and weather forecasts for the day. This prediction enabled the optimum deployment of resources as follows.

(a) *Registration:* Sports medicine physicians provided advice and medical

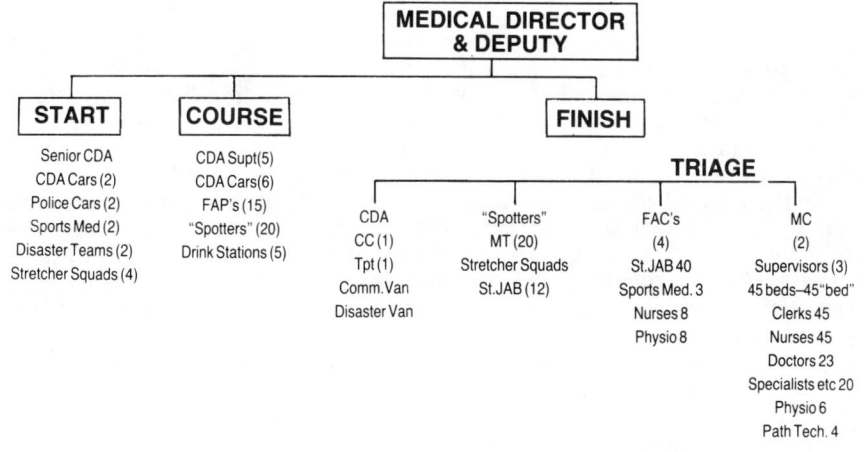

Fig. 15-2. *Organization of medical support for the Sydney* Sun *"City-to-Surf."*

identity cards to runners who had medical problems (10). StJ members provided dressings for minor injuries and petroleum jelly to prevent chafing. Surplus clothes were placed in numbered plastic bags to be conveyed to the finish area. Portable toilets were provided.

(b) Start: A senior CDA Superintendent was at the start to coordinate the activities of 2 disaster teams (DT), 4 StJ stretcher bearer squads, 5 CDA transport cars, and 2 police cars had there been a major disaster near the start. Sports medicine physicians were available to advise runners who had medical problems whether to start, when to slow down or stop, about the need to take drinks at all drink stations, and how to obtain first aid and medical attention. The starter also advised runners, while warming up, of the need to take safety precautions to avoid illness and injury to themselves or others. Drinking water and portable toilets were provided in the park adjacent to the start.

(c) Course: Fourteen static first aid posts (FAP), located in minibuses along the course at approximately 1-km intervals, were staffed by StJ members to treat minor injuries. Two mobile FAP staffed also by sports medicine physicians were in the start area and followed the run together with two CDA ambulances and one CDA bus to pick up stragglers. "Spotters" (approximately 20 doctors, physiotherapists, and students) were located at strategic positions along the course to identify runners who were becoming exhausted or who required first aid or medical care. Five senior CDA Superintendents were located along the course to coordinate the activities of "spotters," first aiders, and the 10 CDA transport cars on call in the vicinity. Casualties who collapsed along the course were taken to a medical center/first aid center (in a Scout Hall) approximately 300 meters (m) from the finish. Five drink stations supplied water and half-strength "Staminade" (an electrolyte/glucose drink), at approximately 3-km intervals along the course. Portable toilets were also provided.

(d) Finish: In the finish area 10 "spotters" and 12 StJ stretcher bearer squads identified, then assisted or carried those who required medical attention to either one of 2 medical centers (one in the Scout Hall and the other in the pavilion adjacent to the finish line). A large drink station was located beyond the finish line, adjacent to the clothes collection point and a satellite first aid center. Toilets and shower facilities were provided in the pavilion.

Casualties brought to the pavilion were directed after triage to the first aid center or assisted to the medical center. On entry to each medical center two members of StJ recorded race number, time of admission, and time of discharge. From a computer listing of race numbers, names were checked and recorded. In the medical centers, provision was made to treat up to 90 casualties. On admission the protocol of management was followed.

In the medical centers the allocation of staff was: 1 clerk per bed to record data on the clinical notes, and 1 volunteer hospital disaster team (one doctor and two nurses) to treat up to 4 casualties simultaneously. In addition, there were anesthetists, intensivists, cardiologists, orthopedists, and physiotherapists available as required. Pathology laboratory technicians were available to process blood samples taken before the commencement of treatment.

On discharge each casualty was given printed advice stating the nature of illness, the complications which occur, and an invitation to attend an inner city hospital to report progress and have further blood taken for analysis on two occasions, 2 days and 9 days after the event.

One CDA coronary care ambulance and one CDA car were situated at the bathing pavilion and at the Bondi Ambulance Station (adjacent to the Scout Hall), available to transport casualties from the medical centers to hospital, if required. The CDA Disaster Communication van and emergency equipment vans were located at the ambulance station.

5. PROTOCOL FOR MANAGEMENT OF COLLAPSED CASUALTIES: A protocol of management, with minor modifications, has been used since 1978 (14). The essential elements of the protocol include: (a) cardiopulmonary resuscitation, (b) prompt transfer to an on-site medical center, (c) initial and progressive documentation by the clerk, (d) thermal resuscitation and other treatment, and (e) discharge instructions.

The medical center clerks (usually medical, physiotherapy, or nursing students) recorded: full name, age, sex, race number, blood specimen number, admission time, presenting symptoms, clinical history, training history, initial and progressive vital and other physical signs, details of treatment (intravenous fluids, cold packs, etc.), diagnosis, and discharge declaration (nature of illness, fitness to leave, invitation to report complications and to give blood for further investigations 2 and 9 days after the event, permission to use data for research).

First aid center clerks (usually StJ members) recorded: race number, presenting symptoms and signs, types of injuries, treatment, and discharge details (referral for further care, etc.).

6. RESEARCH AND EVALUATION: The protocol of management and documentation of casualties were designed to provide accurate data for later analysis and evaluation. After the run the clinical records were correlated with the pathology and other data to evaluate the effectiveness of management and to prepare an annual report and recommendations for improvement for submission to the organizing committee. The data were analyzed and formed the basis for future advice to runners, organizers, and medical teams as well as for scientific reports for public presentation and publication.

7. DISASTERS NOT RELATED TO RUNNING: A few kilometers from the start of the 1984 Sydney *Sun* "City-to-Surf" run, a helicopter carrying a television camera crew crashed out of control into a playing field a few meters away from the densely packed runners. The only casualties were the pilot and camera crew. Fortunately none was seriously injured.

Auckland *Star* "Round-the-Bays" 12-km run; up to 80,000 Entrants

The event commences in a park in the downtown area of Auckland and follows a course over a causeway and alongside several bays to a park 12 km from the city. There were no casualties reported in 1,200 runners in the first event in 1974 when the medical support team consisted of 1 doctor and 2 StJ members. The event was held in March (late Autumn), one month before the commencement of winter sports. By 1977 (17) there were 20,000 entrants. As a result of unseasonable and unfavorable weather conditions (atmospheric temperature 22°C, relative humidity 85%, and no recorded air movement), 60 male runners (0.3% of entrants) collapsed with heat exhaustion, 40 within 20 minutes after the first casualty collapsed. Sixteen cases were transferred to hospital; 5 were admitted. One serious case (8) remained for 6 weeks; the others were discharged within 3 days. The medical support team comprised 30 members including 5 doctors and 18 StJ members, 4 ambulances deployed at 4 first aid posts along the course, and a first aid center at the finish under the control of a medical director.

In 1978 (17) the weather conditions were more favorable for the 25,000 entrants (atmospheric temperature 20°C, relative humidity 74%, and wind velocity 8 m/s). As a result of the previous year's experience, the medical support team was increased to 184 members including 34 doctors, 28 nurses, 74 first aiders, and 9 ambulances deployed in 7 static and mobile units along the course and at the finish. Eight heat casualties (0.04% of entrants) were taken to hospital; 4 required admission. In addition, 488 runners were treated for minor injuries (1.95% of entrants).

In 1980 (16) approximately 40,000 runners competed in favorable weather conditions (atmospheric temperature 15.3°C, relative humidity 59%, and calm air). The medical support team consisted of 170 members, 20 ambulances deployed in 4 static first aid posts, 2 static medical aid posts, 1 mobile medical unit along the course, and an Army Field Hospital at the finish. All 6 heat casualties were thermally resuscitated (rectal temperatures reduced to <38° C) before transfer to hospital. None required admission. Approximately 170 were treated for minor injuries.

By 1984 (personal communication) the number of runners had grown to an estimated 80,000, and the medical support team was expanded to 300 members deployed in 7 static and mobile first aid posts and 3 medical units supported by 22 ambulances (static and mobile) and 1 helicopter rescue unit. Medical communications were provided by 4 radio networks.

In 1985 over 1,000 cases of minor injury (mainly chafing) were treated in 2 of the first aid posts, but the incidence of heat exhaustion was low—only 3 cases were recorded. One 43-year-old male died of myocardial infarction after unsuccessful attempted resuscitation.

Comprehensive administrative instructions and a protocol of treatment of casualties were distributed to all medical units and discussed at 2 pre-run seminars attended by medical team members. Adequate equipment and large quantities of water and electrolyte solutions were provided at the 10 aid stations. The 4-month program of education of runners conducted by *The Star* was aimed at improving the fitness of runners and creating an increased awareness of the need and means to avoid heat exhaustion. In 1978 the finishing times of runners were not recorded in order to reduce the atmosphere of competition, in an endeavor to reduce the pace of running and the incidence of heat exhaustion. However, the incidence of heat exhaustion did not appear to be affected by this maneuver.

Melbourne "Big M" 42-km Marathon; 4,000 Entrants

It was reported (6) that in the 1979 event the temperature rose to 29°C and that there were approximately 600 heat casualties (15% of approximately 4,000 runners). As a result of this unexpected disaster, the Australian Sports Medicine Federation conducted comprehensive investigations on runners competing in the 1980 "Big M" (6, 7). This is the only reported comprehensive investigation of runners competing in marathons in Australia. The essential findings of this study were as follows:

At 0800 hrs on October 12, 1980 (Spring), approximately 4,000 runners started the event in overcast mild (11 to 16°C) weather conditions. Ninety-seven athletes, approximately 2.6% of finishers, sought treatment at 8 medical stations. Seventy-two percent of these were 20 to 39 years of age. Ten casualties suffered from "dehydration," but "there were no cases of frank heat exhaustion or heat stroke." The absence of heat exhaustion was probably due to the overcast mild weather conditions (6). In addition, there were no cases of asthma or cardiac problems. Most of the treatment was provided by physiotherapists and StJ members. There was no reference to education of runners. Details are not available for the runs conducted before and after 1980.

Perth *Daily News* "City-to-Surf" 12-km Fun Run; 4,000 Entrants

The first event in 1975 attracted 500 runners. Up till 1982 the event was held in April (late Autumn) when the weather conditions were described as "extremely hazardous," and up to 5 heat casualties (at least 0.17% of runners) were admitted to hospital each year. Since 1983 the event has been conducted in September (early Spring) when expected weather conditions were "more favorable." Up to 2 competitors each year (approximately 0.07% of runners) were taken to hospital, but only 1 required hospitalization overnight (personal communication).

All first aid, medical, and emergency support was organized by the medical support coordinator, a member of the Australian Sports Medicine Federation, and a senior member of StJ. More than 30 StJ members provided 1 ambulance (with others on call), staff in 9 first aid posts along the course, a major first aid station at the finish, and 1 mobile first aid station. Drinks (water only) were provided at the start and finish and at 4 stations along the course.

On the entry form each runner completed a medical questionnaire to provide information about previous medical history, present illness, and medication. The details were reviewed by the medical support coordinator who contacted the runner if he considered the runner to be at risk. A list of those with medical problems was compiled in numerical order according to chest numbers and distributed to doctors ("spotters") along the course. Should a runner collapse, the chest number was checked against the list so that appropriate treatment was instituted promptly.

The *Daily News* published a number of articles over a period of several months advising runners on training, diet, clothing, and how to avoid heat exhaustion. In addition, the paper published a 34-page booklet, "Running for Fun," which included medical advice and a 12-week detailed training schedule. Post-race debriefings were considered unnecessary. Bloomfield in 1981 (3) analyzed 950 questionnaires completed by those who finished the event in 1980. (The total number of finishers was not stated but was probably less than 3,000).

The ages of competitors ranged from 10 to 60 years. The largest group was 30 to 39 years of age. Males represented 79% and females 21% of those who responded. More than 30% trained for at leat a year, and 29% trained for 6 to 26 weeks. Only 16% had trained for 1 week or less. More than 50% participated for fun, 30% for the challenge, 25% as part of training, and 18% to get fit. Only 2.3% ran as members of a team.

Wang Australian 42-km Marathon (Sydney); 5,000 Entrants

The third event was held in 1985. There was full first aid coverage by StJ with first aid posts and drink stations at the start, at 5-km intervals, and at the finish, in accordance with the International Amateur Athletic Federation regulations. In addition, there was an on-site medical team including doctors, physiotherapists, chiropractors, and masseurs, with adequate equipment. Reported casualties were minor. Pre-run instructions and seminars were provided (personal communication).

Sydney *Yellow Pages* 14-km "Bridge-to-Breakers;" 1,000 Entrants

First aid posts—3 on the course and one at the finish—were manned by StJ. The on-site sports medicine team included doctors and physiotherapists. Reported casualties included a few minor injuries, 3 heat casualties (0.3% of starters), and 4 with asthma (personal communication).

Xerox New South Wales 42-km Marathon (Sydney); 600 Entrants

The fourth event was held in 1984. First aid cover, provided by StJ, included first aid posts and drink stations at 5-km intervals and at the finish. The on-site medical team included doctors and physiotherapists. No major casualties were reported (personal communications).

DISCUSSION

Organization

The stated objective in conducting fun runs and marathons is to promote long-term regular exercise as part of a healthy lifestyle to improve cardiorespiratory endurance and to reduce cardiovascular disease. That is, those in the target group are the less fit members of the community who are more prone to suffer the ill effects of overexertion and who should be protected by adequate organization and medical support when they are induced by promoters to compete.

The Sydney *Sun* "City-to-Surf" and Auckland *Star* "Round-the-Bays" have comprehensive organization, administrative instructions, and protocols of management of casualties based on previous experience. They would provide adequate medical support for even abnormal and unexpected circumstances.

Most other events have some form of less comprehensive organization and may find it difficult to cope with abnormal and unexpected circumstances. There is a clear need for the medical director to be appointed to the organizing committee of each event and to assume full control of the medical support team.

The organizing committee should ensure that the event is held under expected favorable weather conditions and that all reasonable safety precautions should be taken (competitor, traffic, and crowd control; drink stations; toilets; communications; and medical support).

Most entry forms included some form of a waiver of liability by the promoters. In the Perth *Daily News* "City-to-Surf," questions relating to illness and medication were included on the entry form, and the relevant information was distributed to doctors on the course. Such action had been considered, but rejected, by the organizers of the Sydney *Sun* "City-to-Surf" on the basis that they might be liable if the information was omitted, overlooked, or not observed by the large numbers of first aiders and others on the course. As an alternative, at registration, the runners were provided with medical identity cards containing similar information, which was pinned to the chest number. In addition they were requested in a "Medical Advice to Runners" handout to carry appropriate medication, particularly for diabetes, asthma, or cardiovascular disease.

Education of Runners

In most events runners were provided with some form of medical advice which was included in "Instructions to Runners" distributed prior to the events. In addition, training programs and general medical advice were published in the newspapers that sponsored events and given at pre-run seminars for competitors. The electronic media in some cities broadcast interviews to warn runners of the hazards of running and of how to avoid problems. The starters of some events broadcast general advice about the run over the public address system, gave special warnings if there was an increased risk of heat exhaustion or hypothermia, and announced what facilities were available (drink, toilet, first aid, medical).

Education of Medical Support Teams

The Sydney *Sun* "City-to-Surf" and Auckland *Star* "Round-the-Bays" medical support team members received pre-run briefings of administrative instruction, protocols of management, and documentation of casualties. We believe that post-run debriefing sessions are equally important, as recommendations can be made to the organizers for improvements to be implemented in future events.

Education of Organizers

Runners in the Sydney *Sun* "City-to-Surf" were provided with a "Comments card" on which they advised the organizers of their opinions, problems, and suggestions for the improvement of future events. These have been found to be most informative and valuable. Many improvements have resulted from these suggestions.

Medical Support

In most cases, medical support has been adequate provided the weather conditions were "average." When the weather conditions have been unexpectedly unfavorable—high atmospheric temperature and relative humidity or little wind—the medical support sometimes has been inadequate. As a result of the potentially tragic occurrences in the 1971 Sydney "City-to-Surf," the 1977 Auckland "Round-the-Bays" run, and 1979 Melbourne "Big M" marathon, the organizers made significant changes to the organization and medical support provided in subsequent events. By moving the event to times of more favorable expected weather conditions, the incidence of heat casualties has been reduced in both the Sydney *Sun* and Perth *Daily News* "City-to-Surf" runs.

It is clear from the Sydney *Sun* "City-to-Surf" and Auckland *Star* "Round-the-Bays" experiences that the most important factors in providing adequate medical support are comprehensive administrative instructions, a protocol of management, and documentation of casualties. Several types of voluntary medical support have been found successful. The Sydney *Sun* "City-to-Surf" has used teams based on sports medicine members (1972 to 1977), on one hospital (1978 to 1982), and on disaster teams from several hospitals as provided by the New South Wales Disaster Medical Plan (1983 to 1985). StJ has provided first aid in all events. The Auckland "Round-the-Bays" used a combination of private practitioners, hospital medical staff, a mobile medical unit, an Army Field Hospital, a helicopter rescue squad for medical care, and both StJ and Red Cross members to render first aid.

In other events in Australia, medical support was provided by members of the Australian Sports Medicine Federation or hospital teams and private practitioners, and first aid by StJ and in some cases by Red Cross members.

We consider that all casualties should be treated in on-site medical facilities capable of delivering intensive care and that the extent of the medical support should be determined by previous experience, allowing a generous safety margin to cover unforeseen eventualities such as extreme weather conditions and disasters not related to running. The helicopter crash in Sydney in 1984 provided a dramatic warning of such a possibility when mass participation events are held.

VOLUNTEER MEDICAL SUPPORT TEAMS AND AMBULANCE SERVICES—SYDNEY *SUN* "CITY-TO-SURF:" The recruitment of volunteer hospital disaster teams in 1983 (9) was a question of necessity and not one of choice. Since then it has been shown that the experience in coping with a genuine disaster situation, as distinct from treating simulated casualties in a practice exercise, was of value to the disaster teams. In addition, it provided the CDA with the opportunity to deploy its Disaster Communications Center and emergency equipment vans as part of a disaster practice conducted officially by the Department of Health's New South Wales Disaster Medical Planning Committee, to the extent that it has now become the major disaster exercise for the year.

The organizers responsible for the medical support of mass participation events such as the Sydney *Sun* "City-to-Surf" should consider the possibility of and prepare for disasters which are not directly related to running. Had the helicopter crashed a few meters to the north in the 1984 run, into the runners or spectators, the full disaster organization could have been put into immediate operation and many lives would have been saved. Any doubts which may have existed as to the wisdom of using hospital disaster teams and their equipment in the Sydney *Sun* "City-to-Surf" were dispelled after the 1984 event. By utilizing the New South Wales Disaster Medical Planning Committee to coordinate the off-duty volunteers, disaster teams were drawn from hospitals in such a way that no major areas or hospitals were left depleted of necessary staff and equipment.

The Sydney *Sun* "City-to-Surf" also provides an opportunity for students (medical, nursing, physiotherapy) who act as clerks and "spotters" under the supervision of experienced intensivists or sports medicine physicians to observe at first hand the behavior and management of heat casualties as well as the management of a disaster situation—an increasingly prevalent possibility in our society.

It may be argued that the deployment of such human and material resources is not justified in an event which attracts only 30,000 to 35,000 entrants. However, we believe that the improved lifestyle and fitness necessary for runners to compete and the experienced gained by those who provide the medical support more than justify the manpower required to conduct the Sydney *Sun* "City-to-Surf" with optimum safety for the runners—more than 350 medical team members and approximately 1,500 run officials, representing a ratio of one per 20 runners.

Research and Evaluation

We have demonstrated that the protocol of management and documentation of casualties should be in a form that can be subjected to ongoing analysis and evaluation in order to increase our knowledge of medical problems in fun runs, particularly of heat exhaustion, and to improve the effectiveness of our medical organization and management of casualties. Perhaps some authority such as sports medicine organizations should undertake the task of coordinating the collection of such research data from all major events.

SUMMARY

The importance of providing adequate medical care in endurance events in Australasia is gaining recognition. The Sydney *Sun* "City-to-Surf" experience is provided as a model which incorporates most of the best features of other events.

There is a need for a medical director to organize the comprehensive planning and briefing of all who provide medical support. The basis of such planning should be the ongoing analysis and evaluation of data provided by accurate recording of observations and other information. Volunteer disaster teams, experienced as intensivists but inexperienced in the Sydney *Sun* "City-to-Surf," have effectively managed scores of collapsed casualties simultaneously when provided with comprehensive administrative instructions, an effective protocol of management, and a means of accurately recording observations.

The experience of participating in the medical support of the Sydney *Sun* "City-to-Surf" and similar events can be an invaluable exercise for the disaster organizations as well as providing all members with an appreciation of how to cope with a disaster situation. The presence of such teams ensures that other disasters unrelated to running could be managed without delay.

CONCLUSIONS

The experience of the Sydney *Sun* "City-to-Surf" and the Auckland *Star* "Round-the-Bays" indicates that effective treatment of medical emergencies, particularly heat exhaustion, can and should be conducted in fully staffed and equipped on-site medical facilities. The nature and extent of such medical support should be determined by previous experience and scientific research.

REFERENCES

1. American College of Sports Medicine, Prevention of thermal injuries during distance running. Position stand. *Med. Sci. Sports Exerc.* 16:ix–xiv, 1984.

2. Bassler, T. J. Heat stroke in a "run for fun." *Br. Med. J.* 1:197, 1979.
3. Bloomfield, J. The Perth "City-to-Surf" Fun Run 1980. *Sports Coach* 5:9–13, 1981.
4. Bryson, L. G. and A. Seymour. Popular marathons. *Br. Med. J.* 288:1613, 1984.
5. Consensus Conference—Popular marathons, half-marathons, and other long distance runs: Recommendations for medical support. *Br. Med. J.* 288:1355–1359, 1984.
6. Duras, P. I., J. W. Russell and A. Kretsch. Illness and injury during the 1980 Big M Melbourne Marathon. *Aust. J. Sports Med. Ex. Sci.* 15:35–39, 1983.
7. Kretsch, A., R. Grogan, P. Duras, F. Allen, J. Sumner and I. Gillam. 1980 Marathon study. *Med. J. Aust.* 141:809–814, 1984.
8. Nicholson, R. and K. W. Somerville. Heat stroke in a "run for fun." *Br. Med. J.* 1:1158, 1979.
9. Richards, R. and D. Richards. Exertion-induced heat exhaustion and other medical aspects of "City-to-Surf" fun runs. *Med. J. Aust.* 141:799–805, 1984.
10. Richards, R. and D. Richards. Prevention of exercise-induced heat stroke. In: *Sports Medicine for the Mature Athlete.* J. Sutton and R. Brock, eds. Indianapolis: Benchmark, 1986.
11. Richards, R., D. Richards and R. Whittaker. Method of predicting the number of casualties in the "City-to-Surf" fun runs. *Med. J. Aust.* 141:805–808, 1984.
12. Richards, D., R. Richards, P. Schofield and V. Ross. Biochemical and haematological changes in Sydney's *The Sun* "City-to-Surf" fun runners. *Med. J. Aust.* 2:449–453, 1979.
13. Richards, R., D. Richards, P. Schofield, V. Ross and J. R. Sutton. Reducing the hazards in Sydney's *The Sun* "City-to-Surf" runs, 1971 to 1979. *Med. J. Aust.* 2:453–457, 1979.
14. Richards, D., R. Richards, P. Schofield, V. Ross and J. R. Sutton. Management of heat exhaustion in Sydney's *The Sun* "City-to-Surf" fun runners. *Med. J. Aust.* 2:457–461, 1979.
15. Richards, R., D. Richards, P. Schofield, V. Ross and J. R. Sutton. Organization of *The Sun* "City-to-Surf" fun run, Sydney. *Med. J. Aust.* 2:470–474, 1979.
16. Roydhouse, N. "Round-the-Bays" 1980 medical report. *N. Zealand J. Sports Med.* 8:14–16, 1980.
17. Roydhouse, N., H. Karn and L. Johnson. "Round-the-Bays" 11.92 Km fun run for 25,000 entrants. *N. Zealand J. Sports Med.* 6:4–10, 1978.
18. Sutton, J. R., M. J. Coleman, A. P. Millar, L. Lazarus and P. Russo. The medical problems of mass participation in athletic competition. The "City-to-Surf" race. *Med. J. Aust.* 2:127–133, 1972.

16

Medical Support For Marathons In The United Kingdom: The London Marathon

DAN S. TUNSTALL-PEDOE, M.D.

St. Bartholomew's Hospital

SUMMARY

The medical support and problems faced by the organizers and providers of this medical support are described for the London Marathon, the largest full course marathon in the world, with more than 20,000 entrants. The problems of the London Marathon are compared with those of smaller, less prestigious races in the United Kingdom. The aim of medical support for an event of this type is to deal with the large number of trivial problems quickly and efficiently, thus returning runners to the race or their families with minimum delay, but also to be capable of dealing with the less common major medical problems of hypothermia, hyperthermia, hypovolemic collapse from severe dehydration, and cardiac events at the finish. The London Marathon's medical philosophy is to contain as much as practicable of its medical problems and refer to hospital only those runners requiring hospital diagnostic or therapeutic facilities. In 1985, of 2,300 casualty contacts on the course, only 5 were sent on to the hospital; from the 466 at the finish, only 1 was sent; and none was admitted. In 5 years with 69,442 runners, there have been no deaths, and only 2 runners have spent more than 1 night in hospital as a consequence of running the London Marathon.

INTRODUCTION

A brief description will be given of the medical arrangements for the London Marathon including some of the casualty statistics along with some com-

---

Acknowledgements

I would like to thank all of the St. John and other medical staff who help with the London Marathon and the production of these statistics.

ments on other races in the United Kingdom. Unfortunately, data do not exist on medical arrangements for European marathons as a whole.

Popular marathons and road races of the type seen in North America for more than a decade are a more recent phenomenon in the United Kingdom and Europe where the traditional type of race predominated until quite recently.

The Traditional Marathon and Club Athlete

The traditional race used to attract a small number of experienced athletes all belonging to established running clubs many of which have in the last few years been celebrating their centenaries. The runners had many seasons' experience of track, cross-country, and road running. The event would be unlikely to field more than 100 runners, and logistic and medical support would be minimal. Drink stations were infrequent and the drinks were often the runner's favorite concoction distributed at 5-mile intervals from 10 miles onwards in marked bottles. The medical support consisted of 1 or 2 voluntary ambulances plus a mobile medical officer in his own car with no radio contact with the first aid ambulances. They would all be available at the finish. The runners themselves expected little in the way of medical support, except perhaps to "raid" the First Aid facility before the start to pad out an uncomfortable shoe, repair it or cover some callosity, or get some petroleum jelly. Logistic support was usually provided by fellow runners or their families, and the whole race was run on a financial shoestring.

The runner was usually running as part of a team to score points or gain a personal position. His self-esteem would make him most unwilling to become a casualty as he would lose face with the rest of his team. He also reckoned that he knew far more about blisters and cramps than any doctor or first aider.

The Popular Marathon and Novice Runner

The advent of the mass popular marathon, half marathons, and similar events has transformed the scene. Most runners may well be novices at the event, many having taken up running in their 30s, 40s, or even later. Few belong to a club or have any real contact with experienced club athletes and their training, and fitness is extremely variable. These runners need and expect to be protected from themselves by adequate first aid and medical coverage at the event, and I believe a medical advice sheet should be sent to each competitor beforehand. The medical advice sheet is of some importance in putting the onus of being fit for the event on the individual runner rather than the organizers, particularly as the runners have disparate motives in running a popular marathon and may well suffer from diseases of middle age such as ischemic heart disease.

These runners may be taking part:

1. To prove they can do it. They will be happy to finish, however slowly, and are not likely to push themselves too hard unless they are unprepared or have been ill.
2. To run faster than the last time and do a personal best. This group also includes many of the traditional club runners who may well push too hard for the conditions and become casualties.

3. To deny illness. There is an interesting tendency for marathon races to attract disabled runners of various kinds. A Norwegian with a heart transplant ran the 1985 London Marathon. Various cardiac, respiratory, and other patients regard a marathon as the ultimate rehabilitation graduation test.
4. To raise money. In the United Kingdom, marathon races have been used by volunteers to raise money for worthy causes. Some £5,000,000 is raised for charities by the London Marathon with particular celebrities such as Jimmy Savile leading the way. These sponsored runners may have thousands of pounds riding on them. They are under considerable pressure to finish the course; this results in special problems should they be unwell.
5. Sheer exhibitionism. The British are an undemonstrative, rather conventional breed. The London Marathon, with 500,000 spectators along the course and millions watching television, gives a fantastic opportunity for exhibitionism of a harmless sort. Mickey Mouse, Superman, Spiderman, a Pantomime Horse, and Gorilla have all run the London Marathon, surviving the risks of heat exhaustion in their all-embracing costumes and often raising money for charities as well.

The popular marathons are large media events with considerable commercial sponsorship, without which they might well not survive. A large part of the planning of these events is geared towards the media and commercial interests, and medical priority and the safety of the runners may be neglected in the early planning stage unless there is medical input.

THE LONDON MARATHON

The London Marathon is the largest road race over the full marathon distance attracting more than 80,000 aspiring entrants, of whom over 20,000 are accepted and about 17,500 run (Table 16-1). It is run over a relatively flat course (slightly downhill for the first 5 miles) in early spring. The roads are closed for the occasion and the course takes in some of the main tourist attractions of London, including Tower Bridge, the Tower of London, the Embankment, Big Ben, and the Houses of Parliament. It finishes on Westminster Bridge, and the finish area is adjacent to County Hall.

Selection and Entry

The race is open to anyone over the age of 18 who wishes to take part. No fitness or medical qualification is required for entry, but each entrant signs a legal liability waiver exonerating the marathon authorities from blame for any misfortune that may afflict him or her (which, luckily, has not been tested in court). Initially, entry was on a first postal receipt basis, then on the basis of queuing all night. Because of some anomalies, a lottery system was devised for subsequent races.

Starting in 1981 with 7,700 entrants, the race became the largest full course marathon in 1982 with 18,000 entries (Table 16-1) and an astonishingly high percentage of finishers (96.4%), according to the official start and finish numbers. In subsequent years, at my insistence, runners with accepted entries have been able to exchange these in the week before the marathon for a prom-

TABLE 16-1. *London Marathon statistics from 1981 to 1985*

	1981	1982	1983	1984	1985
ACCEPTED ENTRIES	7,747	18,059	19,735	21,142	22,274
TOTAL FEMALES	330	1,393	1,677	3,210	2,283
%	4.3	7.7	8.5	15.2	11.0
NOVICES %	50	51.9	34	30	28
TOTAL FINISHERS	6,418	15,758	15,776	15,649	15,841
UNDER 3 HOURS	1,294	1,795	1,991	1,889	2,761
TOTAL CASUALTY CONTACTS	586	1,300	1,606	2,078	2,905
TO HOSPITAL TOTAL	11	34	19	15	6
FROM FINISH	0	15	2	2	1
DETAINED IN HOSPITAL	3	5	0*	0	0

*"rogue" runner collapsed with cardiac arrest and an inferior infarction on his way home from the London Marathon. He was resuscitated and survived but did not pass through the marathon medical facilities. Like his running, he is an unofficial statistic.

ise of a guaranteed entry the following year. This facility, copied from New York, is to discourage sick runners from taking part. (Fig. 16-1). It has undoubtedly reduced the percentage of entrants who run but has also helped to reduce the number of serious problems reaching the hospital (Table 16-1).

Medical Support for the London Marathon

The planning of the London Marathon begins almost a year ahead. The Medical Director is part of the planning committee and has been involved since the inception of the race in 1980.

ST. JOHN AMBULANCE BRIGADE: There is close liaison with St. John who supply the vast majority of the personnel including all the first aiders. The Metropolitan police will not work with any other first aid organization. They have close links with St. John and have reciprocal arrangements for catering, etc. As Medical Director, I was told that there was no point in planning groups of volunteers for the aid stations—the police would not work with anyone except St. John!

MARATHON COURSE AID STATIONS: The aid stations en route are planned between the police and St. John. They are positioned in such a way that the mobile vehicles and ambulances can evacuate casualties without any disruption of the race. The St. John medical stations should ideally be readily visible from the throng of runners, and for this purpose are best placed 100 to 200 meters or so downstream of the drinks stations so that everyone knows where the medical stations are, but in practice they are often not positioned there and vary greatly in visibility. Each station is normally manned by a particular St. John unit or units (e.g., from Guildford), all of whom know each

Marathons, half marathons, and long distance runs

MEDICAL ADVICE TO RUNNERS

If you have any medical problems, discuss these with your general practitioner. This advice sheet supplements anything he or she says. See your doctor if you have *any* medical problem which makes it risky for you to run or take part in the marathon.

Training

Muscular aches and pains occur most commonly after an increase in training.
- Increase training gradually so that you do not suffer prolonged exhaustion.
- Intersperse days of heavy mileage with one or two days of lighter training, so that your body can replace its muscle glycogen.
- If you have flu, a feverish cold, or a tummy bug, **do not** train until fully recovered. Then start gently and build up gradually.
- Do not attempt to catch up on lost mileage after illness or injury. This may cause further damage.
- *To reduce risk of injury* train on soft surfaces (parkland, footpaths, etc) when you can, especially on days of light training. Vary routes and run on varying cambers—hills, etc. *Always face the oncoming traffic*, especially in the dark.

If you cannot run 15 miles comfortably a month before the marathon you will not manage a marathon in safety, or enjoy it. *Please do not run on this occasion.*

Diet

- Eat what suits *you*.
- Large doses of supplementary vitamins and minerals (such as iron) are not essential and produce no benefit if you are on a good mixed diet, but additional vitamin C in small doses is reasonable when fresh fruit and vegetables are in short supply.
- Training helps you to sustain a high level of muscle glycogen. Before you run the marathon decrease your intake of protein (meat) and increase your intake of carbohydrate (pasta, bread, potatoes, cereals, rice and sweet things), especially for the last three days, which is when you should be reducing your mileage and resting. (Unless you reduce the protein you will not eat enough carbohydrate.)
- Carbohydrate (glycogen) depletion and then loading does not help all runners and can make your muscles very heavy.

Fluids

You must replace fluids lost in sweat; otherwise your body becomes dehydrated and less efficient.
- Drink plenty of fluids after training and during races, especially in the first half of the marathon.
- Alcohol is dehydrating. A pint of beer produces more than a pint of urine. Spirits have a worse effect. So take plenty of non-alcoholic drinks, especially before the race and in hot weather.
- *Drink enough to keep your urine pale straw colour and abundant.*

Clothing

- *When training in the dark be seen.* Wear white clothing and reflective flashes or bandoliers. *Run facing the traffic.*
- Wear comfortable clothing. Natural fibres such as wool and cotton are kinder to the skin than artificial fibres. Trendy shorts with sewn on trimmings can rub your groins until they bleed.
- Find shoes that stay comfortable for long periods.

On the day

- *Do not run if you feel unwell* or have just been unwell. Most medical emergencies occur in people who have been unwell but do not wish to miss the start. If you feel feverish, have been vomiting, have had severe diarrhoea or any chest pains, or otherwise feel unwell, it is unfair to you, your family, and the marathon support staff to risk becoming a medical emergency and you are unlikely to do yourself justice.

There are many other marathons. If you surrender your certificate of entry to the marathon office you will be guaranteed a place next year.
- If you have any medical problem which might lead to an emergency, such as fits, diabetes, put a cross on the front of your number (well away from the bar code) and write details on the reverse of the number, especially your medication.
- Wear appropriate clothes for the weather. On a cold wet day you can become very cold if you slow down or walk. A hat and gloves prevent heat loss and are easily carried.
- If it is hot, wear loose mesh clothing, *start slowly*, run in the shade, and drink whenever you can.
- Start the race well hydrated (urine looks pale) and drink regularly as you lose a lot of fluid "insensibly." This will help you feel better late in the race and may prevent cramp.

At the finish

- *Do not stand about* getting cold. Go straight to the baggage area and change into warm dry clothing.
- Do not trust your clothing to someone else. Use the baggage system, get dressed, and then go to the reunion area. Foil blankets do not stop you from becoming cold.

Medical aid

Train sensibly. Follow this simple advice and you will probably not need medical aid. The medical aid posts are generally situated 50 to 100 metres downstream of the drink stations and at the finish.
- If you drop out make for an aid station.

Make sure your relatives know your running number.
Enjoy your running and *keep this advice sheet.*
[Signed Medical Director]

Guidelines produced by a consensus conference, convenor Dr D Tunstall Pedoe, Cardiac Department, St Bartholomew's Hospital, London.

Fig. 16-1. *The London Marathon Medical Advice Sheet. This sheet (slightly modified) is sent to every entrant at the time of acceptance (5).*

other. Not all stations have doctors, but St. John has its own doctors and nurses distributed along the course with the units. All have radio communication with a central control and can report evacuation of casualties. They work closely with the several thousand police along the course. In 1984 a large aid post was positioned on the Isle of Dogs (at about 17 miles), using accommodation there; increasingly, non-St. John physiotherapists and podiatrists are working alongside the St. John staff on the course as well as at the finish medical area.

NON-ST. JOHN STAFF: DOCTORS, PHYSIOTHERAPISTS, AND PODIATRISTS: St. John is a voluntary first aid organization which is run like a paramilitary presence. In 1981, they had virtually no experience of the problems of mass popular marathon races and the then Commander was very intolerant of any suggestion that non-St. John doctors and sports medicine personnel could work alongside them. In 1981, they agreed to 6 doctors, physiotherapists, and podiatrists working in the finish area, and over the last 5 races I have increased the number to 50 non-St. John sports medicine experts who work alongside St. John and are now much more readily accepted.

The physiotherapy service is planned by a chief physiotherapist (Rose MacDonald) who works at the Crystal Palace Sports Complex and is an expert on musculoskeletal problems (3). The podiatrists and chiropodists are organized by a chief podiatrist (Ralph Graham) who, like Rose MacDonald, recruits his staff from contacts; they give their considerable services free (2). All the non-St. John staff are fully qualified and registered in their own profession.

A group of doctors interested in sports medicine was recruited by the Medical Director and works alongside St. John at the finish area.

THE FINISH MEDICAL AREA—A FIELD HOSPITAL: The Finish Medical Area is at County Hall, adjacent to the Bridge on which the race finishes. Several large rooms plus a corridor area are sealed off as the medical area. The area is planned carefully between the Medical Director and the St. John Chief Nursing Officer, Katherine Stretton, as a field hospital with 150 camp beds, an intensive care area for intravenous fluid administration and resuscitation, a large room for female runners, and other rooms for men. A one-way flow of casualties is arranged, with triage at the entrance divided into 3 categories: ICU, Campbed, and Walking Wounded.

No one is allowed into the medical area unless they are casualties, St. John staff, or have a medical pass from the Medical Director. The casualties are clocked in and out so that it is possible to know by their race numbers which casualties are still in the medical area. There is an information desk.

Apart from the County Hall medical area or field hospital, it was found in 1982 that additional medical stations were required nearer the baggage reclaim buses and at the relatives' reunion area, as late collapses occurred. Many of these casualties could not be brought back against the stream of runners to County Hall, and a large number were therefore sent on to hospital rather than receiving medical care from the marathon medical services. These extra medical posts, which have instructions to bring their sicker casualties back to the intensive care section of the County Hall medical area, have almost totally eliminated the need to evacuate casualties from the finish to the hospital (Table 16-1).

Casualty Cards: A casualty card was designed specifically for the marathon (Fig. 16-3). It is used in addition to the St. John casualty reporting (see Results below).

First Aid Advice Sheet: A first aid advice sheet was composed by the Medical Director for the first London Marathon as there were so many first aiders and doctors who knew nothing about the types of problems they were likely to encounter. This was distributed to the St. John staff and also to the hospitals en route. The advice sheet has been updated and modified as a result of a conference on medical services for popular marathons and forms part of the recommendations of that conference (5). It is reproduced in Fig. 16-2.

Marathons, half marathons, and long distance runs

FIRST AID AND CASUALTY MANAGEMENT

Running 26 miles 385 yards (42·2 km) on roads puts a severe stress on muscles, joints, the skin of the feet, and anywhere that can be chafed and may lead to considerable loss of extracellular fluids in insensible loss—from respiration and sweating as well as into muscles as oedema. Muscle stores of glycogen can be totally depleted. The effects of these stresses and the failure of normal homoeostatic (corrective) mechanisms may produce the conditions described below. These are more likely to occur in inexperienced runners, who form a large proportion of the entrants for mass marathons and fun runs.

Runners making contact with first aid staff may be classified as: *Social contacts*—that is, those requesting vaseline, a shoelace, a sticking, plaster or even a drink or sponge, who want to help themselves, and *Medical or casualty contacts*, who require aid from the staff. The casualty contacts may be subdivided into those with topical, musculoskeletal, or constitutional problems.

Topical conditions include blisters, skin chafing, wasp stings, subungual haematoma (toe nail bruise), scrapes from falls, etc.

Musculoskeletal conditions include cramp, pulled muscles, fatigue fractures, knee and ankle problems, backache, etc. The most common problem is muscle cramp, a disabling condition often associated with fatigue and dehydration. It can occur with both hyperthermia and hypothermia. Extend the adjoining joint to stretch the affected muscle which is knotted up; this is often best achieved by helping the runner to stand up. Recurrent cramps are helped by rehydration and warmth if the runner is cold. Water or dilute electrolyte drinks are acceptable so long as the drinks have been freshly made up according to instructions. *Do not give salt or a strong saline drink.* The runner may be able to continue after an attack but if cold and wet he or she should be warned of the risks of hypothermia.

Constitutional conditions include collapse, vomiting, headaches, etc. Hypothermia and hyperthermia can look similar and may occur on the same day. *Every confused or collapsed runner with signs of peripheral circulatory collapse must have a rectal temperature recorded* (at a depth of 7 cm (3 in) from the anal margin).

Hypothermia or exposure

Hypothermia is most likely on a cold wet day in poorly clad runners but can occur with cold alone in slow moving runners who are not generating enough heat to maintain body temperature, especially those who start too fast and become exhausted. They feel cold, suffer muscle cramps, look cyanosed, and may be confused.

Diagnosis is based on a properly taken *rectal* temperature of less than 36°C. Oral or axillary values are useless and misleading. Strip all wet clothing off the runner, dry him, and put him in warm surroundings with dry clothing and blankets. Hypoglycaemia (see below) interferes with shivering so warm sweet drinks may help. If the temperature is less than 34°C check the rectal temperature periodically.

Hyperthermia, heat stroke, or heat collapse

Diagnosis of hyperthermia is based on a rectal temperature of 40°C or over 10 minutes after running. Although commoner on hot humid days, hyperthermia can occur even in temperate conditions if homoeostatic mechanisms break down (through dehydration, toxins, drugs). Marathon runners raise their core temperature as they have to dissipate a large amount of heat. This core temperature usually drops rapidly at the end of the race but occasionally may rise higher and be accompanied by cramps and mental confusion. Paradoxically skin temperature may be cool and the skin dry. Profuse sweating with severe generalised muscle cramps is also possible. If the temperature is over 40°C start tepid sponging, fan, and give intravenous fluids. If the temperature does not then fall arrange rapid transfer to hospital and sponge and fan en route.

Hypovolaemic collapse

Marathon runners can lose several litres of extracellular fluid, which results in dramatic hypotension when they stop running, leading in some cases to syncope. The pulse will feel weak and may be imperceptible at the wrist (feel carotid pulse). The runner will feel faint and dizzy and may vomit. Blood pressure is very low but is conserved by peripheral vasoconstriction (causing cyanosis), and secondary collapse can occur 20 to 30 minutes after finishing, when this vasoconstriction turns to vasodilatation, if blood volume has not expanded sufficiently in the meantime. The worst cases are those in whom there is gastrointestinal loss of fluid from vomiting or diarrhoea in addition to loss from sweat.

The simple case is self limiting and responds well to rest and oral rehydration with the legs raised for 30 minutes or so. Intravenous rehydration is indicated if there is continuing fluid loss from persistent vomiting or diarrhoea, mental confusion, or obvious deterioration. *The rectal temperature must be taken.*

Hypoglycaemia

Severe hypoglycaemia is rare, but it may present as mental confusion, possibly aggression, sweating, and tremor. It may complicate hypothermia as it inhibits normal shivering. It should respond rapidly to an electrolyte glucose drink, sugar, or confectionery.

Caveats

General—Runners are independent minded and may resent being treated as casualties, and they will often have diagnosed their own problem (correctly). They may wish to dress their own blisters or tell you how to do it. Please be patient with them. If they insist on continuing make sure they understand that they must reach the next aid station, or, if it is cold and wet, the next transport point (Underground Station in London) because their slow running will make them liable to hypothermia. If they are obviously confused and disorientated get a medical officer to try to convince them that they should not continue.

Medical—Marathon running produces profound electrolyte fluxes and release of intracellular enzymes. Electrocardiographic and serum enzyme results may suggest myocardial damage, and urine may contain blood, protein, sugar, haemoglobin or myoglobin—all as a result of the stresses of marathon running. Marathon runners have been admitted to hospital and kept as inpatients on the basis of these findings, which, under these circumstances, may not indicate disease.

Guidelines produced by a consensus conference, convenor Dr D Tunstall Pedoe, Cardiac Department, St Bartholomew's Hospital, London.

Fig. 16-2. *The first aid advice sheet. This is distributed to the St. John personnel and the hospitals en route (5).*

RESULTS

The results of the medical support for the London Marathon are shown in Tables 16-1, 16-2, and 16-3. Table 16-1 shows that although there has been a steady increase in the percentage of experienced runners taking part, (now almost 75% are not novice marathon runners), there has also been a steady increase in casualty contacts with St. John. However, since the peak of 1982, improvements in the medical service have resulted in a dramatic fall in the number of casualties sent on to the hospital. This fell from 34 in 1982 to 6 in 1985. This fall in hospital transfers could have various causes: 1) The runners could be better prepared. 2) The opportunity to not run but get an entry for the following year if lame or ill must prevent some problems.

However, it is undoubtedly true that the organization of the medical services and the increased confidence of the St. John staff have meant that many potential hospital cases have been adequately treated at the first aid centers and thus saved the runner a hospital visit and the hospitals, work.

The load on individual aid stations is very variable. Over the last 3 years there has been peak demand at about 18 miles. The enormous peak this year (Station 14 in Table 16-2) at 18.5 miles was the result of the extreme visibility of this aid station which also had a large notice near it saying, "8 MILES TO GO." Rumor has it that there was a very attractive nurse who was also quite visible aiding runners with cramps and chafed groins! Certainly, stations 13 and 15 had nothing like the work load, and future planning must aim to spread the load more evenly between the aid stations.

TABLE 16-2. *Runner casualty statistics on the course, 1985. C/S is approximate ratio of casualties to staff*

STATION	SITE	CASUALTIES	STAFF	C/S	TO HOSPITAL
1	START	14	12	1	
2	START	17	23	1	
3	3 miles	6	10	0.6	
4	6.5	5	17	0.3	
5	7.5	49	18	3	
6	8.5	1	12	0.1	
7	10.5	26	22	1	
8	12	49	16	3	
9	13	13	21	0.7	
10	14	52	24	2	
11	15.5	132	31	4	
12	16.5	135	27	5	
13	17	86	18	5	
14	18.5	1,059	41	26	3
15	20	219	49	4	
16	21	71	22	3	
17	22	82	28	3	
18	23	64	29	2	1
19	24	170	17	9	1
20	24.5	16	21	1	
21	25	137	30	4	
22	25.5	26	16	2	
23	26	14	22	0.7	
COUNTY HALL FINISH		466	273	2	1
TOTAL		2,905	799	(3.5 AV)	6

(71 members of the public also treated, 2 at Station 6)

The Difficulties of Accurate Diagnosis and Casualty Statistics

The St. John dignoses are shown in Table 16-3, the most common problems in 3a, and the complete list of diagnoses on the course in 3b. These do not include statistics from the 466 casualties at the finish. As will be appreciated, these are not precise medical diagnoses and do not even include the diagnoses listed on the First Aid Advice Sheet (Fig. 16-2). The bulk of the casualties in a marathon are seen as fleeting encounters with trivial problems. Whereas the topical problems, blisters, grazes, chafing, are easily diagnosed and recorded by first aid staff, the accurate diagnosis of musculoskeletal problems is impossible (4). Although a casualty card was specifically designed for the recording of marathon medical problems (Fig. 16-3), it has met with a variable response from the different St. John units. They have their own methods of recording casualty data which are used for all their functions and are expected on marathon day to use their own methods in parallel with and at

TABLE 16-3a. *St. John course casualty totals—the most common diagnoses*

Diagnosis	Total on Course		Casualty Station with Largest No.	
Cramp	1,654	14	18.5 miles	(697)
Sore groins	226	14		(139)
Blisters	169	14		(59)
Leg pain	137	14		(45)
Chafing	117	14		(76)

TABLE 16-3b. *Classification of diagnoses with totals*

TOPICAL	528 CASES
Sore/bleeding groin	226
blisters/sore feet	169
chafing/vaseline	117
sore breasts/axillae	13
cuts/grazes	2
nose bleed	1
MUSCULOSKELETAL	1,863 CASES
Cramp	1,654
strain/sprain ankle-knee	137
strain/sprain elsewhere	64
backache	14
muscular pain unspecified	2
CONSTITUTIONAL	48 CASES
Feeling cold	18
stomach upset or pain	6
diarrhea/vomiting	6
exhaustion/collapse	4
dehydration	4
headache	3
breathlessness	2
confused/dizzy	2
excessively hot	2
requested Paracetamol	1

CONFIDENTIAL

(see over)

Running No. .... Aid Station No. ....

Time In .... Time Out ....

Classification (check one or more)

1. Social contact ☐
2. Casualty Topical ☐ (blister, bruise, chafe etc.)
3. Musculo skeletal ☐ (cramp, knee pain etc.)
4. Constitutional ☐ — P.T.O.

2., 3., 4 Diagnosis ....
or reason (1.)

Treatment (2. or 3.) ....

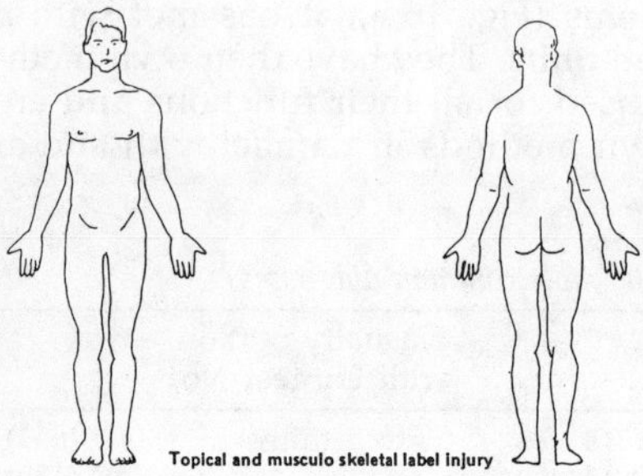

Constitutional Complaint ....

RECTAL TEMP MUST BE TAKEN IF CONFUSED OR COLLAPSED.

EXAMINATION (tick where appropriate)

Mental state ☐ normal, ☐ confused, ☐ comatose

Circulation pulse ☐ good vol, ☐ feeble, ☐ fast, ☐ slow.

Skin ☐ dry, ☐ sweating, ☐ flushed, ☐ pale, ☐ cyanosed.

Rectal temp (if appropriate) ....(if repeat record below)

Blood pressure (if appropriate) ....(..................)

Other comments ....

....

TREATMENT GIVEN First aid, Physiotherapy, Podiatry, Medical

Progress

DISPOSAL (tick as appropriate)

Ambulance ☐, Retired ☐, Continued marathon ☐, Unknown ☐

Additional comment if any (Name and address if unregistered) ....

....

ASSURE RUNNERS THAT DETAILS ARE CONFIDENTIAL to M.O.

Definitions.

Social contacts treat themselves, (request plaster etc.)

Topical injuries blisters, chafing, scrapes, stings, toe nail injuries etc.

Musculo skeletal cramp, all joint and muscle or tendon pain.

Constitutional collapse, headache, vomiting, diarrhoea, fits, confusion etc.

Fig. 16-3. *The London Marathon casualty card.*

a higher priority to the marathon cards. Perhaps not surprisingly, the marathon cards, initiated by an outsider to St. John (the Marathon Medical Director) and more than doubling the paper work, have not been filled in very assiduously, particularly where a unit has been under pressure. The problems can therefore be listed as follows.

1. NON-PRESENTERS: Gross underestimates of trivial problems. Not every runner with a blister or chafing or an attack of cramp will get first aid for it. His chances of seeking aid will increase with the density and visibility of the facilities provided and decrease with his own self-sufficiency. Equally, he may have more than one problem, only the most important one being recorded by the St. John statistics.

An attractive nurse or physiotherapist in a very visible situation may well alter the race casualty statistics dramatically by encouraging the non-presenters to become casualties, as probably happened at Station 14.

2. DOUBLE RECORDING: Closer analysis of St. John statistics from some stations reveals the same runner's number on 2 or even 3 casualty cards; in a very busy situation this type of error may occur, particularly where a runner has several problems and there are specialists such as physiotherapists and podiatrists who will fill in their own cards. The same problem may also be double-recorded at the same station. A runner may, of course, stop with the same blister or other problem at several different stations along the course for further treatment and swell the total number of casualties seen. The St. John records make this almost impossible to trace, whereas the Marathon casualty cards, if properly completed, can be analyzed for this error. Unfortunately, this error is not allowed for by the press who may headline, "One in six runners needs assistance."

3. UNDER-RECORDING: If a first aid station becomes overrun, treatment has to take priority over recording. Station 14 had insufficient casualty cards for the number of casualties. Three thousand cards were distributed but no one foresaw such a disproportion in casualty experience of the different stations.

4. MISDIAGNOSIS: First aiders are not trained orthopedic specialists. All they can reasonably do is record the site of the pain and whether the runner could continue the race. They perhaps could be expected to record whether a runner has a cramp or a pulled muscle, but surprisingly, not a single muscle pull is recorded on their own statistics, although the more detailed marathon cards have not been fully analyzed. Similarly, there is no way of diagnosing the number of fatigue fractures arising in the London Marathon except by subsequent postal enquiry.

5. ROGUE RUNNERS: A certain number of runners either had no running number and joined along the course, swelling the potential field of casualties, or were runners running under false colors, having been given a running number by an official entrant who could not compete. In both cases, first aiders are likely to be given false personal information and the runners will not have received the advice sheets including the Medical Advice Sheet sent to all the official entrants. These cheats complicate the official race statistics.

These examples will illustrate the fascinating aspects of marathon casualties. The London marathon medical support does not aim to pamper the runners with medical luxuries, such as massage for all at the finish or, as in New York, psychotherapists at the start. What it aims to do is make the marathon a safer event, prevent problems, and deal swiftly with as many as possible to save the hospitals from what many regard as self-induced injuries.

COMPARISON OF THE LONDON MARATHON MEDICAL SUPPORT WITH OTHER MARATHONS IN THE U.K.

A comparison was made in 1983 of the medical arrangements for 108 British open-entry marathons by Williams and Nicholl (7). Unfortunately, no comparable data exist for European marathon races, but there is nothing to suggest that the same principles do not apply. Certainly from anecdotal information, medical arrangements can be virtually non-existent as in the traditional British event, or be of the highest standards. Williams and Nicholl found a wide disparity in medical arrangements in the 108 British marathons, with the London having the largest degree of medical support. They found that the number of static first aid posts varied from 0 to 28 (median 9), with some marathons having only mobile medical posts. The first static post could be located as far as 10 miles into the race. Resuscitation equipment also varied, with oxygen being commonly available in ambulances, but intravenous fluids and defibrillators being available at 55% and 31% of events, respectively. Facilities varied with the size of the event, 67% having fewer than 1,000 runners and only 5 having 5,000 or more.

The number of casualty contacts increased with the density of the medical support, with mean contact rates of 75 per 1,000 runners for races with fewer than 10 posts (S.E. ± 15.4) and mean rates of 107 per 1,000 for those with more than 10 stations (S.E. ± 14.4). The authors found a total of 160 runners taken to the hospital from these races, giving a hospital contact rate of 1.6 per 1,000 entrants. There were 2 deaths from presumably 100,000 entrants. The authors claim that there was no relationship between the hospital contact rate and the size of entry, density of first aid posts, or the sophistication of the first aid offered. This conclusion seems to be in direct contrast to the London Marathon experience (6) where, with the increasing sophistication and experience of the staff along the course as well as at the finish, the rate of hospital referral has dropped dramatically from 34 (2 per thousand runners) in 1982 to 6 (0.3 per thousand runners) in 1985. These numbers refer to same day attendances at the hospitals designated to receive casualties by ambulance from the marathon and other hospitals on the route and do not count runners' visits to hospitals off the course or throughout the country on the following day.

The medical aid requires a significant budget. St. John has nearly 1,000 staff at the London Marathon with 40 ambulances, and their expenses amount to about £7,000. Additionally, blankets and stores of some magnitude are required, so that the total medical budget for the London Marathon is about £8,000 or 50 pence per entrant. Anyone planning such a venture must allow at least this much.

CONCLUSIONS

The London Marathon has set the standard for medical care for marathons in the United Kingdom, and the result of experience gained with the London and other races was used in drawing up "Recommendations for medical support for popular marathons, half marathons, and other long distance runs" published in the British Medical Journal (5). The medical advice sheet to runners, which may well prevent many problems, has been widely copied for entrants to other U.K. marathons, and the First Aid Advice sheet has also been widely distributed.

Whereas before the London Marathon none of the voluntary first aid organizations had significant experience with mass popular marathons, the fact that the London Marathon makes use of St. John units from a large part of Southern England, that they have had lectures on marathon medical problems from the Medical Director, and have received copies of the First Aid Advice Sheet (Fig. 16-3) means they are much better prepared when called upon to give medical support for other marathons and long distance runs.

"Distance running is a socially sanctioned and relatively harmless method for gratifying potentially dangerous narcissistic and masochistic tendencies."

The aim of the medical teams should be to make running even less harmful and perhaps less gratifying for the masochist.

REFERENCES

1. Brotherwood, R. W. Marathons and St. John. *Br. J. Sports Med.* 18:281, 1984.
2. Graham, R. Podiatrist's advice for marathon casualty management. *Br. J. Sports Med.* 18:286–287, 1984.
3. MacDonald, R. Physiotherapy management of marathon musculoskeletal casualties. *Br. J. Sports Med.* 18:283–285, 1984.
4. Tunstall-Pedoe, D. S. Marathon medicine. *Br. Med. J.* 288:1322–1323, 1984.
5. Tunstall-Pedoe, D.S. (ed.). Popular marathons, half marathons, and other long distance runs: Recommendations for medical support. Recommendations of a consensus conference. *Br. Med. J.* 288:1355–1359, 1984.
6. Tunstall-Pedoe, D. S. Marathon medicine. *Br. J. Sports Med.* 18:238–240, 1984.
7. Williams, B. T., and J. P. Nicholl. Medical arrangements in 108 open-entry British marathons, 1983. *Health Trends* 16:68–70, 1984.

17

Providing Medical Services For Fun Runs and Marathons in North America

STAFFORD W. DOBBIN, M.B., C.C.F.P.

Greater Niagara General Hospital

This paper identifies the problems faced by marathon medical directors (MMDs) in the provision of adequate marathon medical services (MMS). The practical solutions to such problems as promoting public awareness of safe running techniques, handling mass casualties, and identifying the high-risk runner before injury occurs often require decisions to be made by race organizers (ROs) and municipalities rather than physicians.

Today's non-elite, non-qualifying popular marathon is an exercise in casualty medicine rather than sports medicine, and the general principles which apply are those of good disaster planning and pre-hospital emergency care. Directors of sports events such as these should plan to treat all their own casualties rather than impose burdens on local hospitals. Treatment should be brought to the athlete/runners rather than expecting them to run on to pre-arranged aid stations. This requires total access to the entire course by MMS vehicles in an emergency vehicle lane with no other vehicles allowed on the course.

Principles of pre-race selection and on-course medical intervention should apply, and all registrants should complete adequate pre-race medical questionnaires. This article recommends the use of atomized spray and fanned air in association with cooled intravenous fluids for the treatment of heat syndrome. There is a need for regional and national sports bodies to refuse sanction or certification to any race whose historical data do not suggest the likelihood of acceptable temperatures. Sanctioning should also include the name

---

Acknowledgements

Don Mitchell and Norm Schwendler of the Buffalo Marathon Association, and its founder Jesse Kregel; Betty Lou Rienzo and her inestimable typewriter; and the Staff of the Greater Niagara General Hospital Marathon Medical Team. The heat unit described in the text was engineered by James Ralston, Medical Coordinator of the Buffalo-Niagara Falls Marathon, from an idea by Dr. Francois Croteau, Medical Director of the Montreal Marathon.

of the MMD and an outline of the MMS design. The adverse publicity for recreational exercise as a whole attendant upon a critical injury during a marathon requires no less than the above.

There are two methods by which an RO can gain official recognition for his road race in North America. The first is to have the race sanctioned by a regional track and field association. The second is to have the course certified. There are 2,036 certified road races in the USA. Of these, 175 are marathons; 778 are 10-kilometer (10K); 232 are 5K. An RO gets certification by obtaining sanction from one of the 60 regional branches of The Athletic Congress. The course is then measured and the results acknowledged by the National Running Data Center in Arizona. Regional track and field associations do not report sanctioned events nationally; there may be up to 5 times as many sanctioned races as those numbered above. In Canada there are 7 nationally certified road races; 1 territorial and 10 provincial bodies sanction and certify their own events.

In neither country are the recording of the marathon medical director (MMD), or the marathon medical services (MMS), or details of runner care part of the sanction or certification process except for national elite events. Yet nearly all ROs apply for sanction, as the cost is minimal and the benefits significant. Most joggers/runners come into contact at least once with a sanctioned event which would provide them an opportunity to receive public education in safe running techniques. Critical injury could be avoided if such education existed.

The popular non-elite, non-qualifying road race became prevalent in North America in the 1970s. The New York City Marathon was first run in 1970 and Buffalo-Niagara Falls in 1974. Starters and finishers for the last named are shown in Table 17-1, correlated with race day temperatures. MMS for this event were intensified after 1978 when 60 runners were admitted to local hospital emergency departments who implemented the hospital disaster plan for more than 25 casualties from one incident. This inexcusable incursion of athletes into already busy emergency departments is still a primary reason for establishing on-site MMS which treat all injuries and transfer to hospital only for admission and follow-up (4). Avoiding multiple hospital registrations provides a saving to the taxpayer usually far in excess of the MMD budget (3).

The contacts and casualties for a non-elite event on the Niagara Falls course

TABLE 17-1. *Skylon Marathon 1974 to 1984. Entered, started, finished, and dropped out data per year with race temperatures. For larger road races, the percentage of drop-outs would translate into very high casualty loads. The runners complete the last 16 miles of the course toward the North.*

	ENT	ST	FIN	D/O	%	TEMP	HUM	Wind (m.p.h.)
1974	430	352	285	67	19.0	43°	79%	8-S
1975	960	718	612	106	14.8	68°	70%	17-S
1976	1136	946	869	77	8.1	43°	70%	10-N.W.
1977	2210	1982	1680	302	15.2	54°	87%	10-W
1978	2680	2565	2076	489	19.1	67°	43%	20-W.S.W.
1979	3412	2430	2252	178	7.3	45°	69%	20-N.W.
1980	2510	1977	1722	255	12.9	63°	63%	20-S.W.
1981	2270	1689	1519	170	10.1	44°	76%	8-S
1982	2120	1867	1589	278	14.9	38°	70%	20-W.N.W.
1983	1544	1394	1193	201	14.4	48°	61%	12-N.W.
1984	1462	1330	1154	186	16.1	50°	96%	3-S

are seen in Table 17-2 and similar data for an elite event in Table 17-3. The collection of such data over a few years quickly provides a formula for the calculation of likely casualties. Such a formula is essential to the provision of adequate equipment and manpower under varying race conditions (14, 15).

TABLE 17-2. *1981 Skylon Marathon breakdown of medical activity on the course and at the field hospital. This race included a sudden cardiac death among the aid station volunteers, in spite of resuscitation efforts.*

Temp—44°, Humidity—76%, Wind—8 m.p.h., South	
Number of registrants:	2270
Number of starters:	1689 (74.4%)
Numbber of no-shows:	581 (25.6%)
Number of finishers:	1519 (89.9%)
Number of drop-outs:	170 (10.1%)
Number of drop-outs to pace:	89 (52.4%)
Number of drop-outs to medical:	81 (47.6%)
MEDICAL DROP-OUT TRIAGE	
—Orthopedic:	54 (66.7%)
—Podiatry:	18 (22.2%)
—Holding, ICU:	9 (11.1%)
MEDICAL FINISHERS TRIAGE	
—Orthopedic:	43 (36.4%)
—Podiatry:	37 (31.4%)
—Holding, ICU:	38 (32.2%)

TABLE 17-3. *1984 U.S. Olympic Marathon Trial breakdown of medical activity on the course and at the field hospital*

Temp—65°, Humidity—60%, Wind—Light and swirling	
Number of qualifiers:	202
Number of starters:	159 (78.7%)
Number of no-shows:	43 (21.3%)
Number of finishers:	108 (53.5% of qualifiers)
	(67.9% of starters)
Number of drop-outs:	51 (32.1%)
Number of drop-outs to pace:	36 (71.6%)
Number of drop-outs to medical:	15 (29.4%)
MEDICAL DROP-OUT TRIAGE	
—Orthopedic:	14 (93.3%)
—Podiatry:	1 (6.7%)
—Holding, ICU:	0
NUMBER OF FINISHERS TO MEDICAL:	32 (29.6%)
MEDICAL FINISHERS TRIAGE	
—Orthopedic:	5 (15.6%)
—Podiatry:	7 (21.9%)
—Holding, ICU:	20 (62.5%)
NUMBER OF STARTERS WHO FINISHED FIT:	76 (47.8%)

TABLE 17-4. *Race Organization*

BUFFALO-NIAGARA FALLS INTERNATIONAL MARATHON

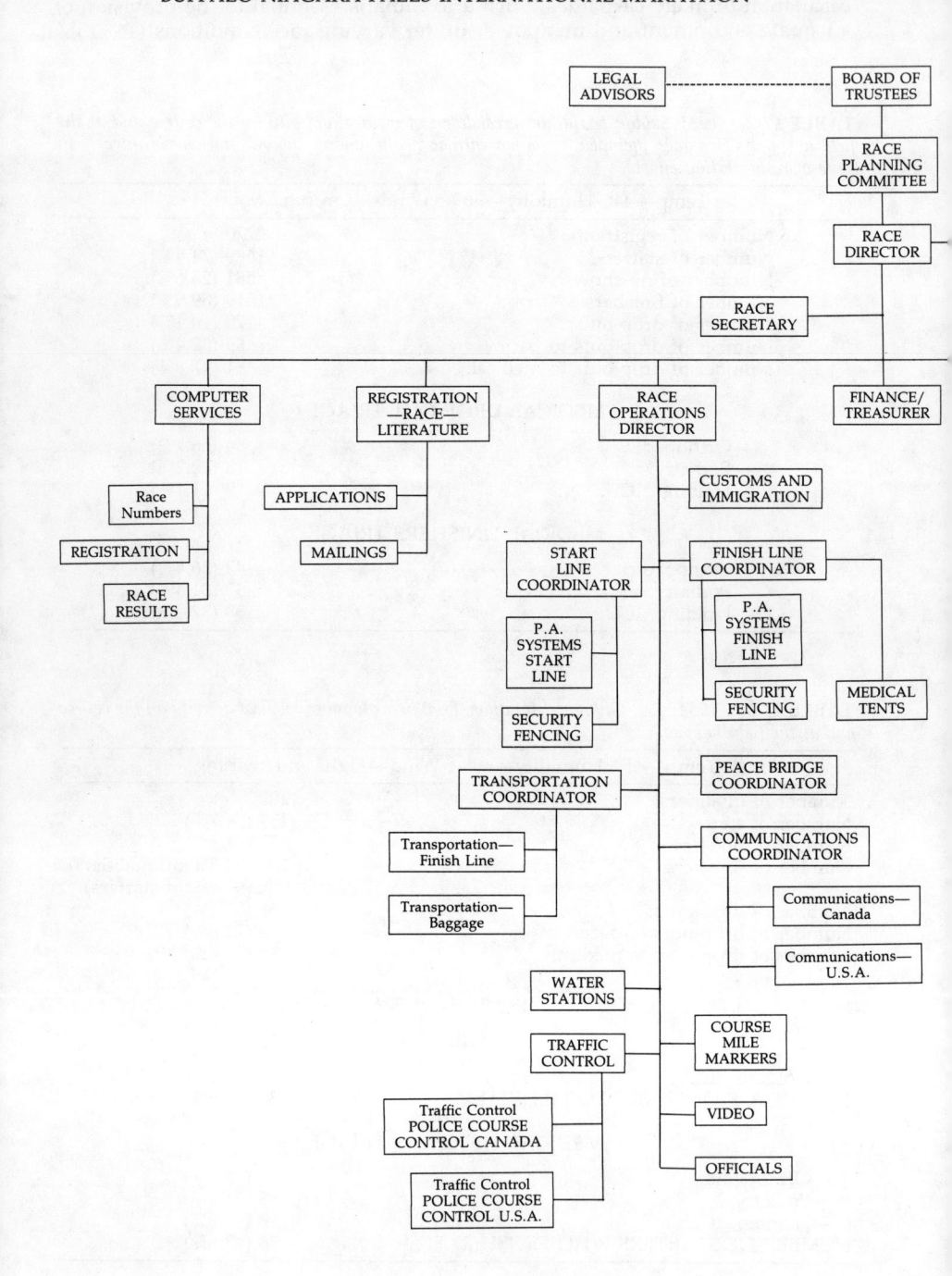

- BOARD OF TRUSTEES
  - LEGAL ADVISORS (advisory)
  - RACE PLANNING COMMITTEE
    - RACE DIRECTOR
      - RACE SECRETARY
      - COMPUTER SERVICES
        - Race Numbers
        - REGISTRATION
        - RACE RESULTS
      - REGISTRATION—RACE—LITERATURE
        - APPLICATIONS
        - MAILINGS
      - RACE OPERATIONS DIRECTOR
        - CUSTOMS AND IMMIGRATION
        - START LINE COORDINATOR
          - P.A. SYSTEMS START LINE
          - SECURITY FENCING
        - FINISH LINE COORDINATOR
          - P.A. SYSTEMS FINISH LINE
          - SECURITY FENCING
          - MEDICAL TENTS
        - TRANSPORTATION COORDINATOR
          - Transportation—Finish Line
          - Transportation—Baggage
        - PEACE BRIDGE COORDINATOR
        - COMMUNICATIONS COORDINATOR
          - Communications—Canada
          - Communications—U.S.A.
        - WATER STATIONS
        - TRAFFIC CONTROL
          - Traffic Control POLICE COURSE CONTROL CANADA
          - Traffic Control POLICE COURSE CONTROL U.S.A.
        - COURSE MILE MARKERS
        - VIDEO
        - OFFICIALS
      - FINANCE/TREASURER

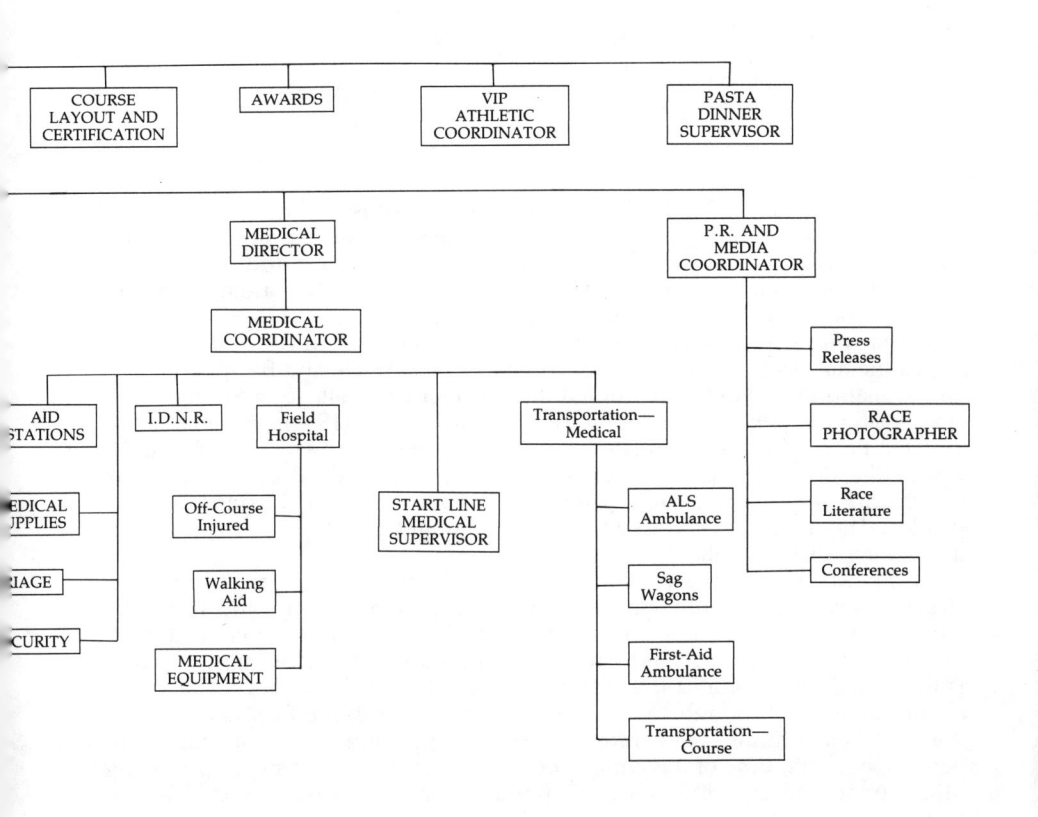

```
COURSE                AWARDS          VIP                PASTA
LAYOUT AND                            ATHLETIC           DINNER
CERTIFICATION                         COORDINATOR        SUPERVISOR
```

```
                MEDICAL                                P.R. AND
                DIRECTOR                               MEDIA
                                                       COORDINATOR
                MEDICAL                                         ├── Press Releases
                COORDINATOR
                                                                ├── RACE PHOTOGRAPHER
AID         I.D.N.R.    Field      Transportation—
STATIONS                Hospital    Medical                     ├── Race Literature
EDICAL          Off-Course      START LINE    ALS               └── Conferences
PPLIES          Injured         MEDICAL       Ambulance
                                SUPERVISOR
                Walking                       Sag
IAGE            Aid                           Wagons

CURITY          MEDICAL                       First-Aid
                EQUIPMENT                     Ambulance

                                              Transportation—
                                              Course
```

MEDICAL SERVICES FOR FUN RUNS AND MARATHONS

TABLE 17-5. *Medical Planning Group*

Medical Director
Secretary/Treasurer
Police Chief
Fire Chief
Communications Director
Sponsor's Representative
Media Representative
Finish Line Coordinator
Coordinator: Aid Stations and Spotters
Water Station Coordinator
First Aid Coordinator
Pick-up Vehicles Coordinator
Equipment Manager
Computer Data Director
Directors of Local Hospital Emergency Departments

During the late 1970s in Buffalo-Niagara Falls, this planning of MMS resolved into 3 basic strategies: 1. Educating runners in safe running techniques and in cooperating with MMS. 2. Handling mass casualties and critical care. 3. Identifying high-risk runners before injury occurs. The organization required to plan for these different goals is complex. And, while the running boom has produced a similar boom in medical literature on running, surprisingly little has been written on MMS (1, 16, 19, 23). Noble and Bachman (1979) and Williams et al. (1981) are quoted in the American College of Sports Medicine Position Paper on Prevention of Thermal Injuries (1984). More recently, Tunstall-Pedoe (21) has stimulated a comprehensive review by different agencies in the *British Journal of Sports Medicine* (5, 21). Medical planning alone, however, is not enough without the direct involvement of ROs and municipalities. This is often lacking even in high budget events with turnovers of many thousands of dollars.

Good MMS require a professional organization, with a recognized infrastructure involving all other aspects of the race organization, and reporting mechanisms which include police, ambulance, hospital emergency departments, first aid agencies, and City Hall. The Buffalo-Niagara Falls structure is listed in Table 17-4 and the Planning Committee in Table 17-5. The group should be flexible enough to accommodate such modifying factors as elite or non-elite fields, number of runners, urban or rural course, time of year, number of spectators, time of day, and prevailing weather. The basis for providing MMS for non-elite, non-qualifying, popular road races is, in fact, disaster planning.

Public/Runner Education in Safe Running Techniques

Public and runner education is complicated by the different goals of the runners. As Maron and Horvath pointed out, road races consist of: a) runners planning to win. b) runners of lesser training and/or ability planning to achieve personal bests. c) runners just hoping to complete all or some of the course. d) runners hoping to preclude serious illness by participating (11). Most road races supply some advice on training and avoidance of injury in their confirmation or registration packages. Many shorter and often more dangerous races give advice immediately before the start, which is useless. Education of the runner is of dubious benefit if education of the ROs fails to provide safe running conditions. For instance, advice from the journals recommends cancelling races when the wet bulb-globe temperature (WBGT) exceeds 25° (1, 5, 23). This is impractical (17). Races can be cancelled only on the day of the race, and this almost never occurs. Not only is RO intransigence to medical demands a factor, but if some runners arrive at the start they will probably run anyway. There is little solace to MMD in a runner sustaining critical injury as a bandit rather than as a registered runner. The solution is for medical organizations and sports bodies to support MMDs in becoming part of the sanction/certification process, and insist that sanction is granted only if ROs submit historical data to suggest the likelihood of acceptable temperatures on race day. The sanction process should also include the name of the MMD and an outline of his MMS, co-signed by the RO.

The Handling of Mass Casualties and the Treatment of Critical Care

Dealing with mass casualties and providing critical care treatment require all the elements of good disaster planning: communications; access to the site (i.e., emergency vehicles on the course); control of the site (the entire course); identifications and registration of casualties; triage; treatment (at an on-site field hospital); and transfer. Most road races supply medical aid stations at fixed points, but the principles of pre-hospital emergency care should apply here. Treatment should be brought to the casualties rather than asking them to run a further distance before getting help.

All vehicle drivers should possess 1:25 ordinance survey maps marked with all marathon and medical facilities. Advanced life support ambulances patrolling the course in unison with pick-up vehicles which deliver to a field hospital triage area work well if coordinated by good communications directed by an on-course medical director. And this is where the MMD should operate rather than at the finish; most difficult decisions must be made on the course. But this system infers the availability of vehicle access lanes. Good MMS should insist on free passage both ways for emergency vehicles—the only vehicles permitted on the course after the front runner. On-course vehicle personnel work in association with spotters, ham radio cyclists, aid station nurses, therapists, and podiatrists. All these personnel should have experience in assessing road runners and handling casualties. Data are collected on all contacts, casualties, and transfers. Information is fed to an Identification and Registration desk in the reunion area for family and friends.

Suspending race services after a set time, (e.g., 5 hours) is not helpful, as it encourages slow runners to start out too fast, and MMS personnel rarely leave the event with runners still on the course. Slower runners can, however, be turned into an adjacent park to complete the distance in laps without disturbing the municipality (14). Ham radio cyclists are essential for monitoring the latter stages of the race when emergency vehicles are working at full capacity.

All on-course volunteers should have taken a recent CPR course which, with the patrolling advanced life support (ALS) ambulances, will guarantee basic cardiac life support within 4 minutes and advanced cardiac life support within 8 minutes anywhere on the course. In races run under hotter conditions, patrolling vehicles should include mobile heat units with cooling systems, i/v fluids, and monitoring devices on board. As noted below, successful resuscitation of hyperthermic episodes requires immediate onset of cooling procedures (7, 8, 24). The field hospital operates as a casualty clearing station with triage, intensive care area, holding area, podiatry, and orthopedic services. Transfer protocols are arranged with the nearest suitable hospital emergency department. Runners should be kept under observation after the race in a reunion area to check for afterload injury (6). Aid stations should be provided at showering and changing venues.

Identifying The High-Risk Runner Before Injury Occurs

Preventing injury by identifying high-risk runners requires pre-race information on each runner which can be computerized and communicated to spotters and vehicles. In non-elite, popular road races, MMS should include intervention by medical staff for runners who appear compromised. This should include checking rectal temperatures, blood pressure, pulse rate, respiratory rate, and mental state. Significant findings should result in disqualification and transportation to the finish line triage. Runners should be informed that aggressive or emotional behavior is an early sign of heat injury and will be interpreted as such by MMS if encountered in runners they are attempting to assist (5).

ALS ambulances carry ECG equipment for cardiac patients. Handicapped athletes should be assessed no differently from other runners; facilities should be available for dealing with wheelchairs (12). General high-risk principles apply to all runners who are unacclimatized or undertrained, and they should be so advised at the start, especially in hot weather. Similarly, in hot weather, all cardiac, overweight runners, past heat victims, and those who have fever or have taken certain drugs or alcohol should be advised to take transportation home or complete only part of the distance (1, 5, 7, 9, 16). In 1984, New York was a good example of a race which encountered freak weather conditions and in which many runners should have been actively discouraged from participating. The value here of accurate reporting of past medical histories is obvious.

Some road races include room for medical histories on the back of the number bib but again, this is only of benefit after injury has occurred. In contrast, elite events demand a different approach. Elite runners cannot be stopped for assessment without disqualifying their entire performance. Since the 1980 U.S. Olympic Trials, Buffalo-Niagara Falls has used mental state assessments in elite events. An identified MMD drives alongside the runner in an ambulance and asks details of home and business telephone numbers and addresses. These give a quick evaluation. If there is obvious impairment, the runner is stopped for more detailed checkup. The conversation should be recorded on tape to justify the withdrawal after the athlete has recovered. Elite road racers probably deserve the same musculoskeletal self-determination as rugby or hockey players and should not be disqualified for musculoskeletal reasons even though appearing compromised to TV audiences. Certain road races have implemented these Buffalo-Niagara Falls protocols in the last few years at non-elite events, but intervention at non-elite runs should be permitted on appearance alone and the runner should be mandatorily stopped for full assessment. Definitely impaired runners who refuse to cooperate should be physically detained by prior arrangement with race security personnel.

Specific Treatment of One Type of Critical Care Situation

HYPERTHERMIA: illustrates the application of the critical care treatment. Pre-race planning includes:

1. Withholding of regional and national sanction unless historical data for the day of the race suggest likely acceptable temperatures.
2. Withholding of regional and national sanction if the race MMS do not fall within acceptable guidelines.
3. Medical past histories as part of registration.
4. Emphasis on RO and municipal cooperation with MMS.
5. Spotters and pick-up systems.
6. ALS vehicles and mobile heat unit vehicles.
7. Fully equipped and staffed finish line field hospital.
8. Transfer protocols to local emergency and critical care units.
9. Pre-race selection to exclude children under 18, (1, 2, 9), cardiacs, the

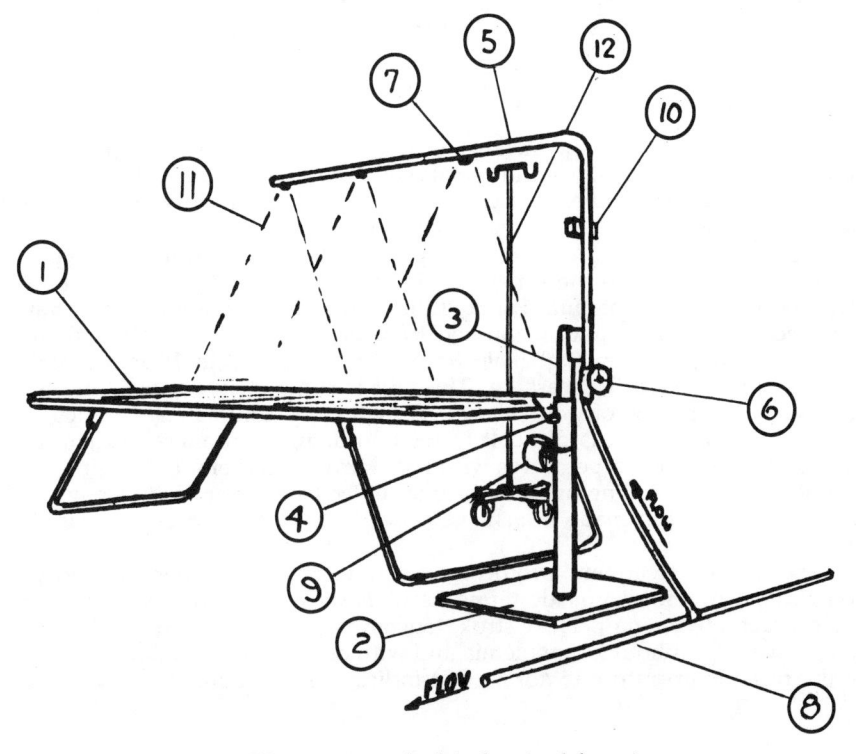

1. Water resistant bed (galvanized frame)
2. Spray system support stand
3. Spray height adjusting tube
4. Height tube locking handle
5. Rigid galvanized water pipe
6. Water control valve
7. Water spray nozzle
8. Water hose
9. Cooling fan
10. Digital probe thermometer
11. Water spray area (80°)
12. IV stand

Fig. 17-1. *Cooling System for Hyperthermia in Runners*

grossly overweight, past heat victims, runners with fevers, those who have taken alcohol and certain drugs, and possibly elderly runners.
10. Runner education on clothing, fluid intake, acclimatization, training, and cooperating with MMS with confirmation packages, and registration packages delivered no later than 15 minutes before the start of the race.
11. Water stations at start and early in the run on both sides of the road.
12. Large cups with tops and straws (17).
13. Flag system in place to warn runners of temperature changes; readings should be taken each half-hour and communicated to all medical units (16). Pick-up and ALS vehicles should be equipped with loud hailers to call readings.
14. Runners to weigh in at the start; weight is recorded on number bib and scales are available at aid stations in checking for more than 3% loss of weight (24).
15. Rectal thermometers at all medical units and rectal probes on heat units.

Treatment of episodes which occur despite the above includes immediate cooling; taking of vital signs and rectal temperature; cooled i/v fluid replacement with dextrose/saline, or bicarbonate if metabolic acidosis is likely (24); blood sampling for urea, electrolytes, creatinine, CPK, SGOT, SGPT, and LDH; and control of convulsions with diazepam or chlorpromazine. The type of cooling probably reflects the experience of the particular MMS personnel. Buffalo-Niagara Falls uses atomized spray from above a three-quarter conduit frame with webbing support and air fanned from below (Fig. 17-1) (22). This unit can cool an 80 kilogram (kg) male from 42.5° to 38.5° C in 15 minutes. Restraints are provided if necessary. The unit is completely portable and easy to place in a van for on-course use. Ice baths, by contrast, are difficult to maneuver on-course; it is difficult to restrain delirious runners in them and difficult to measure temperatures with rectal probes in them. But again, there is little point in quibbling over the niceties of ice baths over sprinkler systems if no effort has been made to achieve prevention by good pre-race planning (13).

Establishing treatment protocols and flow charts for thermal injury is complicated by the diagnostic terms used. Heat stroke and heat exhaustion are not definite enough. Heat stroke encompasses a variety of clinical conditions with or without hypovolemia and with or without dry skin. The height of the rectal temperature is not a good indicator for treatment or prognosis.

Conclusion

The recommendations of this article are that physiological and biochemical solutions to medical problems encountered during fun runs and marathons should be addressed through more intensive medical planning and the insistence on full cooperation from ROs, municipalities and national and regional sanctioning bodies. The latter groups should support MMDs in refusing to sanction events which are run in likely adverse conditions and without acceptable standards of MMS. Very few sponsors will maintain support for unsanctioned events. The medical community should realize that the non-elite, non-qualifying popular road race requires medical planning different from elite races or other sporting events. The position of popular marathons should be recognized as being representative, at least in the eyes of the media and thence the general public, of the whole field of recreational exercise. The adverse publicity generated by critical injuries and road races has a negative effect on many high-risk individuals (and their often equally high-risk children), for whom recreational exercise might be a worthwhile lifelong commitment. The media must be made to realize that road running is not a panacea for disease, that individuals with existing disease may encounter critical injury while running, and that despite the best efforts of MMS, a few of those injured will not survive, (10, 18, 20).

REFERENCES

1. A.C.S.M. Position Statement. Prevention of thermal injuries during distance running. *Med. Sci. Sports Exerc.* 16:ix–xiv, 1984.
2. Amer. Acad of Paediatricians. Climatic heat stress and the exercising child. *Phys. Sportsmed.* 11:155–159, 1983.
3. Brotherwood, R. W. Marathons and St. John. *Br. J. Sports Med.* 18:281, 1984.
4. Bryson, L. G., and A. Seymour. Popular marathons. *Br. Med. J.* 288:1613, 1984.
5. Consumers Conference. Popular marathons, half marathons and other long distance runs: recommendations for medical support. *Br. Med. J.* 288:1355–1359, 1984.
6. Dimsdale, J. E., L. H. Hartley, T. Guiney, J. N. Ruskin, and D. Greenblatt. Post exercise peril. *J.A.M.A.* 251:630–632, 1984.
7. Hanson, P. G. and S. W. Zimmerman. Exertional heat stroke in novice runners. *J.A.M.A.* 242:154–157, 1979.
8. Hart, L. E., B. P. Eiger, A. G. Shimizu, P. J. Tandan, and J. R. Sutton. Exertional heat stroke: the runner's nemesis. *Can. Med. Assoc. J.* 122:1144–1150, 1980.
9. Kains, J. P., S. DeWit, P. Close, C. Melot, J. Nagler, and P. VanRooy. Exertional heat stress disease. *Acta Clin. Belgica* 38:315–322, 1983.
10. Koplan, J. P. Cardiovascular deaths while running. *J.A.M.A.* 242:2578–2580, 1979.
11. Maron, M. B. and S. M. Horvath. The marathon: A history and review of the literature. *Med. Sc. Sports.* 10:137–150, 1978.
12. Marshall, T. Wheelchairs and marathon road racing. *Br. J. Sports Med.* 18:301–304, 1984.
13. Mash, L. H. Treating thermal injury: disagreement heats up. *Phys. Sportsmed.* 13:134–144, 1985.
14. Nicholl, J. P. and B. T. Williams. Popular marathons: Forecasting casualties. *Br. Med. J.* 285:1464–1465, 1982.
15. Nicholl, J. P. and B. T. Williams. Injuries sustained by runners during a popular marathon. *Br. J. Sports Med.* 17:10–15, 1983.
16. Noble, H. B. and D. Bachman. Medical aspects of distance race planning. *Phys. Sportsmed.* 7:78–84, 1979.
17. Porter, A. M. W. Marathon running and adverse weather conditions: A miscellany. *Br. J. Sports Med.* 18:261–264, 1984.
18. Siscovick, D. S., N. S. Weiss, R. H. Fletcher, and T. Lasky. The incidence of primary cardiac arrest during vigorous exercise. *N. Engl. J. Med.* 311:874–877, 1984.
19. Sutton, J. R., M. J. Coleman, A. P. Millar, L. Lazarus, and P. Russo. The medical problems of mass participation in athletic competition. The "City-to-Surf" race. *Med. J. Aust.* 2:127–133, 1972.
20. Thompson, P. D. and J. H. Mitchell. Exercise and sudden cardiac death: Protection or provocation? *N. Eng. J. Med.* 311:914–915, 1984. (Editorial).
21. Tunstall Pedoe, D. Marathon medicine. *Br. Med. J.* 288:1322–1323, 1984.
22. Weiner, J. S. and A. Khogalim. Physiological body cooling unit for treatment of heat stroke. *Lancet.* 1:507–509, 1980.
23. Williams, R. S., D. D. Schocken, M. Morey and P. F. Koisch. Medical aspects of competitive distance running. *Postgrad. Med.* 70:41–51, 1981.
24. Wyndham, C. H. Heat stroke and hyperthermia in marathon runners. *Ann. N.Y. Acad. Sci.* 301:128–138, 1977.

18

Road Racing Medical Management

JACK E. TAUNTON, M.D.
R. S. MCLEAN, M.P.E.

University of British Columbia

INTRODUCTION

The medical coverage of any road race plays an integral part in the well-being of all participants. With the ever-increasing popularity of distance running, proper medical supervision is of considerable importance. It is vital that knowledge of any potential running-related injury is well understood and that all appropriate preventative measures are provided.

Physicians, physiotherapists, first aiders, and other medical personnel may have minimal direct experience with the specific medical problems which arise during road races.

The purpose of this chapter is to provide guidelines for medical personnel involved in arranging medical coverage for distance races. It is of the utmost importance that a medically safe environment is provided for participating runners.

ORGANIZATION

Prior organizational meetings to secure personnel, equipment, and supplies, as well as a medical seminar for the personnel, are very useful.

Medical Facilities

A central medical station or field hospital should be positioned at the finish line; the length of the race course will determine the number of first aid stations on the course itself.

In the Vancouver International Marathon, which is a 2-loop course, we utilize 4 medical aid stations positioned adjacent to a fluid station. Most 10-kilometer (km) races require 2 medical aid stations and the finish line field hospital.

Noble and Bachman (3) suggest a list of required equipment that should be at this central medical facility. A modified list is presented in Table 18-1.

The field hospital should be equipped to handle potential emergency and life-threatening situations. These could be due to pre-existing medical conditions or the result of environmental or race conditions. It is important to remember that the medical personnel may have to treat spectators as well as participants.

Ideally, this facility should be located at the finish line area to serve as many individuals as required. We have divided our field hospital into a triage area, a minor treatment area (i.e., blisters and cramps), and an intensive care area. Propane heaters have been useful in races run in colder areas. Large quantities of ice are required for muscle strains, ligament sprains, and for cases of hyperthermia. Zip-lock plastic bags (500 per 1,000 runners) are useful for the ice. Portable toilets (4 per 1,000 runners) are necessary at the field

TABLE 18-1. *Recommended Equipment for Field Hospital (for each 1,000 runners)*

No.	Item
10	Stretchers
4	Sawhorses
10	Blankets
200	Space Blankets
10	Intravenous Setups
	-5% D/NS
	Ringer's Lactate
	2/3–1/3
2 each	Inflatable arm and leg splints
2 cases	1 1/2 inch tape and prowrap
2 cases each	Elastic wraps (2 in., 4 in., and 6 in.)
2 cases	Sheet wadding
	Underwrap
2 cases	4 × 4 inch gauze pads
	Bandaids—assorted sizes
	Steristrips
	Blister kits
	"Second skin"
	Adhesive knit
	Petroleum jelly (skin lube)
	Ice in small plastic bags
	Small instrument kits
1/2 case	Surgical soap
2	Oxygen tanks
2	ECG monitors with defibrillators
100	Towels
1 box	Paper towels
2 boxes	Alcohol swabs
4	Portable toilets
200 cups each	Fluids
	—cold drinks (water, electrolyte and soft drinks)
	—hot drinks (coffee, tea)
6 doz.	Glasses
6	Stethescopes
6	Blood pressure cuffs
6	Rectal thermometers (high/low)
	Clip boards and medical chart paper for recording

hospital in addition to the large number required at the start and finish lines.

In the Vancouver International Marathon field hospital, we have found that we require for each 1,000 runners: 10 tables, 25 chairs, a minimum of 25 stretchers, and 4 wheelchairs. We have also used successfully 2 "hot tubs" at the field hospital for hypothermia care.

The personnel required for each 1,000 runners in the Vancouver Marathon are:

Coordinators (5)—Chief Medical Officer
　　　　　　　　—Intensive Care Coordinator
　　　　　　　　—Triage Coordinator
　　　　　　　　—Course First Aid Coordinator
　　　　　　　　—Ambulance Coordinator
Physicians　　　—20 at field hospital
　　　　　　　　—2 per medical aid station
　　　　　　　　—1 per ambulance
Nurses　　　　 —10 at field hospital
Therapists　　　—20 at triage area (field hospital)
　　　　　　　　—2 per medical aid station

Communication with nearby hospitals as well as the first aid stations on the course is of utmost importance. Radio communication is necessary throughout the course and should be relayed to the field hospital. Easy, unobstructed ambulance access to the field hospital is essential.

Depending on the number of runners, at least 1 ambulance should be stationed at the field hospital. It is suggested that 2 ambulances be on the course for a race of 1,000 people and an additional ambulance be dispatched for each additional 1,000 runners. Ideally, 1 ambulance should follow the last runner on the course; all emergency vehicles must be in constant radio communication with the central medical facility.

All personnel must be clearly identified (e.g., red hats, arm bands, or special jackets). Through personal experience and observation at many road races, it appears that the medical aid station situated at the finish line is the busiest; that is where most injured runners seek medical attention. Therefore, it is important that this medical facility be isolated from the crowd and yet be easily accessible to the runners. Movable walls, barricades, or ropes are recommended to keep unauthorized or uninjured individuals out of the medical area, thereby eliminating unnecessary congestion. An information board kept up to date on the status of the athletes in the field hospital has been useful. An identification tag on each patient in the field hospital aids in record keeping.

The medical aid stations on the course should also be maintained by qualified personnel who should have on hand the supplies recommended in Table 18-2, (modified from Ref. 3). All medical stations should be in tents and should have radio communication with the ambulances and finish line field hospital.

MEDICAL EMERGENCIES

Due to the large number of persons participating in road races, a variety of medical emergencies could occur. As a result, it is necessary that the medical personnel be prepared to give quick and effective treatment.

TABLE 18-2. *Recommended Equipment for Aid Stations (for each 1,000 runners)*

No.	Item
5	Stretchers (10 at 10 km and beyond)
5	Blankets (10 at 10 km and beyond)
10	Space blankets
6 each	Elastic wrap (2 in., 4 in. and 6 in.)
1/2 case	4 × 4 in. gauze pads
1/2 case	1 1/2 inch tape
1/2 case	Surgical soap
1/2 case	Petroleum jelly (skin lube)
2 each	Inflatable arm and leg splints
	Small instrument kits
	Bandaids—assorted sizes
	Blister kits
	"Second skin"
	Adhesive knit
1 box	Alcohol swabs
2	Intravenous setups
6 large	Thermoses of cold and hot fluids
3 doz	Glasses
1	Portable toilet
1 chest	Ice in small plastic bags
1	Athletic trainer's kit

1. Myocardial Infarction

With the ever-increasing number of older individuals entering road races, as well as those with a medical history of heart disease, the chance of a cardiac arrest occurring must be recognized. Personnel qualified to use a defibrillator are necessary at any major road race. Further equipment and drugs which may be required by attending physicians to effectively administer prolonged advance cardiac life support must also be available.

2. Hyperthermia

It appears that the incidence of hyperthermia is the most common serious problem found in road races. If neglected and/or treated improperly, a life-threatening injury could develop. Proper training, hydration, and runner education should help prevent the development of various stages of heat injuries. The American College of Sports Medicine published a detailed position stand on the prevention of thermal injuries during distance running (1).

    (a) Heat Cramps
  —with excess sweating, many people suffer from heat cramps;
  —ingestion of fluids and foods such as bananas and oranges appears to help alleviate these symptoms;
  —stretching and ice massage are also helpful.

    (b) Heat Exhaustion
  —symptoms include fatigue, nausea, headache, irritable, cool and clammy skin, usually active sweating, weak and rapid pulse, and dyspnea;
  —treatment involves the cessation of activity and immediate cooling and rehydration.

(c) Heat Stroke
- —this is a medical emergency;
- —symptoms include weakness, exhaustion, marked alterations of mental status, usually moist, warm, flushed skin, rapid and bounding pulse; sweating may or may not be present; breathing is usually deep and fast;
- —immediate cooling of the body temperature to 39°C, followed by closely monitored passage cooling is recommended (2).

The only way to truly distinguish between heat exhaustion and heat stroke is by mental status; the absence or presence of sweating is not an indicator, and there is no absolute diagnostic rectal temperature.

Environmental conditions, as well as other factors, greatly affect the participating runners. Hyperthermia develops when the body's rate of heat production is greater than its ability to dissipate the heat produced (4). It is important to realize that even though the ambient temperature may be cool and the day windy, it is still possible for runners to experience hyperthermia.

Sweat loss obviously increases with prolonged exercise and can account for a total body water deficit of about 6 to 10% of body weight (7). The resulting dehydration reduces the sweating rate and predisposes the runner to the development of heat injuries. It is important, therefore, to educate the runners about problems which could occur and encourage them to ingest fluids—preferably cool water—dress appropriately, and be aware of the physical signs and symptoms of heat injuries.

3. Hypothermia

Weather conditions play a major role in any athletic event, but particularly so in long-distance road races. Moderately cool days can play havoc with the thermoregulatory system of runners—body heat is lost and the core temperature can begin to decrease. Therefore, an understanding and recognition of the signs and symptoms of the developing injury is very important.

Due to a combination of strenuous activity, cool and wet climate, and the increase of muscular fatigue, the rate of exercise may decrease to a point at which the body heat loss to the environment exceeds the metabolic heat produced. The result is an impairment of neuromuscular responses and exhaustion. Early signs and symptoms are shivering, disorientation, and muscular weakness. As the core temperature continues to drop, the victim may eventually lose consciousness.

The physical demands placed on the body, in combination with inclement weather, improper clothing, and poor runner education, can all predispose a runner to thermal injury. The medical personnel must be well educated and aware of these problems and be ready to handle such potentially life-threatening injuries.

Emergency procedures involve monitoring vital signs, immediate rewarming, use of the respirator if required, use of intravenous fluids, and preparation to transport the victim to the nearest hospital.

4. Hypovolemic Collapse

Some runners experience syncope immediately after crossing the finish line and require rapid medical attention; however, it is important to understand that a relapse may occur up to 30 minutes after the finish of the race (5). Long distance runners can lose several liters of extracellular fluid, resulting in hypotension; the situation is further complicated if the runner also experiences increased gastrointestinal loss of fluid through vomiting or diarrhea.

It is important to monitor this individual. Rehydration is required immediately. If further loss continues through persistent vomiting and diarrhea, intravenous fluids may be necessary.

5. Blisters and Others

By far the most common injuries observed in any race are blisters, chafing, abrasions, and other orthopedic or podiatric problems.

The aid stations on the race course will probably treat these running-related injuries as well as the central facility; therefore, all medical areas must be well stocked with bandaids, blister kits ("second skin" and adhesive knit), thick petroleum jelly, and ice.

RUNNER EDUCATION

Marathon clinics and symposia available to the participants months in advance of the actual race can help greatly in the education of potential race participants.

Talks on proper training methods, acclimatization, fluid consumption, and signs and symptoms of common running-related injuries all make the runners increasingly aware of factors that could predispose them to injury.

Information on specific medical problems should be included in each runner's pre-race packet as well as a map of the course, indicating the position of all medical aid and water stations.

On race day, runners should be made aware of the weather conditions and the risk of thermal injuries by the use of color-coded flags (Fig. 18-1). They should also be aware of *all* the medical aid stations, water stations, and any potential hazards. It is a good idea to have an individual with a history of medical problems include a description of the specific problem and instructions on the back of the registration number along with his or her name, address, phone number, and name of the person who should be notified in case of an emergency.

COMMUNICATIONS SYSTEM

Ideally, the medical communication network should be separate from that of the race organization; however, many times it is more convenient, not to mention economical, to maximize the radio operators' participation. Radio operators should be stationed along the course at designated positions, at each peripheral medical aid station, and in a follow-up vehicle trailing the final runner. Radio operators can also assist as spotters at busy intersections. The central medical facility must have coordinated radio communication and vehicles ready to be dispatched if notified by one of the aid stations along the course.

Possible resources for finding radio operators are local ham radio organizations as well as area military units.

HEAT INJURY RISK

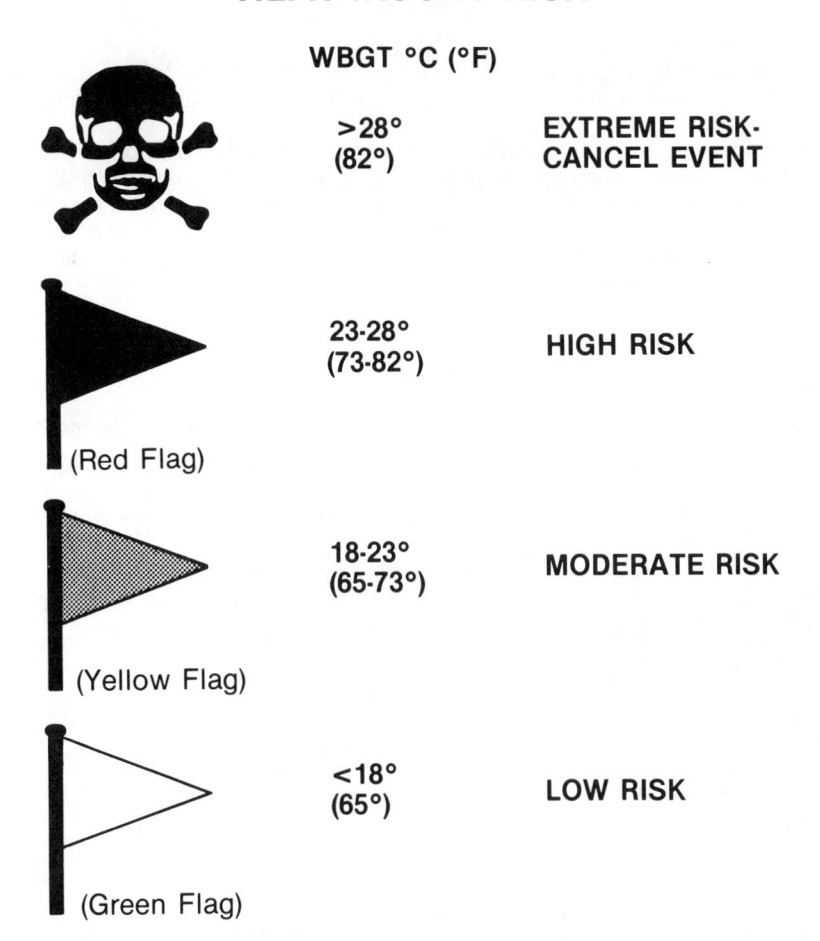

WBGT °C (°F)

☠	>28° (82°)	EXTREME RISK- CANCEL EVENT
(Red Flag)	23-28° (73-82°)	HIGH RISK
(Yellow Flag)	18-23° (65-73°)	MODERATE RISK
(Green Flag)	<18° (65°)	LOW RISK

Fig. 18-1. *Color-Coded Flags to Indicate the Risk Of Thermal Stress*
1. RED FLAG: High Risk: When WBGT is 23 to 28°C
   This signal would indicate that all runners should be aware that heat injury is possible and any person particularly sensitive to heat or humidity should probably not run.
2. AMBER FLAG: Moderate Risk: When WBGT is 18 to 23°C
   It should be remembered that the air temperature, probably humidity, and almost certainly the radiant heat at the beginning of the race will increase during the course of the race if conducted in the morning or early afternoon.
3. GREEN FLAG: Low Risk: When WBGT is below 18° C
   This in no way guarantees that heat injury will not occur, but indicates only that risk is low.
4. WHITE FLAG: Low Risk: When WBGT is below 10° C
   Hypothermia may occur, especially in slow runners in long races, and in wet and windy conditions.

*** This scale is determined for runners clad in running shorts, shoes, and a T-shirt. In warmer weather, the less clothing the better. For males, wearing no shirt or a mesh top is better than wearing a T-shirt because the surface for evaporation is increased. However, in areas where radiant heat is excessive, a light top may be helpful. ***

CONCLUSION

It is important that medical facilities are provided to ensure the safety and well-being of all participants. Advance preparation for all potential medical problems can ensure that the medical personnel and system will operate effectively and smoothly.

The increased number of runners in road races and marathons forces the race committee to provide proper medical coverage. The medical director is responsible for runner education, the recruitment of physicians, physiotherapists, and other medical personnel to work cohesively towards the safety of all runners. Ambulances, medical equipment at the central and peripheral aid stations, and water stations must all be properly coordinated.

REFERENCES

1. American College of Sports Medicine, Position Stand on Prevention of Thermal Injuries During Distance Running. *Med. Sci. Sports Exerc.* 16:9–14, 1984.
2. Costrini, A. M. Metabolic manifestation of heatstroke and severe heat exhaustion. *Am. J. Med.* 66:296–302, 1979.
3. Noble, H. B., and D. Bachman. Medical aspects of distance race. *Phys. Sportsmed.* 7:78–84, 1979.
4. Sutton, J. R. Heat Illness. In: *Sport Medicine*, R. H. Strauss (ed.) 307–322. Philadelphia: W. B. Saunders, 1984.
5. Tunstall-Pedoe, T. Marathon medicine. *Br. Med. J.* 228:1355–1359, 1984.
6. Williams, R. S., D. D. Schocken, M. Morey, and F. P. Koisch. Medical aspects of competitive distance running. *Postgrad. Med.* 70:41–51, 1981.
7. Wyndham, C. H., and N. B. Strydom. The danger of inadequate water intake during marathon running. *S. Afr. Med. J.* 43:893–896, 1969.

19

Advanced Age and Altitude Illness

ANNE C. BALCOMB, M.D.

Tekoona, Toogong, via Cudel, N.S.W.

JOHN R. SUTTON, M.D.

McMaster University Medical Center

ADVANCED AGE AND ALTITUDE ILLNESS

Reports from media, governments, and health workers stress that we are becoming an aging society. The percentage of the population over 60 is increasing, and early retirement is common, resulting in increased leisure time for the elderly. Is this leisure time being used effectively? Masters groups encourage and emphasize the advantages of continued activity with increasing age. In one study, older adults were asked what they were planning or would like to do in the years ahead. The most common reply was travel (2). Many travel plans include tours to exotic regions at altitude: the Incan ruins in Peru, the Himalayas in Nepal, the Rockies in Canada, or the United States. These locations necessarily involve hiking and unaccustomed activity.

Do Many Older Adults Travel to Altitude?

Compilations from high altitude studies, trekking companies, and anecdotal accounts indicate that a considerable number of older people already participate in altitude-related activities. We realize that these are only rough estimates and do not take into account many activities including skiing, climbing, and trekking which may involve ascent to altitude.

Hackett et al. studied (6) tourist-hikers en route to Everest base camp in 1975. The researchers found the mean age of trekkers to be 33 ± 11.6 years, with an age range of 18 to 71 years. Sixteen percent of these trekkers were over the age of 45.

Mountain Travel Incorporated of California provided the data based on 1,670 clients participating in adventure travel programs in 1984 (Table 19-1). Seventy-seven percent of these programs are high-activity trips which include trekking or climbing, and 31% go to altitudes over 4,572 meters (m) (15,000 feet). Over 30% of their travelers were over the age of 50. The Ameri-

TABLE 19-1. *Figures from Mountain Travel, Inc. based on 1,670 clients participating in adventure travel programs in 1984*

Age Group	% of total
19	2
20–29	13
30–39	29
40–49	23
50–59	17
60–69	13
>69	3

can Alpine Institute provided data from their Peru/Bolivia treks over 3,658 m (12,000 ft.) for the 3-month period, July through September 1985. Seven and one-half percent of their trekkers were over the age of 50.

Other trekking companies contacted did not have figures available but estimated the majority of clients to be in the 30-to-50-year age range with significant numbers over 50 years. Reasons given for this age breakdown were that these age groups had both the available money and leisure time. The number of people trekking to altitude appears to be increasing each year.

Many anecdotal cases exist such as that of the backpacking octogenarian, Hulda Crooks, who is planning her yearly ascent of Mt. Whitney for 1986 when she turns 90 in May. Mt. Whitney is the highest peak in the contiguous U.S.A. at 4,404 m (14,494 ft.). An inspirational aspect of Mrs. Crook's story is that she did not begin her exercise program in earnest until she was 70 years old. She has climbed Mt. Whitney 22 times. Hulda also runs in local races and about every month in the summertime climbs one of the mountains of Southern California "just to stay in shape." Her guide on these climbs is Sam Fink, a mere 83 years old, who has been climbing for over 50 years. Hulda believes that good health is within the reach of most people, but states that, "If the mind doesn't tell the body what to do, it won't do anything."

Another great climber, Albert McCarthy, was 49 years old when he led the first perilous ascent of Canada's highest peak, Mt. Logan (6,050 m) in 1925. In 1985, a 52-year-old American, Dick Bass, climbed Mt. Everest (8,848 m).

What Are the Medical Problems of Altitude Exposure?

As far back as 37 BC in China (5), descriptive reports exist of illness occuring on ascent to altitude. Over the centuries it has slowly emerged that there are specific illnesses which occur exclusively on ascent to high altitude. Today these are referred to as altitude illnesses. They range from the common and trivial to the uncommon but potentially fatal. Table 19-2 (21) lists the terms in common use for various presentations of high altitude illness.

ACUTE MOUNTAIN SICKNESS (AMS): Acute Mountain Sickness (AMS) is the name given to a collection of symptoms which occur commonly in those going to high altitude (3,000 m or more). Onset is usually within 6 to 96 hours after ascent. AMS in mild cases is characterized by various combinations of headache, insomnia, anorexia, nausea, dizziness, and lassitude which rather resemble having a bad hangover. Everything tends to be worse at night and in the mornings; getting up becomes more of a task than usual. Although an unpleasant inconvenience, the symptoms are usually self-limiting, clearing in

TABLE 19-2. *Altitude Illness*

Acute Hypoxia—Mental impairment and deterioration, progressing to coma after rapid exposures to altitudes, usually above 5,800 m.

Acute Mountain Sickness—Headache, anorexia, nausea, vomiting, weakness, insomnia; usually occurs above 2,500 m; onset 2 to 4 hours after arrival at altitude, but may be delayed for 24 hours or more; usually self-limiting; very common.

High Altitude Pulmonary Edema (HAPE)—characterized by dyspnea at rest, much worse on exercise; cough, audible rales, subject may have white or pink frothy sputum and cyanosis; usually occurs above 3,000 m, is relatively uncommon but requires early treatment and rapid descent if possible.

High Altitude Cerebral Edema (HACE)—Severe headache, ataxia, irritability and any abnormal behavior, drowsiness, hallucinations, progressing to coma and death; may be associated with abnormalities in limb tone, urinary incontinence, papilledema; sometimes cranial nerve palsies and tremor are associated.

High Altitude Retinal Hemorrhage (HARH)—Flame shaped hemorrhages or 'dot and blot' hemorrhages; may occur in more than 50% of subjects going over 5,000 m; rarely causes any symptoms; if visual symptoms do occur, hemorrhages are often in the macular region and descent is advised.

Subcutaneous Edema or Generalized Edema—Common, but may not be altitude-specific: no specific treatment required.

Subacute Mountain Sickness—Failure to recover from acute mountain sickness, with mild disability persisting from several days to weeks; no immediate danger, but descent is suggested.

Chronic Mountain Sickness ("Monge's disease")—This occurs in people living at high altitudes for many years; consists of deterioration in performance and mental function, fatigue associated with pulmonary hypertension, and inappropriate polycythemia; descent is advised.

Other Altitude-related Problems, Thromboembolic phenomena and Cold injury—Conditions may worsen at altitude; sickle cell trait, hematological, cardiac, and pulmonary diseases.

High Altitude Deterioration—Irritability, weight loss, fatigue, and insomnia; affects work performance; generally occurs above 6,000 m where permanent adaptation is not possible.

---

1 to 3 days with rest and fluids. However, a small percentage may rapidly progress to life-threatening high-altitude pulmonary edema or high-altitude cerebral edema.

In 1913, Dr. T. H. Ravenhill was physician to a small mining company high in the Andes near the Chilean-Bolivian border. He wrote the following detailed description which beautifully outlines the nature and time course of AMS (16). His description has not been bettered:

> It is a curious fact that the symptoms of puna (AMS) do not usually evince themselves at once. The majority of newcomers have expressed themselves as being quite well on first arrival. As a rule towards the evening, the patient begins to feel rather slack and disinclined for exertion. He goes to bed, but has a restless and troubled night, and wakes up next morning with a severe frontal headache. There may be vomiting; frequently there is a sense of oppression in the chest, but there is rarely any respiratory distress or alteration in the normal rate of breathing so long as the patient is at rest. The patient may feel slightly giddy on rising from bed, and any attempt at exertion increases the headache, which is nearly always confined to the frontal region. . . . The headache increases towards evening, so also does the pulse rate; all appetite is lost, and the patient wishes to be alone—to sleep if possible. Generally, during the second night he is able to do so, and as a rule

wakes next morning feeling better; the pulse rate has dropped to about 90; the headache is only slight. As the day draws on, he probably feels worse again, the symptoms tending to reappear on any exertion; if, however, he keeps to his bed, by the fourth day after arrival he is probably very much better, and at the end of a week is quite fit again. The most prominent feature in this type of puna is frontal headache and extreme lassitude.

In 1975 Hackett et al. studied 278 hikers at 4,243 m in the Himalaya en route to Kala Patar and the Everest base camp. The researchers found the overall incidence of AMS (both mild and severe) to be 53% (6). They found the incidence of all forms of altitude illness was greater in those who ascended quicker, those who flew to high altitude, and those not taking time to acclimatize. There was no difference in incidence between the sexes, nor did previous altitude exposure or being fit at sea level prevent its occurrence. Severity was also highly correlated with rate of ascent. They concluded that the best prevention is to take time trekking, to acclimatize, and to sleep low.

A second study by Hackett and Rennie (7, 8) in 1977 on the same route with a similar group of trekkers showed a 43% decline in the incidence of AMS. They attributed this decrease to effective education of trekkers, trekking companies, trek leaders, and physicians, who were now aware of the need for incorporating acclimatization days into their itineraries, and of encouraging people to ascend more slowly.

An important point to remember with all forms of altitude illness is that there is marked inter-individual variation in trekkers. Some people just seem to be more susceptible. So far, this predisposition can't be accurately predicted, except that those people who get severe AMS tend to get it recurrently and may be underventilators (14, 22). Ravenhill (16) expressed this point eloquently:

> There is in my experience no type of man of whom one can say he will or will not suffer puna. Most of the cases I have instanced were men to all appearances perfectly sound. Young, strong and healthy men may be completely overcome; stout, plethoric individuals of the chronic bronchitic type may not even have a headache.

Ravenhill was also the first person to attempt a classification of altitude illness. He described 2 very serious and sometimes fatal divergencies from the milder form of AMS, a cardiac form and a nervous form. These correspond to what are generally known today as High Altitude Pulmonary Edema (HAPE) and High Altitude Cerebral Edema (HACE). This terminology is still debated, and the exact relationships between the various illnesses are far from clear. Dickinson (4), for example, suggests that cerebral acute mountain sickness is a better term for HACE as it does not imply a mechanism. The terms above (HACE, HAPE) imply that edema formation is the major process involved in the development of these illnesses. However, no agreement has yet been reached about the exact processes or the relative importance of the mechanisms involved. For convenience we will use the terms HACE and HAPE but recognize that they have limitations.

HIGH ALTITUDE PULMONARY EDEMA. (HAPE): Although described by Ravenhill in 1913, it was not until 1961 that HAPE was clearly differentiated from pneumonia by Charles Houston (11). In one case described by Houston, an individual died from HAPE within 8 hours of the onset of symptoms. A companion wrote the following description in his diary:

The next few hours W. B.'s breathing became progressively more congested and laboured. He sounded as though he were literally drowning in his own fluid, with an almost continual loud bubbling sound as if breathing through liquid. A couple of hours after his death, when we got up to carry on the day's activities, I noticed that a white froth resembling cotton candy had appeared to well up out of his mouth.

HAPE is a very serious illness but fortunately far less common than mild AMS. Incidence figures from most studies are around 1% (6), but vary from .57% to 15% (15, 19). HAPE is uncommon below 3,000 m. The first stages are usually gradual, and involve one or more characteristic symptoms of AMS. In some instances, however, the onset can be quite dramatic and can occur without warning. Respiratory symptoms progressively worsen and soon dominate the clinical picture. These include increasing breathlessness and a dry cough which later produces frothy and sometimes bloody sputum. The picture can rapidly change at any stage to one of stupor, coma, and death. Common findings on examination are cyanosis (often profound), tachycardia, low-grade fever, and crepitations. The chest x-ray of HAPE is characteristic: scattered opacities of pulmonary edema throughout both lungs, with a normal sized heart.

Prevention is similar to that of AMS. Ascent should be slow; strenuous exercise should be avoided in the first few days; and extra fluids, with no extra salt, should be taken. Effective treatment depends on early recognition. Mild cases may recover with a few days' rest, but if symptoms are worsening, immediate descent is imperative. Descent, even if only a few hundred meters, usually results in dramatic improvement, while a few more hours at the same altitude can be fatal. The rapidity with which death can ensue cannot be sufficiently stressed.

HIGH ALTITUDE CEREBRAL EDEMA. (HACE): HACE is less common than HAPE but equally, if not more, deadly. It is unusual below 4,000 m (14,000 ft), although it has led to death at altitudes as low as 3,048 m (10,000 ft). Hackett et al., in two studies of 522 trekkers at Periche in the Himalayas, found the incidence of HACE to be 0.96% (6, 7).

Headache is usually the first and worst symptom of HACE; but as a headache is very comon on ascent to altitude, it is not until other symptoms occur that HACE should be suspected. These other features include extreme fatigue, dizziness, hallucinations, double vision, nightmares, bizarre and irrational behavior, emotional lability, staggering gait (ataxia), difficulty with fine hand movements, and sometimes paralysis. Without descent, these symptoms are followed, often rapidly, by clouding of consciousness, stupor, coma, and death. The major warning signs are ataxia, mental confusion, and hallucinations.

Hallucinations can be visual and/or auditory. They are often vivid and commonly involve an imaginary companion. Houston, in his book *Going Higher* (9), cites the example of one skier who nearly died of HACE. The patient continued to see Marilyn Monroe, live and in color, on the hospital wall after descent.

The higher brain functions such as judgment, difficult decision-making, and appreciation of one's condition tend to be affected first in HACE. This can create further problems for victims, as they often refuse to believe that they are seriously ill and need to descend to a lower altitude.

Prevention of AMS and HAPE is the best management. Effective treatment depends on early recognition and immediate descent. Recovery may occur at any stage but once coma ensues, mortality is over 60% (3). Like HAPE, death can occur rapidly. The two conditions can occur together in the same individual.

OTHER ALTITUDE-RELATED CONDITIONS: Other syndromes which can occur at high altitude are summarized in Table 19-2. Most of these conditions are benign or, as is the case with Chronic Mountain Sickness, are not a problem for the visitor to high altitude.

Does Increasing Age Predispose to Altitude Illness?

The first major epidemiological study of the incidence of AMS was performed by Hackett et al. in 1975 (6). Questionnaires were distributed to 278 unacclimatized hikers passing through Periche, Nepal from October 10 to November 10. The investigators found that both the incidence and the severity

TABLE 19-3. *Comparison of variables in those with and without AMS. (Reproduced with permission from Hackett and Rennie.)*

Variable	No A.M.S.	A.M.S.	P
Age (yr)	35.2 ± 13.3 (19–71)	31.4 ± 9.7 (18–62)	0.029
Male (%)	70	72	N.S.
Female (%)	30	28	N.S.
Previous maximum altitude reached (m)	3770 ± 1300 (700–6000)	3914 ± 1137 (800–7300)	N.S.
Load carried (kg)	9.8 ± 5.5 (0.0–28)	8.8 ± 5.1 (0.0–22)	P = 0.1 (N.S.)
Walked to altitude (%)	52	34	
Flew to altitude (%)	48	66	
Maximum altitude attained (m)	5419 ± 3.56	5293 ± 4.20	< 0.01
Rate of ascent to highest altitude attained from 2800 m (m/d)	355 ± 72 (196–686)	393 ± 88 (212–722)	< 0.001
Rate of ascent to altitude where AMS developed (m/d)	..	397 ± 110 (152–722)	
Average no. of days to maximum altitude from 2800 m	8.1 ± 5.7 (3–14)	6.6 ± 2.0 (2–13)	$<10^{-6}$
Weight-loss as percentage of body weight	2.7 ± 2.8	2.0 ± 2.4	0.07
Weight-loss (kg)	1.9 ± 2.1 (0.0–8)	1.4 ± 1.7 (0.0–5)	P = 0.08 (N.S.)
Upper-respiratory-tract infection during trek (%)	35	38	N.S.

*Mean ± 1 S.D.; N.S. = not significant: P > 0.05.
Figures in parentheses give the range.

of AMS decreased with increasing age (Table 19-3). This finding was constant even when the data were corrected for rate of ascent. They concluded that the old argument that the young are more susceptible to altitude illness because they climb faster could not explain all the differences in incidence observed between the young and the old.

More recent work by both Hultgren et al. (13) and Scoggin et al. (18) adds support to the idea that the young are the most susceptible to development of altitude illness, in particular HAPE.

Hultgren and Marticorena observed that the incidence of HAPE per exposure is far more common below the age of 20 years. Their study was performed in the Andean mining city of La Oroya (3,750 m; 12,303 ft) in central Peru. The population of La Oroya is 40,000. A questionnaire was sent to 100 families who were selected on the basis of their residence in two communities adjacent to the Chulec General Hospital. The incidence of HAPE in these residents was expressed in terms of rapid exposures to high altitude. These exposures were defined as either an initial ascent or re-ascent to high altitude after two or more weeks at less than 1,500 m (4,920 ft). The re-ascent trip to La Oroya involves crossing a pass at Ticlio at 4,694 m (15,400 ft).

An episode of HAPE was defined by the appearance of the usual symptoms (cough, dyspnea, weakness, and fatigue) of sufficient severity to require either hospital admission or supervision of medical treatment by a physician. Chest x-rays were available in 83% of these cases and confirmed the clinical diagnosis of HAPE.

The overall incidence of HAPE per exposure was 6.1%. The incidence was much higher in the group aged 13 to 20 years old. In this group, 17% of ascents resulted in HAPE, and in the group 21 years and older, only 3% resulted in HAPE. Younger subjects also developed more severe episodes than adults.

Limitations of this study are that it was a retrospective study, that most of the cases of HAPE occurred on re-ascent of altitude residents rather than during initial ascent from sea level, and that the lower incidence of HAPE in adults over 21 may be due in part to greater use of precautionary measures and familiarity with the illness. Despite these limitations, these data are probably more reflective of the entire age span than Hackett's study which did not include any children and involved only 7 subjects 18 to 20 years old.

Scoggin et al. carried out a similar retrospective study in Leadville, Colorado, a mining and tourist community at 3,100 m (10, 170 ft). They analyzed hospital admissions between 1970 and 1977 in which a diagnosis of HAPE had been made and compared this with the number of residents of that particular age group in Lake County as determined by the 1970 Colorado census.

The overall yearly incidence of HAPE was found to be 50 per 100,000 people, but for those 1 to 14 years of age it was 140 per 100,000 people. Of the 32 cases that met the diagnostic criteria, all but 3 were less than 21 years old, with an average age of 11.9 years. Scoggin et al. also described 1 case history in which there was a decrease in the susceptibility to develop HAPE with increasing age. The authors suggested that there may be a tendency to outgrow a predisposition to HAPE. Limitations of this study are similar to those of the Hultgren and Marticorena study. Another limitation of this study is that only cases severe enough to warrant admission to a hospital were analyzed.

Thus, the available evidence suggests that far from being a disadvantage, increased age may actually provide protection against developing altitude illness, especially severe illness such as HAPE.

Concomitant Illness

More older people suffer from chronic diseases such as coronary artery disease, chronic obstructive pulmonary disease, and the arthritides. Most travel companies require a medical certificate for those traveling above 3,048 m (10,000 ft) and many require certificates for all travelers older than 60 years. How should the family doctor advise patients when asked, "Is it safe for me to go to altitude?"

There is a normal decline in arterial oxygen pressure with age (20) which will be accentuated by altitude (Fig. 19-1). However, for the healthy elderly person the answer is usually simple, and is found in the description of altitude illness and its prevention. The question regarding one's ability to go to altitude depends more on one's fitness than one's age, although for the person with underlying medical problems, the answers are often not black and white. Few data are available regarding the aggravation of common diseases by ascent to altitude, especially over 3,000 m. Above this altitude the oxygen content in arterial blood begins to fall sharply, especially on exercise.

Specific guidelines as to who should not go to altitude do not exist, and doctors disagree widely in their opinions of certain conditions. Charles Hous-

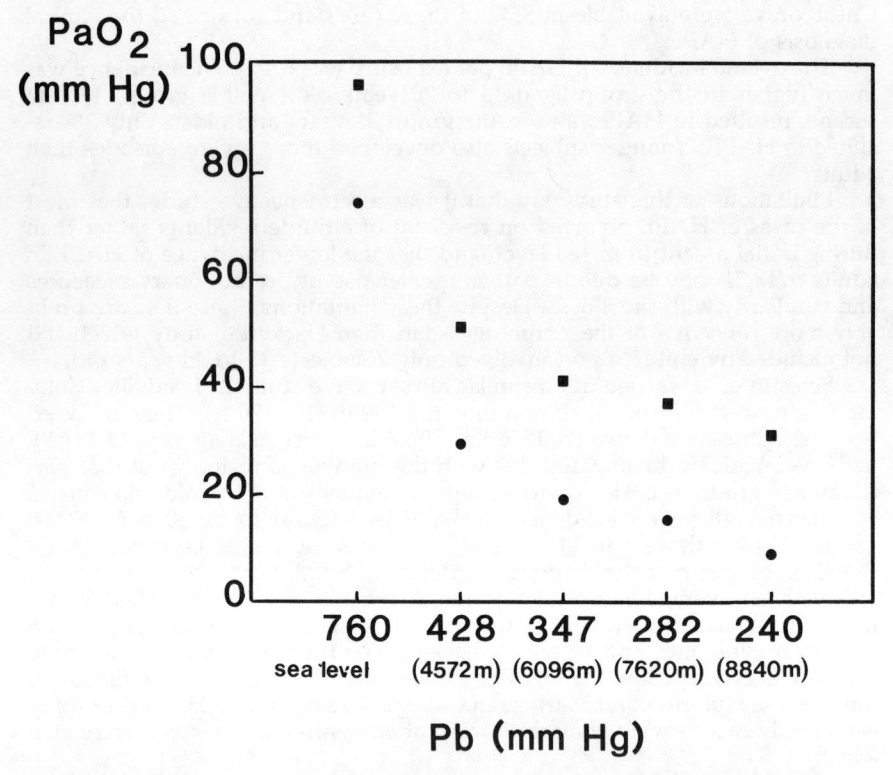

Fig. 19-1. Changes in PaO_2 with altitude. ■—Change in PaO_2 with altitude in subjects aged 18 to 30. ●—Predicted change in PaO_2 with altitude in subjects over 60 years based on sea level data from Sorbini et al. (20) assuming a similar change in A-a gradient and alveolar ventilation.

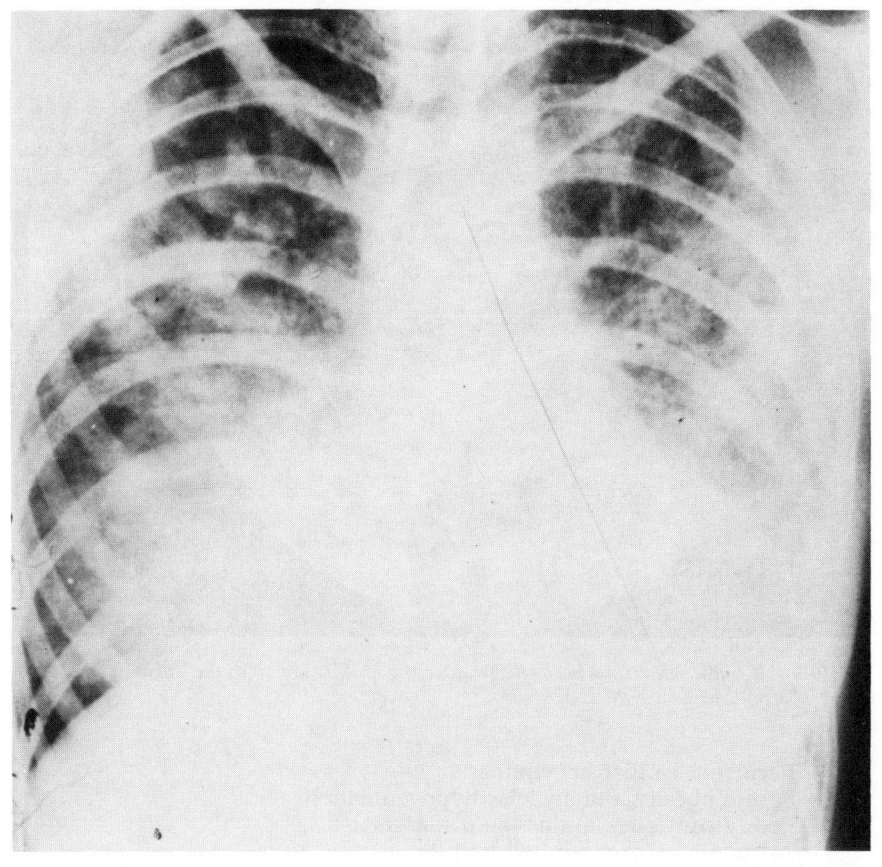

Fig. 19-2. *High altitude pulmonary edema. Chest x-ray of a 26-year-old who developed pulmonary edema in Cuzco.*

ton in his article, "Altitude Illness: The Dangers of High Altitude and How to Avoid Them" (9), provides a sensible working list of contraindications to high altitude travel.

Major contraindications are:

— Repeated attacks of HAPE or HACE
— Myocardial ischemia with frequent angina
— Severe, uncontrolled hypertension
— Congestive heart failure
— Advanced, disabling lung disease
— Sickle cell crisis
— Recurrent thromboembolic episodes

Minor contraindicatioans are:

— Mild angina with myocardial ischemia
— well-controlled congestive heart failure
— well-controlled hypertension

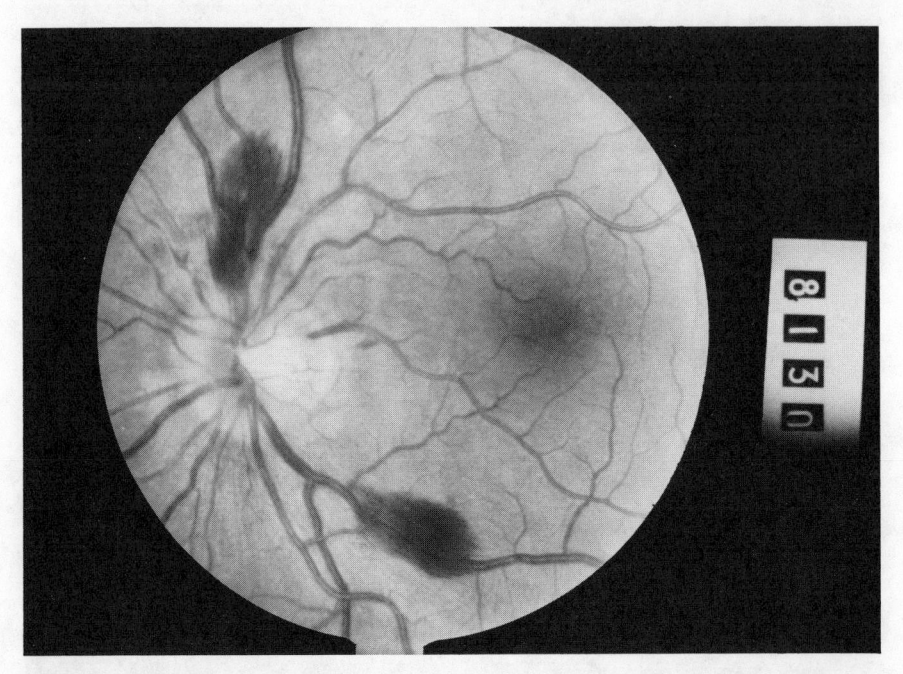

Fig. 19-3. *High altitude retinal hemorrhage occurring on Mt. Logan in the Yukon (photo courtesy of Murray McFadden, M.D.).*

— Recurrent cardiac arhythmias
— Severe obesity and alveolar hypoventilation
— Poorly controlled endocrine disorders
— Anemia and/or sickle cell trait

Because of widespread disagreement and lack of precise information, the practitioner may tend to err on the side of conservatism, wishing to avoid undue risk for the patient. This may lead to such persons foregoing the pleasure of mountain climbing or trekking. Each case must, of course, be considered separately and the advantages and disadvantages discussed for that individual. Further guidelines are found in Rennie and Wilson's article, "Who Should Not Go High" (17). Charles Houston (9) expresses our own sentiments:

> In general, the patient planning such travel who is moderately active at sea level, whose medical problems are under adequate control and who is willing to temper enthusiasm with caution and to be observant of any symptoms and descend if problems develop can be advised to "Go ahead."

The best recommendation that can be given to future travelers to altitude is to plan your trip well. First of all, ensure that you are booking through a respected trekking company. Carefully scrutinize your itinerary to check that sufficient time has been allowed for acclimatization. Recent recommendations (12) for effective and simple acclimatization include limiting ascent to 300 m per day when above 3,000 m, and taking one day's rest for every 600 meters gained above 3,600 m. In general, it is wise to climb high and sleep low.

Flight itineraries should also be scrutinized and the altitude of destinations noted. With air travel you are immediately lifted from sea level to a cabin pressure equivalent to around 2,000 m and your destination may be higher. Examples of this are the flights from Buenos Aires, Rio de Janeiro, or Lima at sea level to La Paz (3,664 m) (the highest international capital in the world). These flights almost guarantee that AMS will develop. Planning an itinerary which allows time to acclimatize with stopovers at lower altitudes is the best solution. For example, an alternate route for one of the above is: Lima to Ariquipa (2,440 m) to Cuzco (3,450 m) to La Paz. This route would allow time for acclimatization and yet still cover the spectacular sights of the Incan ruins. Hackett et al. (6) found a greater incidence of AMS in those who had flown from Katmandu to Lukla (2,800 m), before beginning their trek to the Everest base camp, compared with those who had walked from Katmandu to Lukla. Therefore, even greater care must be taken to ascend slowly if air travel takes you part of the way up.

Trekkers should be as fit as possible for the ascent. Those with medical problems should be encouraged to learn as much as possible about their own conditions, their medications, and the effects of altitude. A common example is the diabetic whose insulin freezes at around 0° C. Insulin should be carried near the body, and the patient should be informed that, even if frozen, the medication will still be active and fine to use when thawed. Most altitude-related problems can be prevented with good planning by trekking companies, physicians, and the traveler.

Altitude should not be seen as a barrier for those of advancing age. Many older people already travel to high altitude and there are few reasons why more should not. In fact, the risks of developing altitude illness may be less than in the young. Older people should be encouraged to remain active and fulfill their retirement dreams. As Robert Burton realized in 1621 (1), the best cure for melancholy is to travel, particularly to high altitude:

> like a long winged hawk . . . so will I, having now come at last into these ample fields of air, wherein I may freely expatiate and exercise myself for my recreation, awhile rove, wander around the world, mount aloft to those ethereal orbs and celestial spheres and so descend to my former elements again.

REFERENCES

1. Burton. R. *The Anatomy of Melancholy*. Part 2, 34–35. New York: Random House Inc., 1977.
2. Carp, F. M. Retirement travel. *The Gerontologist*. 11:73–78, 1972.
3. Clarke, C. High-altitude cerebral edema. *Med. Sport Sci.* 19:103–109, 1985.
4. Dickinson, J. G. High altitude cerebral edema: cerebral acute mountain sickness. *Sem. Resp. Med.* 5:151–158, 1983.
5. Gilbert, D. L. The first documented description of mountain sickness: The China or headache story. *Resp. Physiol.* 52:15–326, 1983.
6. Hackett, P. H., D. Rennie, and H. D. Levine. The Incidence, importance and prophylaxis of acute mountain sickness. *Lancet* 2:1149–1155, 1976.
7. Hackett, P. H., D. Rennie, and H. D. Levine. Rales, peripheral edema, retinal hemorrhage and acute mountain sickness. *Am. J. Med.* 67:214–218, 1979.
8. Hackett, P. H., D. Rennie, and H. D. Levine, Avoiding mountain sickness. *Lancet letter*. 2:938, 1978.
9. Houston, C. S. Altitude illness, The dangers of high altitude and how to avoid them. *Postgrad. Med.* 74:231–248, 1983.
10. Houston, C. S. *Going Higher*. 138–139. Burlington, VT: Queen City Printers Inc., 1983.
11. Houston, C. S. Acute pulmonary edema of high-altitude. *N. Engl. J. Med.* 263:478–480, 1960.
12. Huber, C. J. Preventive medicine for high-altitude trekking. *Can. Med. Assoc. J.* 134:404–407, 1986.

13. Hultgren, H. N., and E. M. Marticorena. High altitude pulmonary edema. Epidemiologic observations in Peru. *Chest* 74:372–376, 1978.
14. King, A. B., and S. M. Robinson. Ventilatory response to Hypoxia and acute mountain sickness. *Aviat. Space Environ. Med.* 43:419–421, 1972.
15. Menon, N. D. High-altitude pulmonary edema. *N. Engl. J. Med.* 273:66–73, 1965.
16. Ravenhill, T. H. Some experiences of mountain sickness in the Andes. *J. Trop. Med. Hyg.* 16:313–320, 1913.
17. Rennie, D., and R. Wilson. Who should not go high. In *Hypoxia, Man at Altitude*, J. R. Sutton, N. L. Jones, and C. S. Houston (eds.). New York: Thieme-Straton, Inc., 186–190, 1982.
18. Scoggin, C. H., T. M. Meyers, J. T. Reeves, and R. F. Grover. High-altitude edema in young adults of Leadville, Colorado. *N. Engl. J. Med.* 297:1269–1272, 1977.
19. Singh, M. B., C. C. Kapila, P. K. Khanna, R. B. Nanda, and B. D. Rao. *Lancet* 1:229–234, 1965.
20. Sorbini, C. A., V. Grassi, E. Solinas, and G. Muiesan. Arterial oxygen tension in relation to age in healthy subjects. *Respiration.* 25:3–13, 1968.
21. Sutton, J. R. Classification and terminology of altitude illnesses. *Sem. Resp. Med.* 5:129–131, 1983.
22. Sutton, J. R., A. C. Bryan, G. W. Gray, E. S. Horton, A. S. Rebuck, W. Woodley, I. D. Rennie, and C. S. Houston. Pulmonary gas exchange in acute mountain sickness. *Aviat. Space Environ. Med.* 47:1032–1037, 1976.

20

Exercise Performance At High Altitude

ROBERT B. SCHOENE, M.D.

University of Washington, Seattle

In the year of the first World Masters Games, it seems fitting that Mount Everest was climbed by a 55-year-old American. This feat flies in the face of a continual flow of youthful elite athletes who climb to the top of their sports. It also defies a number of points of exercise physiology related to both aging and high altitude that would suggest that this climb was not possible. In contrast, if the summit of Everest is to be reserved for elite climbers, then the young ages of elite track athletes are sharply contrasted to the ages of elite Himalayan climbers which span from the mid 20s to 50s.

Although the climber to extreme altitude is a much more heterogeneous, yet no less elite, athlete than the Olympic marathoner, Nordic skier, or swimmer, he or she still requires the proper balance of exceptional qualities such as aerobic capacity, muscle strength, biomechanics, nutrition, ventilatory drives, and motivation. In light of the fact that both aging and high altitude result in less than optimal effects on aerobic capacity, muscle strength, appetite and absorption, ventilatory drives, and motivation, it seemed unlikely that the aging climber could ever make it to altitudes greater than 8,000 meters (m). It will, therefore, be the focus of this paper to discuss some of the factors which contribute to and may predict success or failure in climbers at high altitude. Although we shall frequently refer to extreme altitude, the points also pertain to moderate altitudes where more climbers, both young and old, venture.

Climbing at extreme altitude requires prolonged work output at a relatively low level of intensity for many hours each day, for many days to weeks on end. It has long been known that exercise performance decreases the higher one ascends. Recent data from the 1981 American Medical Research Expedition to Everest (AMREE) emphasize this point and will be expanded further (19). To analyze why this phenomenon occurs, we shall review the various components of the oxygen cascade which may affect work output and impose a limit to performance. Furthermore, if work output is closely related to oxygen consumption, then the oxygen cascade must be analyzed with special reference to the Fick equation, the components of which are affected by adaptation to high altitude: [oxygen consumption ($\dot{V}O_2$) = cardiac output ($\dot{Q}$) × oxygen extraction or arterial-venous oxygen content difference].

TABLE 20-1.

	P_B(torr)	P_IO_2	P_AO_2	P_ACO_2	PaO_2
Sea level	760	149	99	40	95
8848 m	250	43	33	10	26

First, let us consider the decrease in barometric pressure (P_B) that occurs with increasing altitude. West and Wagner (14) reviewed this topic in a theoretical paper about gas exchange on the summit of Mount Everest at 8,848 m. Table 20–1 shows estimates of the oxygen cascade at sea level and 8,848 m.

These figures are, of course, based on a constant fraction of oxygen in our atmosphere of 0.2093, as well as approximate values of P_ACO_2, respiratory exchange ratios, and alveolar-arterial oxygen differences. The important point to be taken from these numbers is that alveolar and, subsequently, arterial oxygen partial pressure depends on the ventilatory response which is reflected by, and inversely proportional to, the alveolar carbon dioxide partial pressure (i.e., the greater the ventilatory response, the lower the alveolar carbon dioxide and the higher the oxygen partial pressure). Data collected on the 1981 AMREE (18) as well as earlier observations support the suggestion that at extreme altitude P_AO_2 is defended between 35 to 40 Torr by decreasing P_ACO_2 with an increased ventilation to extraordinary levels. On the same expedition, Dr. Chris Pizzo collected alveolar gas samples on the summit and found his P_ACO_2 to be 7.5 Torr. More recent direct measurements on the "summit" during Operation Everest II reveal P_AO_2 = 30.5.

Of course, this ability to decrease the P_ACO_2 to such low levels depends to a certain degree on one's inherent hypoxic ventilatory response (HVR). The HVR's of a number of climbers who had ascended to 7,500 m or greater were studied and found to be significantly higher than those of a group of controls as well as a group of endurance athletes (8). These findings suggested that a high ventilatory response at extreme altitude may be helpful in climbing to these altitudes. In a follow-up study in climbers on Mount Everest, Schoene et al. (9) noted a relationship between HVR at sea level, HVR at altitude, exercise ventilation, and performance at extreme altitude. These findings supported the hypothesis of the earlier study. It seems, therefore, that, unlike the elite endurance athlete at low altitude who may benefit from low ventilatory drives and a lower exercise ventilation (1), the climber to extreme altitude may benefit from a brisk HVR.

A brisk HVR is not, however, a prerequisite for climbing to extreme altitude. We have recently collected data on an elite high altitude climber, an Everest summiter without supplemental oxygen. His hypoxic chemosensitivity, studied both on Mt. McKinley as well as at sea level, was found to be quite blunted ($\Delta \dot{V}_E/\Delta SAO_2$ = −0.05 at 4,400 m and −0.2 at sea level) (10). These motivated and talented individuals must invoke other attributes to ascend to the world's highest summits.

Increasing evidence is accumulating, however, which links blunted HVR and hypoventilation to altitude illnesses, and this parameter may play a permissive role in illness at high altitude (3, 5, 6). Presumably, a blunted HVR would result in more profound hypoxemia and relative hypercapnia, both of which may result in greater cerebral blood flow as well as greater pulmonary hypertension. The former may contribute to headache, the most common symptom in acute mountain sickness, while the latter may lead to pulmonary vascular damage and subsequent high altitude pulmonary edema (HAPE). In a recent study on Mt. McKinley, Hackett et al. (3) found climbers to have very blunted hypoxic chemosensitivity, both during and after recovery from HAPE, as compared to controls. Whatever its role, the ventilatory response to high altitudes plays an important part in one's adaptation, performance, and survival in these environs.

West et al. (19) also showed in climbers on Mount Everest that the climber is probably not limited by ventilation per se. Maximum exercise ventilation ($\dot{V}_{Emax}$) was actually lower above 8,000 m than at 6,300 m, suggesting this lower degree of ventilation may be secondary to a low work rate and metabolic demand for ventilation as well as the marked respiratory alkalosis. Respiratory muscle fatigue may also be important. Recent studies on Operation Everest II suggest that peripheral factors in muscle fatigue may be as limiting to exercise as dyspnea.

Limitation to exercise performance probably depends on several other complex phenomena. Maximum oxygen uptake ($\dot{V}O_{2max}$) decreases with increasing altitude (19). A controversy exists as to how important the actual level of $\dot{V}O_{2max}$ is to success at extreme altitude. Clearly, a high $\dot{V}O_{2max}$ is a prerequisite to performance for elite athletes in low altitude competitions such as rowing, middle- and long-distance running, and Nordic skiing, but it is not clear that an extraordinary $\dot{V}O_{2max}$ is necessary for high altitude success. Again, on Mount Everest, West et al. (19) showed that while breathing a low oxygen mixture to simulate 8,848 m, $\dot{V}O_{2max}$ was about 20% of sea level $\dot{V}O_{2max}$. These climbers all had levels of $\dot{V}O_{2max}$ at sea level that were well above the normal range, so that 20% of those values still left them with a value that allowed for at least low levels of work. These findings documented how some exceptional climbers can climb 8,000 m peaks without supplemental oxygen. It is probably prudent to say that individuals with normal $\dot{V}O_{2max}$ levels cannot climb to extreme altitude, but how high this inherent characteristic need be is not clear. A more important factor may be how close to one's anaerobic threshold a climber can perform for prolonged periods of time. In other words, in a sport that requires prolonged submaximal exercise, $\dot{V}O_{2max}$ may not be the important variable. Further work is necessary to clarify this issue.

Another component of the oxygen cascade plays a significant role in limiting performance at high altitude. This component involves the gas-phase and the blood-phase of oxygen transport and is discussed by West and Wagner (17). Whereas, at sea level, ventilation and perfusion relationships ($\dot{V}/\dot{Q}$) and diffusion of oxygen from the alveolus to the pulmonary capillary do not limit oxygen transport to a significant degree, these factors are of primary importance at high altitude. Using the multiple inert gas elimination technique during hypoxic exercise, Torre-Buenos et al. (15), Gale et al. (4), and Wagner et al. (16) demonstrated a mild but probably significant degree of $\dot{V}/\dot{Q}$ heterogeneity in addition to diffusion limitation which imposes further limitation to oxygen transport at the alveolar level. The more significant factor is probably diffusion limitation of oxygen transport at the alveolar level. This phenomenon may occur at sea level in athletes with extremely high cardiac outputs at maximum exercise, but otherwise, is unusual (2). At sea level, the equilibration of alveolar oxygen with pulmonary capillary blood takes place comfortably within approximately 0.25 seconds during the estimated traverse time of approximately 0.75 seconds of the red blood cell across the pulmonary capillary. At extreme altitude, however, full equilibration does not take place. This limit is partly caused by an increased cardiac output and decreased transit time. With the above considerations it seems, therefore, that limitations to performance at altitude are already imposed by low barometric pressure, ventilatory response, V/Q heterogeneity, and diffusion limitation of oxygen at the alveolar-capillary level.

Other considerations remain speculative, but are related to oxygen delivery at the tissue level. First, the ventilatory response at extreme altitude certainly imposes a marked blood alkalemia (18). This condition shifts the oxyhemoglobin curve to the left and increases the affinity of oxygen for hemoglobin, which improves the pick-up of oxygen at the alveolus, but may impair the unloading of oxygen at the tissue level. Recent work in dogs during hypoxic exercise (11) suggested that a left-shifted oxyhemoglobin curve provided a higher arterial and lower mixed venous oxygen content without a significant change in cardiac output. The higher diffusion gradient of oxygen from the blood to the tissues presumably overcomes the greater affinity of oxygen for hemoglobin. The naturally occurring left-shift at extreme altitude in humans and some animals may, therefore, be advantageous. What actually happens at the tissues is not known. Tissue adaptation to exercise as well as to altitude, which includes an increase in mitochondrial density and size and increased capillarity of the tissues, may facilitate oxygen utilization in the tissues. These adaptations decrease the distance which oxygen transverses and may minimize or ablate this potentially detrimental leftward shift of the oxyhemoglobin curve.

Oxygen delivery is dependent on cardiac output which may be impaired at altitude. Again on Everest, West et al. (19) noted a progressive decrease in maximum heart rate from sea level to the summit of Everest. It is not known whether this finding is secondary to myocardial or nodal hypoxic depression, to hypervagal tone, or to a decreased metabolic demand from a low exercise level; but since there is a predictable relationship between cardiac output and $\dot{V}O_2$, it is probably secondary to the last factor. This is supported by recent studies in Operation Everest II which show no impairment of cardiac output as measured by the direct Fick technique for a given oxygen consumption, even on the summit (14).

We, therefore can consider a significant number of barriers to oxygen delivery that is exaggerated by hypoxia of extreme altitude (Table 20-2).

We have, therefore, documented limitations at every level of the oxygen cascade which are grossly exaggerated at extreme altitude and which clearly impair work output. Although it is not clear which of these factors impairs oxygen transport at sea level, it is probably safe to say that the hypoxic environment of high altitude merely accentuates the impairment of exercise performance that occurs at most levels of the oxygen cascade at sea level.

Finally, I would like to consider one other factor which may be the key

TABLE 20-2. *Barriers to Oxygen Delivery at High Altitudes*

A. Gas phase
   Barometric pressure
   Alveolar ventilation
   Ventilation/perfusion mismatch

B. Blood phase
   Diffusion limitation
   Steepness of oxyhemoglobin dissociation curve
   Cardiac output

C. Tissue phase
   Decreased diffusion gradient from blood to tissue
   Limit to adaptation of oxidative pathway
   Perfusion of microcirculation

to it all. Let us consider a human exercising sub-maximally in a state in which lactic acid production is decreased. Also, ventilation is probably not limited. Theoretically, physical performance should not be limited. Why, then, is it so difficult to function at extreme altitude?

A number of climbers in this environment anecdotally related several instances during which their vision and mental acuity decreased while carrying out physical tasks that were excessive. A number of summit climbs have been marked by hallucinations and dimness of both thought and vision. All of these experiences abated when the individuals slowed down their pace or used supplemental oxygen.

I would now like to take some excerpts from a talk given by Dr. Thomas Horenbein at the 1983 Banff Hypoxia Symposium. Dr. Hornbein was a summit climber along the uncharted West Ridge of Everest in 1963:

> I believe that the brain, rather than exercising muscle, is the organ ultimately limiting function at extreme altitude. One wonders whether the cerebral vasoconstriction consequent to acute hypocapnia might also contribute to brain hypoxia. If so, one can imagine being able to work close to maximum for prolonged periods of time without difficulty. Reflecting upon the many decades during which physiologists have searched for the magic predictor of high altitude performance and extrapolating from my own experience during an oxygen-assisted ascent of Everest two decades ago, I am fascinated as a physiologist by the questions of performance at these extremes of altitude even as I am awed at our temerity in attempting to predict who and who will not perform well in such an environment. From all these ruminations, I feel certain of only one attribute without which I cannot imagine success: desire. Physiologically, I suspect there is more than one way to skin a cat, and an endurance athlete with low ventilatory responses may find other virtues to invoke. There ought to be an optimum mix of physiologic attributes, but to separate them from the other elements of a successful event—climbing virtuosity, motivation, and luck—may defy the best efforts of even the most imaginative physiologist. Whatever the elements, a single-minded intensity of purpose seems an important ingredient in many of life's aspirations, the climbing of Everest being but one. (5)

I think it seems safe, therefore, to say that the normal physiological measurements of exercise performance which we physiologists make are interesting, but may be missing the most important organ that will get us to the summit of Everest. Cerebral hypoxia from whatever cause clearly has a most profound depressant effect upon desire and motivation. In keeping with the spirit of the First World Masters Games, I would again like to extract a quotation from Dr. Hornbein's paper (5) that he in turn had borrowed from W. H. Murray:

> Until one is committed, there is hesitancy, the chance to draw back, always ineffectiveness. Concerning all acts of initiative (and creation), there is one elementary truth, the ignorance of which kills countless ideas and splendid plans: that the moment one definitely commits oneself, then Providence moves too. All sorts of things occur to help one that would never otherwise have occurred. A whole stream of events issues from the decision, raising in one's favor all manner of unforeseen incidents and meetings and material assistance, which no man could have dreamt would have come

his way. I have learned a deep respect for one of Goethe's couplets:

> Whatever you can do, or dream you can, begin it.
> Boldness has genius, power and magic in it.

There are no research tools which can measure these intangibles. There are, however, tools of curiosity and joy in one's work and play that lift the human spirit to achievements beyond what can be measured.

REFERENCES

1. Byne-Quinn, E., J. V. Weil, I. E. Sodal, G. F. Filley, and R. F. Grover. Ventilatory control in the athlete. *J. Appl. Physiol.: REEP* 30:91–98, 1981.
2. Dempsey, J. A., P. G. Hanson, and K. S. Henderson. Exercise-induced arterial hypoxaemia in healthy human subjects at sea level. *J. Physiol.* (Lond.) 355:161–175, 1984.
3. Gale, G. E., J. R. Torre-Bueno, R. E. Moon, H. A. Sultzman, and P. D. Wagner. Ventilation-perfusion inequality in normal humans during exercise at sea level and simulated altitude. *J. Appl. Physiol.* 58:978–988, 1985.
4. Hackett, P. H., R. B. Schoene, R. C. Roach, G. Harrison, and W. J. Mills, Jr. Blunted chemosensitivity and hypoxic ventilatory response in high altitude pulmonary edema. *Fed. Proc.* 44:1563, 1985.
5. Hornbein, T. F. Everest without oxygen. In: *Hypoxia, Exercise and Altitude*, J. R. Sutton, C. S. Houston, and N. L. Jones (eds.) 409–414. New York: A. R. Liss, Inc., 1983.
6. King, A. B., and S. M. Robinson. Ventilation response to hypoxia and acute mountain sickness. *Aviat. Space Environ. Med.* 43:419–421, 1972.
7. Lakshminarayan, S., and D. J. Pierson. Recurrent high altitude pulmonary edema with blunted chemosensitivity. *Am. Rev. Resp. Dis.* 111:869–872, 1975.
8. Larson, E. B., R. C. Roach, R. B. Schoene, and T. F. Hornbein. Acute mountain sickness and acetazolamide: Clinical efficacy and effect on ventilation. *J.A.M.A.* 248:328–332, 1982.
9. Schoene, R. B. The control of ventilation in climbers to extreme altitude. *J. Appl. Physiol.: REEP* 53:886–890, 1982.
10. Schoene, R. B., S. Lahiri, P. H. Hackett, R. M. Peters, Jr., J. S. Milledge, C. J. Pizzo, F. H. Sarnquist, S. J. Boyer, D. J. Graber, K. H. Maret, and J. B. West. Relationship of hypoxic ventilatory response to exercise performance on Mount Everest. *J. Appl. Physiol.: REEP* 56:1478–1483, 1984.
11. Schoene, R. B., R. C. Roach, and P. H. Hackett. Blunted hypoxic chemosensitivity at altitude and sea level in an elite high altitude climber. In: *Hypoxia and Cold*, J. R. Sutton, C. S. Houston and G. Coates (eds.) Abstract #7. Philadelphia: Praeger Publishers, 1986.
12. Schumacker, P. T., B. Guth, A. J. Sugget, P. D. Wagner, and J. B. West. Role of hemoglobin P_{50} in O_2 transport during normoxic and hypoxic exercise in the dog. *J. Appl. Physiol.* 58:749–757, 1985.
13. Sutton, J. R., A. C. Bryan, G. W. Gray, E. S. Horton, A. S. Rebuck, W. Woodley, I. D. Rennie, and C. S. Houston. Pulmonary gas exchange in acute mountain sickness. *Aviat. Space Environ. Med.* 47:1032–1037, 1976.
14. Sutton, J. R., A. Cymerman, B. M. Groves, M. K. Malconian, J. T. Reeves, P. D. Wagner, P. Young, and C. S. Houston. Severe arterial hypoxemia at rest and during exercise at extreme simulated altitude—Operation Everest II. *Am. Rev. Resp. Dis.* 133: (In press), 1986.
15. Sutton, J. R., A. Cymerman, P. Rock, P. Young, A. Young, P. Bangs, and C. S. Houston. Maximum ventilation, lactate and perceived exertion at extreme simulated altitude—Operation Everest II. *Med. Sci. Sports. Exerc.* 18:(In press), 1986.
16. Torre-Bueno, J. R., P. D. Wagner, H. A. Sultzman, G. E. Gale, and R. E. Mood. Diffusion limitation in normal humans during exercise at sea level and simulated altitude. *J. Appl. Physiol.* 58:989–995, 1985.
17. Wagner, P. D., G. E. Gale, R. E. Moon, J. R. Torre-Bueno, B. W. Stolp, and H. A. Saltzman. Pulmonary gas exchange in humans exercising at sea level and simulated altitude. *J. Appl. Physiol.* 59:(In press), 1986.
18. West, J. B., and P. D. Wagner. Predicted gas exchange on the summit of Mount Everest. *Respir. Physiol.* 41:1–16, 1980.
19. West, J. B., S. J. Boyer, D. J. Graber, P. H. Hackett, K. H. Maret, J. S. Milledge, R. M. Peters, Jr., C. J. Pizzo, M. Samaja, F. H. Sarnquist, R. B. Schoene, and R. M. Winslow. Maximal exercise at extreme altitude on Mount Everest. *J. Appl. Physiol.:REEP* 55:688–698, 1983.
20. West, J. B., P. H. Hackett, K. H. Maret, J. S. Milledge, R. M. Peters, Jr., C. J. Pizzo, and R. M. Winslow. Pulmonary gas exchange on the summit of Mount Everest. *J. Appl. Physiol.:REEP* 55:678–687, 1983.

Section V
Mind and Eye

21

Psychology of the Masters Athlete: Motivational Considerations

ALBERT CARRON

University of Western Ontario

LARRY LEITH

Lakehead University

Given the potential breadth and depth of "the psychology of the masters athlete," we have chosen to focus on one specific psychological construct—motivation. Motivation, which comes from the Latin word *movere*, to move, is the theoretical construct which is used to represent the selectivity, the intensity, and the persistence which underlie human behavior. Motivation may be the single most important factor influencing the performance effectiveness of the masters athlete.

This suggestion is not intended to minimize the importance of the physiological factors. It has been well documented that with increasing chronological age there are marked changes in physiological function—decreased function in the cardiovascular systems, loss of flexibility, decreased muscular strength and endurance, and impaired neurohormonal control mechanisms (4).

Thus, any discussion of the masters athlete must acknowledge that there are many factors which contribute to or detract from performance effectiveness. Nonetheless, the suggestion that motivation may be the single most important factor influencing performance effectivenss is well warranted. Certainly, in the case of other world class athletes this is true. For example, Ryder, Carr, and Herget (3) examined patterns and trends in world records for sprint and endurance events over the past 50 years. Essentially, they were interested in the question of whether we can reasonably expect a leveling off in performance standards, whether world records are rapidly approaching a ceiling. The conclusion was that they are not. They noted that most world record holders have retired in their prime shortly after achieving their personal best. On the basis of their performance analyses, Ryder, Carr, and Herget concluded that the current limiters of performance are not anatomical, physiological, or biomechanical, but psychological. Moreover, the authors felt that the critical psychological considerations are those affecting daily training

233

and not those in the event itself. Athletes simply cannot maintain their motivation consistently.

In this chapter, a number of techniques which could be used to maintain or enhance motivation of the masters athlete are discussed. Prior to their introduction, however, it is useful to examine how motivation in sport and physical activity should be considered.

A MOTIVATION MODEL

Carron (1) has presented a frame of reference for the analysis of motivation in the context of sport and physical activity (Fig. 21–1). One important aspect of the model presented in Fig. 21-1 is that it emanates from the long accepted view in psychology that behavior (B) is a joint product of personal factors (P) and environmental factors (E), or

$$B = (P,E)$$

It follows directly from this equation that motivated behavior in sport and physical activity is a product of factors within the athlete and factors in the environment.

Another important aspect of this frame of reference is that both personal and situational factors must be considered from 2 perspectives: those that are readily influenced and those that are not. Thus, for example, 2 factors from within the sport situation which can contribute to an athlete's motivation are the presence of an audience and the nature of the practice session. The athlete has little or no control over whether an audience is present (i.e., as a moti-

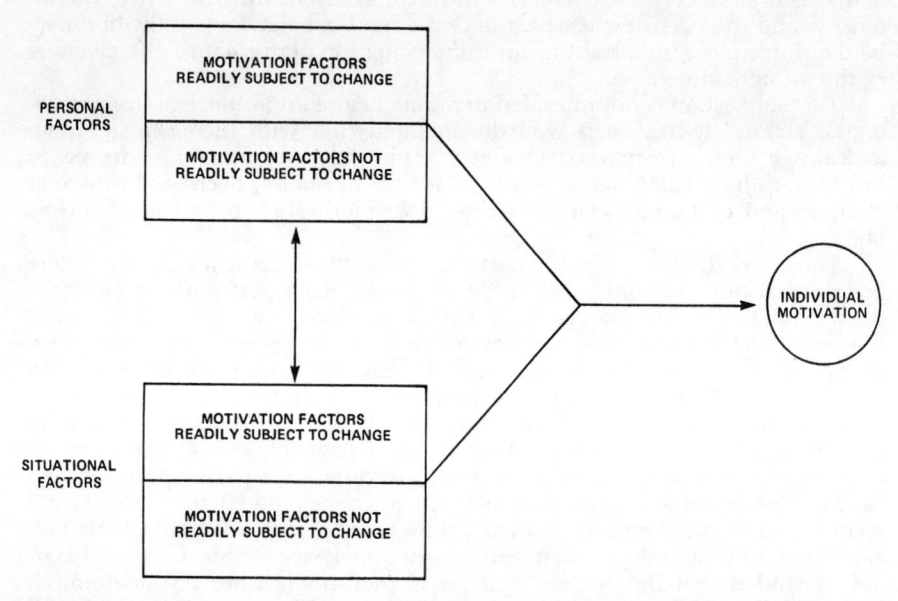

Fig. 21-1. *A model for motivation in sport. Reproduced from Ref. 1 with permission of the editor, 1984.*

TABLE 21-1. *Factors Contributing to Motivation in Sport and Physical Activity*

PERSONAL FACTORS	READILY SUBJECT TO CHANGE	Incentive Motivation Analysis of the Outcome Intrinsic Interest Expectation of Others Self-Confidence
	NOT READILY SUBJECT TO CHANGE	Anxiety Need for Achievement Attention Control
SITUATIONAL FACTORS	READILY SUBJECT TO CHANGE	Token Rewards Goal Setting Practice Session Social Reinforcement Leadership Behavior
	NOT READILY SUBJECT TO CHANGE	Presence of Others Type of Competition Team

vational factor it cannot be readily influenced). The practice session, however, can be readily modified to ensure that variety in situations and experiences is available. This variety, in turn, contributes to motivation.

In the same vein, 2 factors within the athlete that contribute to the overall level of motivated behavior are the personality trait of need for achievement and the degree of intrinsic motivation present. An individual's personality is relatively stable and is only modified slowly over a long period of time (i.e., as a motivational factor, it is not readily modified from day to day or moment to moment). On the other hand, it is possible to readily influence the level of intrinsic motivation of the athlete.

Carron has used this frame of reference to present a wide variety of motivational factors (Table 21-1) and discuss their general implications for coaching and teaching (1). In this chapter, 4 motivational factors particularly relevant to the performance of the masters athlete are examined in detail. Three of these are motivational factors within the athlete's situation which are readily subject to influence—goal setting, token rewards, and the practice session. The other is a motivational factor within the athlete which is also readily subject to influence—the attributions for causation. Each of the motivational factors is treated identically. First, a general summary principle is outlined. Second, a brief explanation and some sample illustrations of that principle are provided. And finally, workshop exercises are set out in order to show how the motivational principle could be utilized.

GOAL SETTING

Principle: Goal setting can be used as a motivator for performance.

Every coach and athlete knows from experience that some motivational techniques work better than others. A thorough review of related research leads to the conclusion that goal setting is one such technique. For example, Locke, Shaw, Saari, and Latham (1981) have summed up the goal setting research findings as follows: "The beneficial effect of goal setting on task performance is one of the most robust and replicable findings in the psychological literature. Ninety percent of the studies showed positive or partially positive effects" (2).

Because goal setting is such a powerful motivator, it is important to realize that its effects can be either positive or negative, depending upon the appropriateness of the goal. Inappropriate goals can lead to serious problems. This often happens when athletes set goals which are too difficult to attain. For example, an athlete may set a personal goal to run the mile in a time of 4:50 by the end of the track season. If that athlete's previous best was 6:00, the goal could be inappropriate. And, setting the goal might lead to overtraining, the development of an overuse injury, and/or frustration and discouragement.

Another example of an inappropriate goal would be if a masters athlete sets a specific goal based upon personal standards which were reasonable 5 years previously. Unless training has progressed over the interim, frustration and a decline in motivation could result.

On the other hand, appropriate goals can lead to positive results. Consider for example, the untrained octogenarian who wants to improve personal fitness. An appropriate goal in this case would be to walk around the block once a day for a week. At the end of that period, the goal could be adjusted upward. This example, of course, parallels the Canadian government's *Participation* model.

Another example of appropriate goal setting would be a masters athlete who wants to improve his or her time for the marathon. Because research has indicated that a runner can expect a 2-second-per-mile improvement in time for every pound of weight lost, the athlete could set a 5-pound weight loss as a goal.

In summary, goal setting is a powerful motivator but it is important that appropriate goals be set. The exercise outlined in Table 21–2 which is patterned after an approach developed by Singer (5) provides practical experience in setting appropriate goals.

TABLE 21-2. *Exercise for Goal Setting*

SELF-ANALYSIS								
Sport Factor				Self-Rating				
Strategy	Poor	1	2	3	4	5	Excellent
Performance Skills	Poor	1	2	3	4	5	Excellent
Physical Development	Poor	1	2	3	4	5	Excellent
Psychological Skills	Poor	1	2	3	4	5	Excellent
GOAL SETTING PROCEDURE								
1) Break down your individual sport into areas of importance. 2) Pick one area in which you would like to improve. 3) Where would you like to be relative to where you are now in regard to that factor? 4) What *specifically* is needed to improve (e.g., time, money)? 5) What is the maximum/minimum that you personally can give to attain this improvement? 6) Set your specific goal(s). 7) Set up a weekly (or monthly) program to attain these goals.								

TOKEN REWARDS

Principle: Token rewards can be used as a motivator for performance.

During the past several years, token reinforcers have enjoyed increased popularity in educational and sport situations. Essentially, a token reinforcer is something that has symbolic value or value because it can be exchanged for a back-up reinforcer of greater value to the individual. In the latter case, the individual is given token rewards (poker chips, points, stars) for appropriate behavior. These tokens can then be traded for something which is more tangible (a T-shirt, a pizza). Token rewards can be used to eliminate undesirable behavior or to enhance desirable behavior. In both cases, individual performance should be improved.

In general, the use of token rewards is a form of contingency management which takes the form "given outcome A, then outcome B." For example, a masters athlete may want to improve his or her weekly running mileage. A token reward system could be set up whereby the athlete received one point for every mile run. The achievement of a set of number of points could then be rewarded—a pizza, an expensive pair of shoes. In this example the token rewards have been used to promote a desirable behavior.

As indicated above, a token reward system also can be used to eliminate undesirable behavior. For example, a tennis player may consistently play exhibition matches rather than spend time practicing on a weak stroke. This player could be placed on a token reward system whereby one point was awarded for each hour spent practicing fundamentals. When a predetermined number of points was accumulated, they could be traded in for time to play exhibition matches.

TABLE 21-3. *Exercise for Token Rewards*

Given . . .	Then . . .
PROMOTING DESIRABLE BEHAVIOR	
e.g., that I train every day this week (1 point/day trained)	. . . I'll treat myself to a pizza Friday night (5 points for a pizza)
ELIMINATING UNDESIRABLE BEHAVIOR	
e.g., that I don't have any alcohol in the next two weeks (1 point per day of no drinking)	. . . then I'll reward myself with that new book on training that I've wanted (14 points for the book)

In summary, token rewards, used as symbols or as a means to a more meaningful reward, can be used to enhance desirable behavior or to eliminate or reduce undesirable behavior. Table 21-3 contains a format which can be used to develop an appropriate contingency management program.

PRACTICE SESSION

Principle: Introducing novelty and changes in the routine of a practice can be used as a motivator for performance.

When an athlete does the same thing day after day, week after week, mental fatigue and boredom invariably set in and the result is decreased motivation for training. Thus, a problem faced by all coaches, particularly those coaching elite athletes (who by nature of their involvement spend a relatively greater amount of time in practice) is to design challenging, stimulating practice sessions. Certainly, research indicates that "motivation can be increased through the introduction of novelty, a change of routine and/or by providing special attention to the athlete" (1).[1]

This principle can be illustrated with the masters athlete who continually runs 60 to 70 miles per week in training. If all of these miles are LSD (long, slow distance), motivation to maintain training at a high intensity will invariably decrease. What is necessary is the introduction of sessions devoted to hill training, fartlek, repetitions, simulated races, or some other form of conditioning activity. Through the introduction of these novel techniques, the athlete's training will become far less boring.

Teams also can profit by capitalizing on this principle. For example, a basketball coach might use the same practice format every day. Consequently, that coach and each athlete would know exactly what skills would be practiced at any given time in the session. The result would be boredom and a loss of motivation. Conversely, the introduction of novel drills, game simulations, and adapted games (e.g., restricting the dribbler to two bounces before passing) would lead to an increased motivation to attend practice and put out maximum effort.

In summary, a change in the routine of practice can act as a motivator to performance. The chart in Table 21-4 can be used to identify training routines currently used as well as modifications which could be used to enhance motivation.

TABLE 21-4. *Exercise to Increase Novelty in a Practice Session*

What I/we do now . . .	Possible modifications . . .
Tennis serves—30 minutes; ground strokes with machine—30 minutes; rally with partner—30 minutes	Adapted touch game—underhand serve puts ball in play, then use service court boundaries. Simulated match play—1 set. Serve into hula-hoops—15 min.

PERCEPTIONS OF CAUSATION

Principle: An athlete's perceptions of the causes of an outcome can serve as a motivator for subsequent performance.

Every athlete analyzes the causes of success or failure after a particular competition—an attempt to determine the reasons for winning or losing. These perceived causes are referred to as "attributions." In a general sense, a causal attribution may be to internal or external factors. Internal attributions are involved when the athlete assumes personal responsibility for an outcome. Lack of effort or inadequate ability would be examples in this regard. External attributions are involved when the athlete perceives that factors in the situation

---

[1]This discussion is essentially a synopsis of Carron. The interested reader may wish to examine that work.

(and outside of personal control) were responsible for the outcome. Blaming the referee, a bad bounce, or poor weather conditions would be examples of this. The important point is that if attributions are not realistic, they may lead to decreased motivation and poorer performance.

One noteworthy example of a faulty attribution is the "learned helplessness" that many national or Olympic teams develop when they compete in international sport. The athletes and their teams develop an inferiority complex in competitions against Eastern bloc countries and the argument is advanced implicitly or explicitly that "we will never beat them because of their . . . coaching, use of steroids, advanced sport technology, superior training facilities, and so on." The major problem with this type of attribution is that it is made to external factors. Thus, it can have a negative impact on motivation. The athletes may decide there is no use concentrating on effort, ability, training, improved techniques, and so on if they are not the primary determinants of the outcome.

In summary, the perceptions an athlete holds of the causes of an outcome can influence motivation for subsequent performance. An attribution to internal factors can increase motivation while an attribution to external factors can reduce motivation. The chart in Table 21-5 can be used to re-examine a previous competition. Identifying personal factors that possibly contributed to the outcome should serve to highlight areas for possible improvement.

TABLE 21-5. *Exercise for Altering the Perceptions of Causation to Internal Factors*

Perceived causes for outcome of event	Origin of cause	Other possible personal causes	Possible areas for improvement
Bad call by referee	external	let myself be distracted	concentration training
Got boxed in during 1500 m race	external	not enough anaerobic work, too slow a start	speed work, fartlek

REFERENCES

1. Carron, A. V. *Motivation: Implications for coaching and teaching.* London, Ontario: Sports Dynamics, 1984.
2. Locke, To come.
3. Ryder, H. W., H. J. Carr, and P. Herget. Future performance in footracing. *Scientific American,* 1976.
4. Shephard, R. J. Physiological aspects of recreational activity. *Recreation Research Review,* 9:48–65, 1982.
5. Singer, R. N. *Sustaining motivation in sport.* Tallahassee, Florida: Sport Consultants, 1984.

22

Cognitive Psychology: A Viable Alternative to Overtraining in Masters Runners

LARRY M. LEITH

Lakehead University

What I would like to do in this brief chapter is present cognitive psychology as a viable alternative to overtraining in masters runners. Specifically, this chapter has the following 3 purposes:

1. to familiarize the runner with general strategies for mental preparation in sport;
2. to suggest the development of mental race strategies;
3. to recommend experimentation with these techniques to improve personal bests and avoid overuse injuries.

Much of the following material is adapted from the *National Coaching Certification Manual* (1), especially the Sport Psychology section. The remainder will apply this information solely to the sport of running.

GENERAL STRATEGIES FOR MENTAL PREPARATION IN RUNNING

Several sport psychological techniques underlie the runners' potential for improving their running with their minds. The most relevant of these will now be examined with specific examples from the world of competitive running.

Relaxation

Much information on the topic of relaxation has been generated in the last few years. Whether the runner is aiming at a championship, a personal best, or merely trying to finish, the tendency exists to get a bit nervous. This nervousness can drain a runner's energy, especially if it results in trouble getting to sleep. If this situation seems at all familiar, you will be happy to learn that certain relaxation techniques have been found to help alleviate the problem. One such method is referred to as progressive muscular relaxation (PMR). With PMR, the runner learns to systematically tense and then relax specific muscle groups. Other techniques such as controlled breathing, belly-breathing, and three-part breathing are available. A runner seeking to explore this area is encouraged to experiment with different techniques to find the one(s) that work best for him or her. Although the most obvious time to utilize this technique is when you go to bed on the eve of the race, it can actually prove beneficial when used throughout the day on a variety of occasions. Other runners may find it helpful to perform before heading to the race site. In summary, while the best time to use relaxation training is an individual matter, it is important to remember that it can help avoid wasting nervous energy which could be better utilized during the race itself. Some evidence also exists indicating that the utilization of relaxation techniques can help the runner avoid tying up or prematurely hitting the wall. The reason for this stems from the fact that a tense runner is a less efficient runner.

Imagery/Visualization

Another value of being relaxed is that it increases receptivity to new ideas and points of view—something like being hypnotized. When in a totally relaxed state, it becomes much easier to picture yourself doing well in a race. With practice, runners can actually learn to see such fine details as the colors of their race numbers or running shorts. More specifically, it also becomes possible to imagine yourself crossing the finish line, setting a personal best, and feeling really satisfied. This helps the runner build up self-confidence and positively reinforces training efforts. Basically speaking, there are two main types of imagery. In dissociative imagery, concentration is on factors not associated with the race itself. Scenery, a luncheon date, or a favorite vacation are examples of dissociative imagery. In actual fact, most runners let their minds wander, especially during long training runs. This serves to reduce boredom and takes the mind off fatigue. Associative imagery, on the other hand, involves concentration on factors that relate to the actual running. Monitoring your body signals as well as position in the race are examples of associative imagery. Once again, these serve to take your mind off fatigue as an issue in itself, thereby helping you deal with the pain.

Mental Rehearsal

Mental rehearsal, another mental preparation strategy, merely expands on the concept of imagery. This technique involves mental practice of the race or its segments. Much research has been done which indicates that the way you imagine an event in advance can play an important role in performance. This mental programming or rehearsal has been utilized by some top runners. Tony Sandoval, for example, has been quoted as saying that he visualized the entire 1980 Olympic Trials Marathon in advance. He went on to describe how he mentally rehearsed the entire race several times. This mental rehearsal was so specific that he reported actually seeing the splits, surges, and other important aspects of the run well in advance of race day. Lee Evans, the 1968 Olympic gold medalist, reported similar use of mental rehearsal. He indicated that his mental rehearsals were so specific that he saw each step throughout the entire race before ever arriving at the stadium. Other elite runners have reported mentally visualizing holding off competitors' surges, and have seen themselves beating their chief rival to the tape time and time again. In summary, this mental rehearsal not only provides the runner with a pre-race plan, but actually suggests successful responses to a variety of possible situations. By mentally practicing successful performances, self-confidence is developed to enable the runner to respond accordingly in the actual race situation.

Simulation

Simulation in running refers to creating situations in practice which are similar to what might be expected in the actual race itself. By performing these simulations, one develops coping behaviors (alternative strategies) which can be utilized in competition. This builds the runner's confidence and fosters the belief that he or she will be able to handle pressure situations when most needed.

Some simple examples of simulation will help clarify the use of this technique. Suppose an upcoming marathon will be run on a point-to-point course that typically experiences a substantial headwind. This being the case, the runner would be wise to follow a flexible training schedule that would allow taking the weekly long run on a relatively windy day. Having practiced some long runs into the wind, the runner would feel more prepared mentally and physically to handle this condition on race day.

Other less obvious examples are also worthy of consideration. Imagine how you might feel if you discovered on the most important race day of your life that your favorite racing shoes were lost or stolen. Worse yet, maybe all of your race gear has accompanied your luggage to the wrong destination. After all, things like this have been known to happen at airports and bus depots. How would you react to this situation? Could you put it out of your mind and still run the race of your life? To a large extent, this would depend upon your mental preparation for this or similar types of occurrences. Simulation has the potential to help in this type of situation. Runners should be encouraged to experiment with different pieces of racing gear in less important races or races run strictly for speedwork. Time trials could also be utilized for this type of mental training. By experiencing this type of situation beforehand, the runner will be much less stressed and affected if it happens unexpectedly on race day.

One last example involves the simulation of holding off an opponent who is trying to pass you. Fartlek workouts are excellent for practicing this technique. Merely imagine an opponent trying to overtake you in a race. Respond by surging and holding off this individual for several hundred yards. Or attempt to break contact with an imagined opponent by picking up your pace as you reach the top of a substantial hill.

Summing up on this point, simulations serve primarily to prepare the runner mentally for stressful situations that may arise on race day. Simulations, as well as the other general strategies for mental preparation in sport, are not different from physical skills—they must be practiced.

THE DEVELOPMENT OF MENTAL RACE STRATEGIES

Another mental technique that will aid the masters runner is the development of a specific competition strategy. The main purpose in planning such a strategy is to develop sufficient information and mental activities to consume totally the time of the competition. The remainder of this paper will focus briefly on three specific portions of an effective competition strategy for masters runners.

Task-Relevant Factors

A substantial portion of any competition strategy should involve concentration on technical aspects of the activity. In running, aspects such as pace, arm carriage, footstrike, fatigue, and positioning are examples of task-relevant factors. It has been suggested that there should be enough task-relevant items to consume at least two-thirds of the competition strategy. By focusing on task-relevant factors, the runner maintains excellent concentration, thereby avoiding errors such as hitting the wall, going out too fast, getting boxed in, or not taking enough fluids.

Cue Words

A fair amount of research has been conducted suggesting that how you think influences how you perform. More specifically, an athlete can speed up performance by merely thinking fast words. During the final kick of a race, the runner is encouraged to think of self-commands such as "faster, faster," "quick, quick," "kick, kick." Research indicates that this will actually pick up your running cadence. Similarly, during endurance phases, the runner should occasionally think self-commands such as "stroke, stroke," "press, press," and "hold, hold." These endurance mood words have been found to have the potential to help the runner over rough spots in the race. Once again, the athlete is encouraged to experiment with different words to find the ones that work best for him or her.

Self-Statements

Self-statements are exceptionally important for endurance activities. Basically speaking, they are positive statements that encourage one to continue with the performance. They have also been referred to as mental pats on the back or positive rewards for what one has accomplished to that point. The best time to use self-statements is either during a monotonous period of the race or when fatigue is increasing noticeably. They also serve a valuable function in what the sport psychologists refer to as segmentation. In marathon running, for example, after the completion of intermediate goals (such as 36 minutes at the 6-mile mark), the runner should use a self-statement such as "way to go, that wasn't so hard—let's do it again," and so on. Statements such as these have been found to improve persistence qualities. Finally, positive self-statements have been found to be very worthwhile in helping the athlete cope with pain. Examples of this would be statements such as "tiredness is a sign to work on," "you have a plan for handling this fatigue," and "keep going, you can make it." Once again, statements such as these have been shown experimentally to help athletes deal with fatigue and cope with pain.

CONCLUSION

In conclusion, this chapter has outlined several general strategies for mental preparation in sport and given a brief overview of some valuable competition strategies that have the potential to benefit the masters runner. It is important to remember that training does not always have to be physical in nature. By experimenting with these techniques, an athlete can still continue to improve without stepping up mileage and risking an overuse injury.

REFERENCES

Level III Theory Manual. *National Coaches Certification Program.* Ottawa: Coaching Association of Canada, 1981.

Orlick, T. *In Pursuit of Excellence.* Ottawa: Runge Press, 1980.

Rushall, B. *Psyching in Sport.* London: Pelham Books, 1979.

Tutko, T., and U. Tosi. *Sports Psyching.* Los Angeles: J.P. Tarcher Inc., 1976.

23

Eyeball To Eyeball—Acute Eye Injuries

THOMAS PASHBY, C.M., M.D., C.R.C.S. (C)

University of Toronto

The recognition of eye injuries requires a basic knowledge of anatomy and physiology of the eye. Basic equipment to conduct an examination is needed. The types of injuries recorded for 2,721 injured eyes are discussed and divided into 3 groups. Some can be treated and the participant returned to play. Others require immediate treatment and referral, while others require referral to ophthalmological care. Prevention of sports eye injuries is essential. This has been successfully managed in Canadian ice hockey and racquet sports. The need for developing standards for eye protectors, the writing of standards, and the certification of products is necessary.

The eye comprises only 0.1% of the erect frontal human silhouette, yet accounts for 1.0% of all injuries related to sports. Eye injuries can end the careers of professional athletes and change the life style and earning power of others.

Prevention is possible as has been proved in Canadian hockey by changing rules and providing certified eye protectors. Unfortunately, sports eye injuries continue to occur and must be recognized, their severity assessed, and proper treatment instituted.

The primary care individual, whether he be the family or team doctor, trainer, or first aid attendant, must have a basic knowledge of ocular anatomy and physiology and be in possession of basic equipment needed to arrive at a provisional diagnosis: a vision card, penlight, sterile eye pads, sterile fluorescein strips, eye shields, tape, sterile Q-tips, and sterile irrigating solution.

Routine examination of the eye is done systematically.

- Soft tissue is inspected for laceration, bruising, and hematoma. The conjunctiva is searched for hemorrhage, laceration, or foreign body. Foreign bodies often lodge under the upper eyelid which must be everted for removal.
- The cornea is examined by oblique illumination for foreign body, laceration, or abrasion.
- The anterior chambers are compared for depth and clarity.
- The pupils are compared for size, shape, and reaction to light.
- The iris colors are compared.

- The structures behind the iris and pupil require examination with an ophthalmoscope by a physician.
- Visual acuity is tested using a reading card and compared with the other eye. Search for contact lenses is made if they are known to be worn.
- Peripheral fields of vision are tested using the confrontation method.
- Ocular movements to the sides, upward, and downward are tested. Any double vision is recorded.
- Both eyes are looked at directly to determine undue prominence (proptosis) or if sunken into the socket (enophthalmos).
- Should there be any doubt about the appearance or function of the eye, referral for ophthalmological assessment is indicated.

Over the past 11 years in Canada I have collected data of over 2,722 sports eye injuries, including 313 blinded eyes. Most injuries are suffered by ice hockey players (38%); however, racquet sports are catching up (30%). Baseball (12%), ball hockey (8%), and football (4%) follow in that order.

Sports vary in popularity from country to country, and the incidence of eye injury for any given sport varies with its type and popularity.

In Canada, ice hockey accounts for more eye injuries than any other sport. In the United States, baseball leads the way, accounting for 27%. In Northern Ireland, hurling causes most sports eye injuries, while in England and New Zealand, squash is the leading cause.

TYPE OF INJURY

Analyzing 2,722 sports eye injuries provided by Canadian ophthalmologists, over 50% are found to be intraocular. Soft tissue (34%), orbital fractures (4%), corneal injuries (9%), hyphemas (27%), other intraocular injuries (23%), and ruptured globes (3%) make up the list.

Soft Tissue Injuries

a) Orbital hemorrhages usually result from blunt trauma. Bleeding into the orbit may cause proptosis. It is wise to check for intraocular damage before lid swelling makes eye examination difficult. An ice pack applied to the eye is helpful. Should extensive hemorrhage occur, the blood supply to the optic nerve may be embarrassed, hence such injuries require ophthalmological consultation.

b) Lid lacerations can be sutured with fine silk. However, if the lid margin or lacrimal apparatus is involved, meticulous closure using a microscope is necessary. Examination of the globe and a record of visual function are necessary.

c) Conjunctival injuries usually require no suturing. Foreign bodies can be removed with a moist cotton-tipped swab. A sterile eye pad is then applied for 24 hours. Eversion of the upper lid may reveal a foreign body which also can be removed with a moist swab. Subconjunctival hemorrhages are alarming to see but, if uncomplicated, require no treatment. An ice cube wrapped in plastic may be helpful if applied early. Visual function is recorded.

Orbital Fractures

These injuries usually result from blunt trauma. The fracture commonly occurs to the orbital floor where the bone is thinnest. As the eye is forced back into the orbit, the floor cracks and the inferior ocular muscles may become caught in the break. At other times trauma to the inferior orbital rim may cause a buckling with fracture of the orbital floor. Limitation of ocular movement causes diplopia and enophthalmos may be evident. Eye function is recorded and tomograms (x-rays) taken. Many recover spontaneously, while others require freeing of the inferior ocular muscles and the insertion of a teflon plate along the orbital floor. Fractures into the sinuses cause crepitus in the orbit. X-rays reveal the presence of air in the tissues. Fractures of the orbital roof require neurosurgical care.

Corneal Injuries

Symptoms of pain, tearing, photophobia, and blepharospasm accompany corneal injuries.
a) Foreign bodies, if superficial, can be brushed off with a moist cotton swab. If embedded, however, they require removal under direct observation using the slit lamp.
b) Abrasions are readily outlined with fluorescein. Such injuries require a record of visual function, then application of a sterile eye pad, followed by recheck in 24 hours.
c) Corneal lacerations require immediate ophthalmological care. A sterile eye pad is applied and the patient carefully transported to the hospital.

Lens Injuries

a) Blunt trauma to the lens may result in a split of the lens capsule leading to cataract formation. Penetrating injuries of the globe may injure the lens directly.
b) Cataract formation may occur immediately or develop gradually over the course of weeks, months, or even years.
c) Subluxation of the lens may occur when the lens zonule is torn. The iris will be seen to jiggle on eye movement (irido donesis).

Traumatic Glaucoma

After eye trauma the intraocular pressure may fluctuate above and below normal for a few days before slowly settling back to normal.
More severe blunt injury to the globe may cause a split in the anterior chamber angle embarrassing the aqueous outflow channels. About 10% of these injuries will lead to glaucoma, early or after many years. These eyes require intraocular tension assessment on a regular basis.
Secondary glaucoma may develop after intraocular injuries such as hyphemas, especially if secondary hemorrhages occur. Surgical intervention may be necessary.

Hyphema

Except for soft tissue injuries, hyhema is the commonest eye injury suffered in sports. More than 700 such injuries have been recorded in Canada. Therefore, it is important that the person rendering first aid recognize this type of injury because referral and hospitalization are usually required. Aspirin should be avoided.

The eye with hyphema will show a haze in the anterior chamber. The pupil is usually irregular in shape and sluggish to the light reflex. Comparison with the other eye will illustrate these findings. Vision is blurred. The eye must be kept quiet to avoid development of secondary hemorrhage (in 15% of cases) with secondary glaucoma. Surgery would then be necessary.

Injuries to the Posterior Pole

A blow to the front of the eye sends a shock wave to the back which, if severe enough, may crush the choroid and retina against the tough sclera. This contra-coup force may result in a choroidal tear which, if it crosses the macular region, results in marked visual loss.

Retinal injuries may cause hemorrhages, even detachments. Early recognition and treatment are essential to restore vision. Blurring of vision and peripheral field loss are recognizable symptoms.

Ruptured Globe

Over 70 ruptured globes have been recorded in our sports eye injury survey. Sticks, pucks, balls, ski tips, bats, and racquets are the injuring weapons. Sight is lost and in most cases the eye must be removed.

PREVENTION

What can be done to curtail these injuries? In 1974 a questionnaire was circulated to Canadian ophthalmologists asking for reports of ice hockey eye injuries treated during the previous hockey season (1972–73). The result totalled 287 injuries including 20 blind eyes. A prospective study was then undertaken for the current hockey season (1974–75). While fewer injuries were reported (257), the number of legally blind eyes rose to 43, an alarming number.

The problem was attacked in 2 ways. Because the hockey stick was the main injuring weapon, new high stick rules were introduced by the Canadian Amateur Hockey Association (CAHA). Simultaneously, work was started at the Canadian Standards Association (CSA) to develop and certify eye protectors (Fig. 23-1). Many of the protectors available were inadequate, so a CSA standard was necessary. As a consequence, manufacturers updated their products to meet this standard and the CAHA mandated the use of CSA-certified protectors by all minor league players under their jurisdiction.

The result has been gratifying. The average age of an injured player before masks were introduced was 14 years; now it is 26 years. The younger players wearing masks are protected; those not wearing masks are still at risk.

At the Hospital for Sick Children in Toronto in 1973, more than 10% of

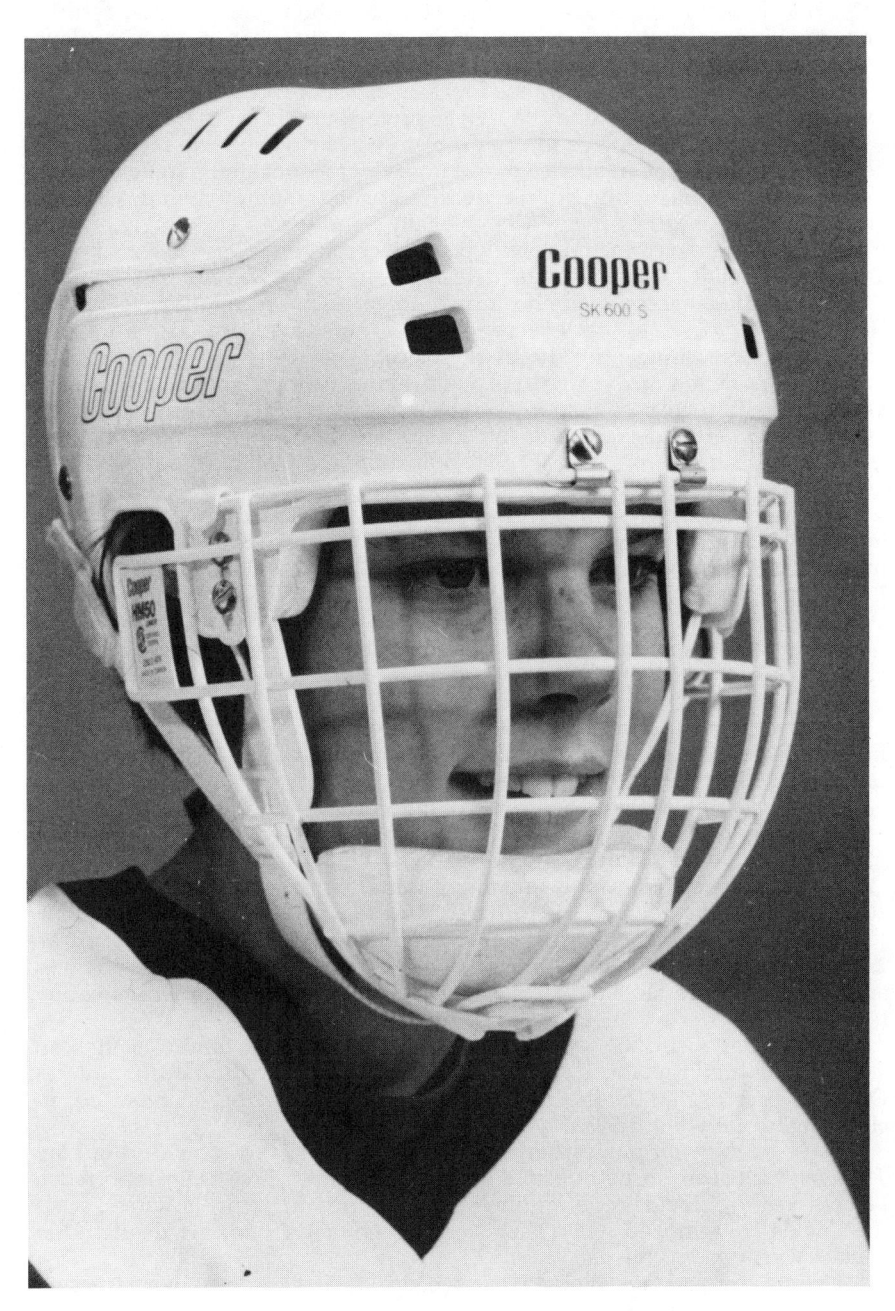

Fig. 23-1. *Hockey helmet and face protector.*

all eye injuries treated were the result of hockey injuries. Five years later, in 1978, that figure had dropped to 3%, none of whom wore a CSA-certified protector. Indeed, not one serious eye injury has been reported of a player wearing a certified protector.

Today our problem is with the older players, many of whom are reluctant to wear a protector. We hope the newer protectors will be more acceptable.

While the ice hockey eye injury problem was being solved, another sport became a concern. The incidence of eye injury in racquet sports increases with their world wide increasing popularity. In Canada our study includes 633 racquet sports eye injuries, including 30 legally blind eyes. Alarmingly, 17% of those injured were wearing an open type of eye protector. These players bought a protector, believing it to be adequate when in fact it was not.

This finding necessitated the formation of a CSA committee to write a standard for racquet sports eye protectors. The unsafe protectors are now gradually disappearing from the marketplace.

The hockey and racquet sport programs have proven that the loss of sight associated with recreational sports can be minimized, if not all but eliminated, by the use of certified protective equipment (Fig. 23-2). Sport regulating bodies and governments must insist that only certified protective equipment be used where available.

Baseball is another sport causing eye injuries. Our survey of 256 injuries includes 15 blinded eyes. Ninety percent are due to impact with the ball. In the United States, baseball is the sport causing most eye injuries (27%). Little League ball players in the United States are now wearing face protectors when at bat.

Ball hockey is popular in Canada, accounting for 173 eye injuries with 19 blind eyes in our survey. The goal tender is most at risk and must wear a mask.

Football, despite the large number of players, seems a relatively safe sport from an eye injury viewpoint. Only 95 injuries, including 4 blind eyes were found in our survey.

Skiing is another sport that can be dangerous. To date, we have recorded 14 eye injuries due to skiing accidents, with 6 blinded eyes. Three of the blinded eyes were due to the ski tip, one to the ski pole and another to the ski lift.

Golf is a pretty tame sport one might think, but 26 eye injuries, including 10 blind eyes have been recorded here. Most (83%) were struck by the ball.

Snowmobiling must be mentioned. Among the 6 eye injuries reported are 2 blinded eyes. Most injuries are caused by collisions with bushes, fences, and trees. Full face shields or ski goggles with polycarbonate lenses should be worn.

War games, using CO_2 powered repeater guns firing 14mm gelatin capsules containing vegetable dyes, are becoming popular with mature athletes. Over the past 18 months in Canada, 26 eye injuries have been reported, including 12 legally blind eyes.

Players are given polycarbonate lensed eye shields to wear during play. These shields seem to be effective as no eye injuries have been reported to players wearing shields covering their eyes. Injuries do occur, however, when the shields are removed when they steam, become dirty, or are displaced by contact with trees or bushes.

Players and spectators must wear eye shields at all times when games are in progress.

No matter what the sport, there is always some eye danger involved and it is wise to take the necessary precautions to avoid being injured. The first

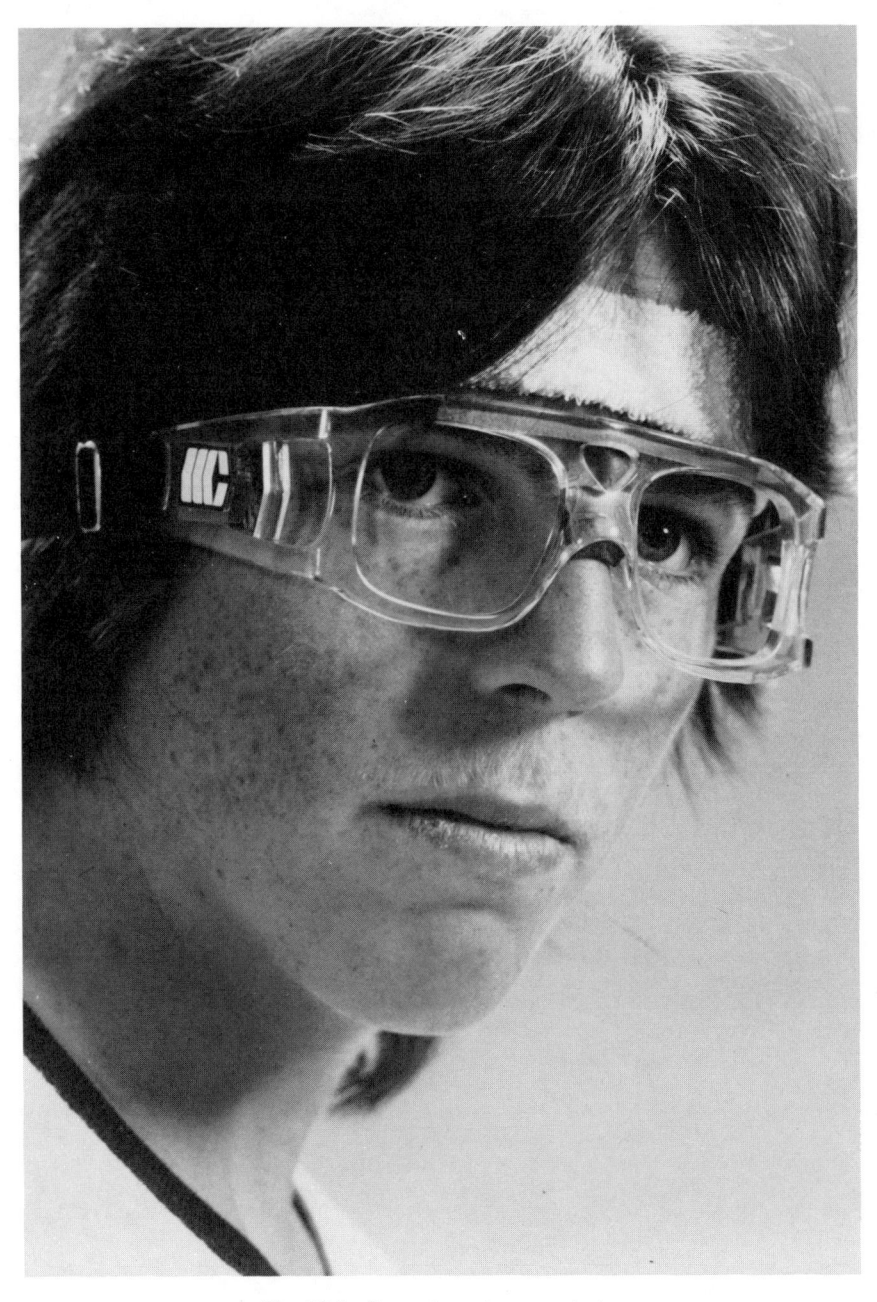

Fig. 23-2. *Racquet sports eye protector.*

rule of the game is to protect the eyes by wearing the proper protective equipment at all times.

REFERENCE

Pashby, T. J., and R. C. Pashby. *Sports Injuries: Mechanism, Prevention and Treatment.* Chapter 30. Baltimore: Williams & Wilkins, 1985.

Section VI
Knee and Shoulder

24

The Masters Knee—
Past, Present, and Future

R. W. JACKSON, M.D., M.S. (TOR.), F.R.C.S. (C)
Orthopaedic & Arthritic Hospital

ABSTRACT

The increased interest in sports and fitness in our society, combined with an aging demographic pattern, has produced an unprecedented number of knee injuries in mature athletes. The injuries include meniscal, ligamentous tears, degenerative articular cartilage changes, and patello-femoral problems. Recent significant changes in diagnosis and treatment of these problems are reviewed and possible therapeutic modalities for the future are considered. A philosophy of continued activity for the older athlete is encouraged.

While some of the knee problems that the older athlete might experience are the direct consequence of injuries that he or she received in the early years of life, we now recognize that new problems can occur, such as those sustained by any athlete, at any age, through participation in sport. This chapter will present some philosophy and some facts regarding present-day treatment of such new and old injuries and some possibilities for treatment in the future.

PAST

Sport began in ancient times as a method of practicing the skills that were so necessary for protection and the provision of food (i.e., hunting and combat). In those early Neanderthal days the average life expectancy was very short and almost any knee injury would have been catastrophic in terms of future function. The masters knee was undoubtedly a non-entity at that time.

In 776 B.C., the first Olympiad was held in honor of Zeus at Olympia. Athletes were beginning to engage in serious competition and one can only presume that knee injuries were occurring. The winners of the Olympics were honored, and consequently, competition was extremely intense. Milo of Croton was the first great Olympic athlete. He won the Olympic wrestling competition on six consecutive occasions (20). Perhaps he might be considered one of the first master athletes—in terms of both ability and age. Milo was also the first to demonstrate the value of progressive resistance exercises as he is reported to have gained his great strength through lifting a male bull daily, from the time of its birth until it reached adult size.

Unfortunately, for many centuries thereafter, a hiatus occurred in both sport and medicine, as there was little activity in either field during the Middle Ages.

Modern sports medicine began in 1854 when a medical doctor named Edward Hitchcock was appointed to Amherst College in Massachusetts as an instructor in physical education (20). In 1899, E. A. Darling at Harvard University published the first paper in English on a true sports medicine topic. It was titled "The Effects of Training—A Study of Fitness in Harvard Crews" (4). In 1906, E. H. Nicholls published an article on the physical aspects of American football (16). Three years later in 1909, he published a follow-up article showing a great reduction in the number of injuries from football after revision of the rules to improve safety and performance (17). These times were often referred to as the bucket and sponge days, as most of the medical care of the injured athletes was delegated to a relatively untrained trainer, whose main therapy was a splash of water from a wet sponge into the unconscious athlete's face.

In recent years, various studies have reported the frequency of injury to the knee joint as from 20% to 43% of all athletic injuries, whether due to contact, endurance, or skill sports.

The most frequently injured structure within the knee has undoubtedly been the meniscus, and in the early days of my career, the standard treatment for a torn meniscus was a total meniscectomy. To do anything less was considered as imperfect treatment and therefore, subject to criticism. However, after a few years of diligently performing total meniscectomies, often using a second incision in order to remove all of the meniscus tissue, I realized that the results were really not very good. When evaluated 2 to 10 years after meniscectomy, only 47% of my cases were totally asymptomatic while 26% had troublesome symptoms and 27% had minor symptoms (3). Fairbank, in 1948, documented the radiographic changes which occur in a knee a few years after total meniscectomy. These included narrowing of the joint space, flattening of the femoral condyles, bony sclerosis and osteophyte formation (6). Most of these changes are easily confirmed by arthroscopic visualization.

The second most commonly injured structure is the anterior cruciate ligament, which in the past was often an unrecognized lesion. Frequently the athlete would complain of a trick knee, and it would simply be treated with some form of a hinged knee brace.

PRESENT

At some point in the past two decades we entered the modern era of sports medicine in which better diagnosis and treatment were augmented by research and education. To many observers, this was closely related to the introduction of arthroscopy, which enabled the doctor to establish the precise diagnosis in knee problems. In addition to the diagnostic potential, a greater insight was gained into prognosis. Arthroscopy also provided a better understanding of the spectrum of pathology that a knee can sustain, and resulted in more rational methods of treatment of that pathology. For example, we were able to appreciate that on occasion, damage to a meniscus was relatively minor and partial meniscectomy, with removal of only the torn, mobile portion, could give results vastly superior to total meniscectomy (18).

Let us now consider the masters knee, and the problems which might plague the older athlete. These problems are exemplified by those experienced by one of the greatest master athletes of all time. Sir Stanley Matthews was knighted by Queen Elizabeth of England on December 31, 1964, for service to his country through the sport of soccer. At 70 years of age, he is still actively involved in soccer, performing regularly in charity exhibition matches, conducting coaching clinics, and personally coaching promising youngsters in the finer aspects of the game. Twenty-five years ago, at the age of 45, he sustained an injury to his right knee. This was never seen or treated by a doctor, and apart from missing a few games and discovering that it was slightly less painful on soft fields, Matthews didn't complain about his knee. He did note, however, that he could never fully extend the knee, but it was stable and painless. This knee has shown slight deterioration over the past 25 years, but has remained functional. However, earlier this year, at the age of 70, he injured his previously normal left knee. The injury occurred while learning a new golf swing. At first, he felt only discomfort in the postero-medial corner of the knee. However, while playing in an exhibition soccer match 2 days later, he twisted on his planted foot and felt sudden, sharp, severe pain in the postero-medial corner of the knee. This injury was disabling, as the knee was now unstable. An arthroscopic examination shortly thereafter revealed the cause of the instability to be a flap-like tear of the posterior horn of the medial meniscus. This was resected, and 3 weeks later he was able to return to his normal activity. Sir Stanley Matthews, therefore, exemplifies the 2 types of problems which may affect the performance of the mature athlete (i.e., an arthritic knee which is the result of an earlier injury, and an acute injury as the result of continued participation in sport).

Do elderly athletes who sustain fresh knee injuries do as well as younger individuals after arthroscopic surgery? To answer this question, we studied 71 knees in patients aged 40 to 74 (mean 52.5 years), with a follow-up of 1 to 5 years (mean 2.6 years) (13). These knees could easily be subdivided into 2 groups. Group I had no degenerative change on the articular cartilage, but did have a torn meniscus. Group II had degenerative articular cartilage changes at the time the meniscal injury was detected and treated. After arthroscopic meniscectomy, both groups were improved, with Group I showing 60% to be asymptomatic and 40% improved with only minimal symptoms. However, Group II, those with degenerative changes already present, did not do quite as well. Only 20% of this group were asymptomatic; 69% were improved but still had mild symptoms, and 11% showed no improvement.

Our conclusions were that traumatic tears do occur in older patients and that age alone does not adversely affect the results. However, degenerative changes present prior to meniscectomy adversely influence the end result. One can speculate that earlier diagnosis and treatment of the torn meniscus might have prevented the degenerative changes occurring and therefore improved the overall statistics. It is important, however, to recognize that arthroscopic meniscectomy can provide significant improvement in any age group, no matter how bad the pathology.

Now, let us consider injuries to the anterior cruciate ligament. This is rarely a primary injury in the elderly athlete. It is, however, a very common injury in the younger age group, and the sequelae of the unrecognized and untreated anterior cruciate injury may seriously and adversely affect the performance of the mature athlete in later life. Any injury which is severe enough to produce a traumatic hemarthrosis carries with it a 75% chance of an anterior cruciate ligament rupture (5, 8, 9, 19). When that occurs, there is also a high probability of associated damage to menisci or articular cartilage. In our study, 75% of knees with torn cruciates had associated meniscal pathology one year after the injury. This percentage rose to 90% in cruciate-deficient knees which went 10 years unrecognized and untreated (15). Similarly, articular cartilage lesions were present in 30% of cruciate-deficient knees seen in the first year after injury and in 70% of cruciate-deficient knees definitively diagnosed 10 years after injury (15). We believe, therefore, that treatment should be directed toward the early restoration of normal biomechanics of the knee joint, thereby providing stability to protect the menisci and the articular cartilages.

Treatment of a torn anterior cruciate includes conservative measures such as bracing, or operative measures in which the torn ligament is either repaired or replaced. The basis of successful non-surgical treatment hinges on the appropriate selection of cases, hamstring exercises, bracing for periods when the individual is at risk, and perhaps most importantly, modification of activity patterns. It is noted that the cruciate-deficient knee is relatively stable in a position of flexion as the hamstring musculature has good mechanical advantage, and can provide appropriate stability. However, as the knee comes into the extended position, the hamstring muscle no longer has a mechanical advantage and stresses such as those generated by quadriceps contraction during deceleration or cutting, can produce forward subluxation of the tibia on the femur. Cruciate-deficient patients are advised, therefore, to avoid cutting and jumping sports and to concentrate on sports in which the knee normally is maintained in some degree of flexion, such as skating, alpine skiing, bicycling, running, or swimming.

I also feel it is important to recognize that there is a spectrum of pathology in relation to the anterior cruciate ligament. The most minimal injury is that of an isolated partial rupture of the anterior cruciate which usually involves the postero-lateral band of that ligament. The most serious injury is a total rupture of the ligament combined with damage to one or more of the secondary restraints (i.e., the menisci, the capsule, or the collateral ligaments). Most of the injuries (81%) are combined lesions, but 19% do occur in isolation (15).

One must also recognize that we are dealing with a spectrum of patients with different athletic demands. The patients vary from the occasional athlete to the recreational, to the competitive, to the professional or elite amateur athlete, with progressively increasing physical demands on the knee.

Consequently, in determining the appropriate treatment, I believe that many factors must be considered (10). If the individual is a professional or elite athlete and the injury is at the extreme end of the severity scale, aggressive surgical treatment would be our treatment of choice. Conversely, if the individual was an occasional athlete or a non-athlete and the severity of the injury was minimal, I would initially consider treating the individual non-operatively. Overall, in fresh injuries, we tend to treat the isolated tears by non-operative measures and the combined tears by aggressive repair and augmentation. In old or previously undiagnosed lesions, I tend to be more conservative, except for the young athletically-oriented individuals. Clinical judgment is obviously needed in making such treatment decisions and in some instances, the initial conservative management is later changed to a surgical repair if the individual is unable to cope with activity modification, exercises, and bracing. Using this approach, 55% of our cases are treated non-operatively and 45% are treated with some operative procedure. The results to date show 60% of all treated individuals return to active, strenuous sports, and 30% return to relatively non-strenuous sporting activities. Only 10% discontinue their athletic efforts because of instability in the knee (15).

Chondromalacia is the most frequent problem affecting the patella and can be produced by a number of etiological factors (11). However, most of these factors can be related to either direct trauma, misalignment, or instability. If the knee is normally aligned and stable, the presence of chondromalacia is usually the result of direct trauma. If the knee has a degree of axial misalignment, an element of instability is introduced. With the addition of excessive activity, a repetitive lateral thrust to the patella on every knee extension produces wearing of the articular surface and the classical symptoms of chondromalacia develop. Misalignment, therefore, is one of the main reasons for the patello-femoral problems we see in younger athletes. As they mature, these symptoms seem to disappear. It is likely that the symptoms seen at age 15 to 30 are due to subchondral bony trabecular micro-fractures, plus the presence of enzymes released by the degenerative articular cartilage. With the passage of time, and as the individual matures, the subchondral trabecular fractures heal, the subchondral bone thickens, enzymes are no longer released, the joint becomes relatively stable; the result is that the symptoms tend to diminish, although crepitus might remain as a constant finding. In general, however, patello-femoral problems do not usually plague the mature athlete.

This leads us to the degenerative knee. Many older athletes have degenerative arthritis of the knee as a result of trauma in their younger years. This is frequently associated with removal of menisci. In some instances, body configuration such as bilateral genu-varus or valgum may be the precipitating cause. Once femoro-tibial degenerative arthritis occurs, the diagnosis is obvious by radiological examination (6). Conservative management usually consists of relative rest, weight reduction, analgesics, non-steroidal anti-inflammatory agents, and the use of soft heels on shoes to cushion the impact loading that occurs with walking or running. Should these conservative measures fail to provide significant relief, or should the individual have severe disability or deformity at the time of initial consultation, one might consider a surgical approach to treatment.

As the initial surgical treatment, arthroscopic evaluation is useful. It has long been known that washing the joint cavity with saline during arthroscopy has a therapeutic value (1, 12, 21). Cartilaginous debris, and presumably degradative enzymes, can be washed from the joint. In a recent study, we found improvement in some 80% of knees for a period of time ranging from 1 to 50 months (mean 14.8 months). Although the improvement may not be sustained, it is a reasonable and rational treatment which can, with minimal morbidity, give relief from the symptoms of degenerative arthritis.

At the time of arthroscopy, one may also encounter a degenerative meniscus or an area of articular cartilage breakdown. Debridement of the meniscus and the articular cartilage in another recent study (follow-up 25 to 112 months) showed 92% improvement following debridement (14). Again, unfortunately, the results of the debridement process may be temporary and the improvement may diminish with time. Arthroscopy does, however, provide an opportunity to evaluate the knee fully and in many instances to provide symptomatic relief of discomfort. It is our philosophy that in degenerative arthritis the damage is usually irreversible and therefore, a cure in the strictest sense of the word is not possible. I believe, therefore, that symptomatic treatment by the simplest methods possible is a reasonable approach to the management of these individuals.

In recent years, an arthroscopic technique called abrasion arthroplasty (which I call fraisage) has become popular as a treatment method for degenerative arthritis. In this procedure, eburnated bone is abraded using a burr, until subchondral bony bleeding is obtained. The concept is that this treatment will promote the egress of fibrocartilage, and ultimate resurfacing of the damaged area. Although some patients do show short-term improvement (7), I believe the long-term results have not confirmed that this treatment is any better than arthroscopic lavage and indeed, in instances where significant varus or valgus deformity is present, the biomechanical imbalance would logically predispose against any significant benefit from such a procedure.

Should the arthroscopic lavage, debridement, or fraisage fail, one would consider further operative procedures. However, in our experience, 76% of the degenerative, arthritic knees did *not* go on to any further operative procedures (14). Only 24% had repeat arthroscopic surgery or some form of major surgery such as a total knee arthroplasty or high tibial osteotomy.

Should significant deformity be present, a realignment and weight transference osteotomy provides a good and reliable method of treatment. For varus deformities, this is commonly done through the upper tibia, and for valgus deformities, the correction is made through the lower femur. Total knee arthroplasty is feasible, but probably should be reserved for patients who are at least 65 years or more of age and who do not place significant physical demands on their knees. Following total knee arthroplasty, patients should be restricted to golf, swimming, bicycling, canoeing and other relatively nonstressful (in terms of the knee) sports.

In all instances, whether one is treating acute or chronic problems, the principles of rehabilitation are essentially the same. One should always strive to maintain general fitness while starting specific rehabilitation of the injured or post-operative knee as quickly as possible. Disuse atrophy should be prevented by protected weight bearing and by mobilization, using hinged casts as early as possible. A principle to remember in the treatment of any knee problem is to avoid the repetitive pounding stress that is imposed by running or heavy lifting. Consequently, rehabilitation should largely concentrate on canoeing, bicycling and swimming.

FUTURE

Finally, I would like to project into the future and speculate on the ways I think knee surgery will evolve in the next 2 decades. We are all aware that prevention of a problem is more desirable than treatment. Consequently, prevention of degenerative arthritis through early diagnosis, conservative surgery, and the education and conditioning of the athlete will continue to be the most important aspect of future management. Should problems occur, however, we will consider several new methods of treatment.

Meniscal repair, rather than resection, will soon be the standard treatment in suitable injuries. Meniscal repair (or meniscorrhesis) is producing excellent results in short-term follow-ups (2). It is now commonly appreciated that the menisci have a good peripheral blood supply which extends approximately one-third of the distance into the substance of the meniscus. Should the tear occur in that vascular region, a repair would seem more reasonable than a resection. This can be done either under arthroscopic control or by open arthrotomy. Also, in the near future, meniscal allografting will be possible. If it seems necessary to remove a torn meniscus, an intact meniscus might be implanted from a cadaver of appropriate size, attached to the patient's vascular rim, and therefore, provide the necessary protection of articular cartilage to avoid degenerative arthritis.

Prosthetic ligaments, particularly for the anterior cruciate, are also on the horizon. Various materials have been tried in the past, none of which has been totally successful. However, it would appear that replacement of the anterior cruciate with the appropriate synthetic material (probably under arthroscopic control) will be commonplace in the near future.

Finally, chondral resurfacing, either regluing the damaged articular surfaces or replacing them with some synthetic material, is not an unreasonable concept although it is very much in the embryonic stage of development at this time. In summary, when a knee is freshly injured or shows the late results of some previous injury and without regard to the age of the patient, one should adopt the policy of *aggressive* arthroscopic diagnosis and temper this by a *conservative* approach to treatment, either non-operative or operative. By making the correct diagnosis, and appropriately treating the injuries that sport might inflict on the knee, we can enable an athlete to continue the pursuit of sporting activities into later life with pleasure, and without pain.

REFERENCES

1. Burman, M. S., H. Finkelstein, and L. Meyer. Arthroscopy of the knee joint. *J. Bone Joint Surg.* 16:255–268, 1934.
2. Cassidy, R. E., and A. J. Shaffer. Repair of peripheral meniscus tears. A preliminary report. *Am. J. Sports Med.*, 9:209–214, 1981.
3. Dandy, D. J., and R. W. Jackson. Meniscectomy and chondromalacia of the femoral condyle. *J. Bone Joint Surg.*, 57A:1116–1119, 1975.
4. Darling, E. A. The effect of training—A study of fitness in Harvard crews. *Boston Med. Surg. J.* 141:205–233, 1899.
5. DeHaven, K. Diagnosis of acute knee injuries with hemarthrosis. *Am. J. Sports Med.* 8:9–14, 1980.
6. Fairbank, T. J. Knee joint changes after meniscectomy. *J. Bone Joint Surg.* 30B:664–670, 1948.
7. Friedman, M. J., C. C. Berasi, J. M. Fox, W. Del Pizzo, S. J. Snyder, and R. D. Ferkel. Preliminary results with abrasion arthroplasty in the osteoarthritic knee. *Clin. Orthop.* 182:200–205, 1984.
8. Gillquist, J., and G. Hagberg, Findings at arthroscopy and arthrography in knee injuries. *Acta. Orthop. Scand.* 49:398–402, 1978.
9. Gillquist, J., G. Hagberg, and N. Oretorp. Arthroscopy in acute injuries of the knee joint. *Acta. Orthop. Scand.* 48:190–196, 1977.
10. Jackson, R. W. Anterior cruciate ligament injuries. In: *Arthroscopy: Diagnostic and Surgical Practice*, Casscells, S. W. (ed.) 52–73. Philadelphia: Lea & Febiger, 1984.
11. Jackson, R. W. *Surgery of the Patello-Femoral Joint. Part III: Etiology of Chondromalacia Patella.* Am. Acad. Orthop. Surg. Instr. Course Text.
12. Jackson, R. W., and D. J. Dandy. *Arthroscopy of the Knee.* New York: Grune & Stratton, 1976.
13. Jackson, R. W., and D. W. Rouse. The results of partial arthroscopic meniscectomy in patients over 40 years of age. *J. Bone Joint Surg.* 64B:481–485, 1982.
14. Jackson, R. W., R. Silver, and H. Marans. *Arthroscopic Debridement of the Degenerative Knee.* Unpublished observations.
15. Maruyama, K., and R. W. Jackson. Presentation at meeting of the International Society of the Knee. Gleneagles, Scotland, 1983.
16. Nicholls, E. H. The physical aspect of American football. *Boston Med. Surg. J.* 154:1–8, 1906.
17. Nicholls, E. H. Football injuries of the Harvard squad for three years under the revised rules. *Boston Med. Surg. J.* 160:33–37, 1909.
18. Northmoreball, M. D., D. J. Dandy, and R. W. Jackson. Arthroscopic open partial and total meniscectomy. A comparative study. *J. Bone Joint Surg.* 65B:400–404, 1983.
19. Noyes, F. R., R. W. Bassett, E. S. Grood, and D. L. Butler. Arthroscopy in acute hemarthrosis of the knee. *J. Bone Joint Surg.* 62A:687–695, 1980.
20. Snook, G. A. History of sports medicine, Part I. *Am. J. Sports Med.* 12:251–254, 1984.
21. Watanabe, M. Articular pumping. *J. Japan. Soc. Orthop. Surg.* 24, 1950.

25

Instability of The Knee In Mature Athletes

DAVID HASTINGS

The Wellesley Hospital

ANATOMY OF THE KNEE

In order to understand the implication of ligament injuries, it is essential to have an understanding of the capsular and ligamentous support of the knee. On the medial side, the medial collateral ligament is essentially a superficial ligament. Most of the support is given by what is called the deep medial ligament or middle third of the capsule and the posterior third of the capsule or the posterior oblique ligament. Anteriorly, the retinaculum is relatively weak to allow full flexion. There is a varying center of rotation for the knee because of its cam shape. This means that the medial collateral ligament is under maximum tension in full extension and maximum relaxation at 90 degrees of flexion, particularly the posterior oblique portion. This is also true of the lateral collateral ligament which is tight in full extension, slightly lax at 30 degrees of flexion, and quite lax at 60 and 90 degrees respectively. If one wishes to immobilize the knee, flexion is the position best designed to put the ligaments at rest and off the stretch. The anterior cruciate ligament originates from the anterior tibial spine. It is surprising that this is relatively posterior in the knee and it inserts over the back of the lateral femoral condyle.

In discussing ligament problems in the mature athlete, I intend to touch on both acute and chronic instability. There are special factors in mature knees which result in different patterns of injury. Of considerable importance is the loss of proteoglycans from the articular cartilage, meaning that this cartilage is more brittle and subject to shear tear and fissuring. For the same reason the menisci are more vulnerable. Ligaments are less elastic. In my experience, medial collateral tears are by far the more common, and the isolated anterior cruciate tear is relatively rare. Because of the loss of trabecular support and subchondral strength, plateau fractures are more common in the mature athlete. This may be one factor that reduces the number of ligament injuries. Degenerative changes simply because of aging and overuse are again more frequent; for this reason, a significant ligament injury in a mature athlete tends to be chronically painful. In general, as we age, our range of motion gets less, and post-injury stiffness is a distinct problem.

For many years diagnostic accuracy in the assessment of knee ligament injuries was poor. It is essential that a correct diagnosis be established. Better teaching and more sophisticated means of examination have improved our accuracy. Nonetheless, examination under anesthesia and arthroscopy should be considered if the slightest doubt exists as to the nature of the injury.

The principle of treatment of acute injuries is to assess the articular surfaces and menisci carefully. This usually requires arthroscopic examination. Careful assessment of the radiograph should be made for the possibility of plateau fracture; tomography is often indicated if there is any doubt. In general, non-operative management of an acute ligament injury is favored. It is wise to avoid major intra-articular reconstruction such as the augmentation of an anterior cruciate tear. Early mobilization of all knee injuries should be encouraged, and the use of continuous passive motion and cast bracing are valuable adjuncts to the overall management picture.

Most chronic instabilities can be managed non-operatively. Motor control can be improved by developing the hamstrings and quadriceps. The athlete can change his activity level. Sports such as swimming, cycling, skating, and skiing can be done with significant chronic ligamentous instability. Appropriate bracing, especially light braces, can be very helpful. Surgery should be reserved for major instability. If there is an angular deformity, osteotomy combined with ligamentous reconstruction should be considered. It is essential that early motion be instituted if any reconstructive surgery is carried out.

I would like to classify the injuries on an anatomical basis. I have grouped these 5 injuries—isolated medial collateral tears, isolated anterior cruciate tears, medial collateral-anterior cruciate tears, medial collateral-posterior cruciate tears, and medial collateral and both cruciate tears—together because they share a common mechanism of injury: valgus either from a direct blow or indirectly, as occurs with a sudden change of direction and deceleration.

Varus forces result in injuries to the lateral complex which may be an isolated lateral collateral, lateral collateral anterior cruciate, lateral collateral posterior cruciate, or a lateral collateral and both cruciates. A direct posterior force may result in an isolated posterior cruciate tear. I have not involved rotation as a major source of ligament disruption as I believe the planar forces are more responsible than rotation, and the recent classification based on rotational instability frankly makes me dizzy. I would like to briefly discuss each of the tears to illustrate their diagnosis and management.

The isolated medial collateral tear is usually the result of a direct force. Under anesthesia this knee will show a definite laxity when a valgus stress is applied, but there will be no anterior or posterior translation of the tibia because of the intact cruciate system. This in turn limits the amount of medial opening, and although there is laxity, this knee can be managed non-operatively. Stress x-ray under anesthesia may show a significant amount of medial opening, but because of the intact cruciate, shows no tibial translation. Minor degrees of laxity (under 4 millimeters in excess of the control knee) can be managed by early mobilization, but athletic activity should be restricted for 6 weeks. Even then the knee should be protected with a brace. I have seen several examples of patients with minor ligament laxity returning to sport with the result that a minor ligamentous injury became a major disruption. Moderate collateral laxity can also be managed non-operatively, even up to 10 to 12 mm of opening in excess of the other knee, providing an associated cruciate tear is ruled out. This is best done by examining the patient under anesthesia and arthroscopy.

Once the diagnosis of an isolated medial collateral tear is made, the athlete is placed in plaster at 90 degrees of flexion. The more mature the athlete, the sooner he should be transferred to a limited extension cast brace, between 1 and 2 weeks post-injury. The extension stop should be at 30 to 45 degrees short of full extension. The patient remains in this for an additional 4 weeks and even following this should be braced by a relatively good support with lateral irons and a strong hinge. Physiotherapy is carried on from the time of injury and consists of maintaining muscle tone and bulk in quadriceps, hamstrings, and hip musculature. As soon as the patient is out of plaster, activities such as swimming, cycling, stair climbing, and light running are encouraged. The only indications for surgery in an isolated medial ligament tear in the mature athlete are those associated with a major bony avulsion, a meniscal tear often on the lateral side, or possibly a lateral plateau fracture.

The isolated anterior cruciate tear is relatively rare in the mature athlete. I feel that this is because the medial ligaments are less elastic and will usually tear before the tension goes on the cruciate. If this injury does occur, however, operative repair is not indicated in the mature age group. Often they can cope with the instability and if there is any degree of flexion deformity, perhaps due to osteoarthritis, the cruciate instability may resolve spontaneously. The problem in this age group, as in the younger age group, is in diagnosis. The symptoms of an audible pop, a sensation of the knee coming apart, and hemarthrosis are valuable clues. The late sequelae of the anterior cruciate syndrome, those of chronic instability with giving way, condylar erosions, meniscal tears, and osteoarthritis are less frequently seen in the mature age group. If they occur, however, bracing should certainly be used as the initial management and in selected cases, operative repair may be required. I recommend the lateral substitution repair popularized by David McIntosh, combined with an intra-articular debridement of osteophytes, chondral fragments, and meniscal tears. Early motion by means of a cast brace is essential in the operative case.

The medial collateral-anterior cruciate tear is the result of a fairly violent blow, usually in a contact sport. Examination under anesthesia shows not only a valgus defect but a major anterior translation of the tibia accentuated by the medial laxity. This results in a block to extension with a valgus stress. As the valgus stress is relaxed and the knee flexed, the tibia will reduce with a jump, a phenomenon that has been termed pivot shift. This knee will also exhibit a strongly positive Lachmann's sign. If an AP stress x-ray with valgus strain is taken, the medial laxity can be clearly appreciated, but of greater significance is a cross-table lateral with the same valgus strain that shows the anterior tibial dislocation relative to the femur. The treatment of this in both the young and mature athlete is operative. In the younger athlete the anterior cruciate is usually reinforced by means of a strip from the quadriceps tendon. This is not advocated in the mature athlete, but certainly meniscal re-attachment and a direct cruciate repair are indicated.

The medial collateral with posterior cruciate tear is usually the result of a direct blow from the anterolateral aspect resulting in some degree of hyperextension or posterior tibial translation combined with a valgus force. The same violent mechanism or a violent valgus injury alone can result in the tear of a medial collateral and both cruciates. Examination of this injury under anesthesia shows the patient to have an increase in hyperextension as compared to the opposite side. Moreover, he shows valgus instability in full extension or hyperextension, a phenomenon not present when one cruciate is intact. Although he shows an anterior and posterior drawer in flexion and extension with the valgus strain, the tibia is not translated anteriorly or posteriorly since there is no cruciate to direct it. The stress x-ray will show a wide opening on the medial side and in the intercondylar area but no anterior or posterior tibial translation on the cross-table lateral. This is indeed a devastating injury and is tantamount to a dislocation of the knee. When a medial collateral tear is combined with cruciate tears, the treatment of acute injury is to do a direct operative repair on all torn ligaments but avoid augmentation of the cruciates. Again early motion is indicated.

Fortunately we do not see a large number of chronic instabilities of this type. The essential treatment, however, would be the same; that is, to attempt a bracing first and if this failed, a reconstruction of the medial collateral ligament by one of the many methods suggested, if possible that of O'Donohue, advancing the tibial insertion distally.

Varus injuries are much less common. The isolated lateral collateral ligament tear does occur and can be managed non-operatively in a limited extension cast brace. The lateral collateral, anterior cruciate ligament does occur in a mature athlete. A 52-year-old man was hang-gliding when he lost control, suffering a tear of his lateral complex where the biceps femoris and lateral collateral ligament avulsed the tip of the fibular head and his anterior cruciate was torn. He was managed by a direct repair of the cruciate and re-attachment of the bony avulsion. He returned to full activities including down-hill skiing within 5 months. A tear of the lateral collateral and both cruciates is usually the result of a violent force and is frequently associated with a peroneal nerve injury. A 35-year-old woman was tobogganing and suffered this major disruption. By some miracle, her peroneal nerve was spared, and she went on to recover remarkable function after a direct repair of all torn structures. In general, the principle of acute injuries on the lateral side involving the collateral and cruciates is to repair the lateral soft tissue support and repair the cruciate without augmentation. A 38-year-old victim of a motor vehicle hit-and-run accident showed the risks of plateau fractures with valgus stress. There was not only a complete collateral and cruciate disruption in both knees, but a lateral tibial plateau fracture as well. This injury must be searched for carefully in valgus injuries in the mature athlete.

The isolated posterior cruciate ligament tear is most likely to occur from a motor vehicle accident, but can occur in Old Timers hockey. This results from a blow to the flexed tibia against a goalpost. One must be aware of the associated patellar and hip injury, especially in the motor vehicle accident group. Most patients retain remarkably good function and it is interesting to see how well those with an isolated posterior cruciate ligament injury can continue in recreational sports. For that reason, I recommend in the mature athlete repairing only bony avulsions and managing the rare isolated posterior cruciate injury without an avulsion by early motion.

I think that it is important to review the special problems in the mature knee. The articular cartilage is more brittle; therefore, fissure tears and subsequent osteoarthritis and meniscal tears are more common. The ligaments are less elastic; therefore, the isolated anterior cruciate injury is less common. One must always look for tibial plateau fractures or even indentations of the femoral condyle because of the mild degree of osteoporosis in this age group. Degenerative changes and stiffness are also more common.

In my experience acute knee ligament injuries are less common in the mature athlete, but when they occur, the medial collateral is the most common type and the anterior cruciate relatively rare. Articular and meniscal injuries are more common in this group, and fracture of the articular surface is definitely a greater risk. Post-injury stiffness is also a greater problem. It is critical to accurately assess the acute knee injury; arthroscopy is very valuable. Tomography may be necessary to rule out a bony injury. In the isolated ligament tear, non-operative measures are favored and even when operative reconstruction is undertaken, major articular procedures should be avoided. Early motion is essential in the immediate post-operative phase.

The mature athlete with chronic ligament instability often has very good motor control. It is also of interest that degenerative change and osteophyte formation might help stabilize the knee. Angular deformity on the other hand is poorly tolerated and should be dealt with surgically. The best management of the chronic knee ligament injury is to build up muscle control and use bracing where indicated. Reconstruction should be done with some degree of reluctance and often combined with osteotomy if there is a major angular deformity and loss of articular cartilage. The surgeon must always be aware of stiffness following any reconstruction in chronic instability and consider the use of adjuncts such as continuous passive motion or cast bracing.

26
Synthetic Materials Used In Intra-Articular Anterior Cruciate Ligament Knee Reconstructions

JAMES H. ROTH, M.D.

University of Western Ontario

Chronic anterior cruciate ligament (ACL) insufficiency may result in recurrent symptomatic giving way of the knee and disability with athletics, work, or even activities of daily living. Many patients are helped with a non-operative treatment regimen of bracing and physiotherapy. Many will modify the athletic or work activities which precipitate their symptoms. However, other patients have symptoms with minimal activity or refuse to modify their lifestyles. It is these patients who require surgical anterior cruciate ligament reconstruction. The masters athlete with a pure ACL tear is more likely to have osteoarthritis; few require ACL reconstruction.

Historically, many techniques utilizing various autogenous tissues have been employed to restore knee stability in patients with chronic ACL insufficiency (5). Our experience with such procedures in animals and humans has been that many have stretched out or failed. The autografts initially undergo degeneration and weakening before recollagenization and strengthening occur. This recollagenization may take up to 2 years before it is complete. During the period of autograft degeneration, it is susceptible to elongation or breakage even with minor stresses, resulting in the return of knee instability.

Autogenous reconstructions require a 6 to 8 week period of cast immobilization because of the autograft degeneration and initial weakness. During this period of immobilization, surface articular cartilage injury and arthrofibrosis frequently develop. This morbidity may necessitate secondary procedures, and may be more disabling than the initial problem of instability.

These 2 major drawbacks of autogenous reconstruction (i.e., initial graft degeneration with frequent loss of restored stability with minor knee stresses, and morbidity of surface cartilage erosion and arthrofibrosis secondary to the required prolonged cast immobilization) have resulted in tremendous interest in developing synthetic materials to be used in ACL reconstructive procedures.

Synthetic material utilized in ACL intra-articular reconstructions falls into one of two major categories: total prosthetic replacements of the ACL and synthetic augmentation devices designed to be fabricated into a composite graft consisting of an autograft and a synthetic device. The total prosthesis must be able to withstand a lifetime of cyclic loading. Various investigators have estimated the loads and strains imparted to the anterior cruciate ligament (3,6). Early fatigue failure or excessive creep deformation could render a prosthetic material unacceptable.

The advantage of biological material over any prosthesis is that it has the ability to repair itself, thus limiting adverse cyclic load characteristics. In theory, the augmentation devices protect the autogenous portion of the autograft until recollagenization and strengthening are complete. Once this occurs, the autograft protects the synthetic device from fatigue failure.

Following are several examples of synthetic materials which have been used in intra-articular anterior cruciate ligament reconstruction of the knee and have failed, or which presently are under investigation.

I—POLYETHYLENE PROSTHESIS

Many materials have been investigated as potential prosthetic ligaments. One of the first used clinically in North America was the polyethylene prosthesis (Fig. 26-1). Most of these prototypes failed due to fatigue failure (8). Biomechanical analysis (6) found the characteristics inadequate for ACL prosthetic replacement and clinical trials were discontinued.

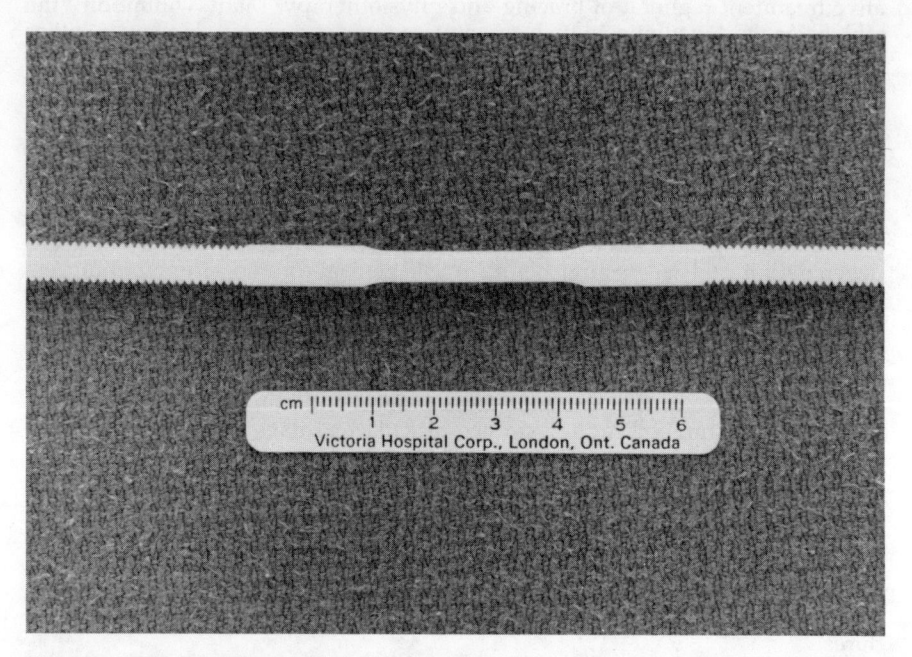

Fig. 26-1. THE POLYETHYLENE PROSTHESIS. *This prosthesis is stabilized to femur and tibial bone tunnels utilizing metal bushings and bone cement.*

II—PROPLAST PROSTHESIS

Proplast is a composite of three materials: a core of polyaramid fiber and fluorinated ethylene polypropylene polymer, a coating of porous low-modulus composite of tetrafluoroethylene (Teflon) and a vitreous carbon (Fig. 26-2).

Strum and Larson (13) reported breakage in 35 of 40 Proplast ACL reconstructions available for review, with an average 13.2 months follow-up. They also noted that 52% of their patients had a satisfactory result despite device failure.

III—CARBON FIBER PROSTHESIS AND AUGMENTATION

Jenkins first reported the use of carbon filament fibers as a ligament prosthesis in 1980 (7). Results of anterior cruciate replacement with uncoated filamentous carbon are unreliable (4, 7, 12).

Weiss and Alexander and co-workers (14) modified the carbon filament with a polylactic acid (PLA) polymer coating (Fig. 26-3) to allow easier handling and to protect the carbon from fragmentation on implantation. The PLA is absorbed over a short period of time. In principle, the carbon mechanically degrades over a longer period of time and the stress which initially is taken up predominantly by the carbon gradually is transferred to the patient's newly formed collagen.

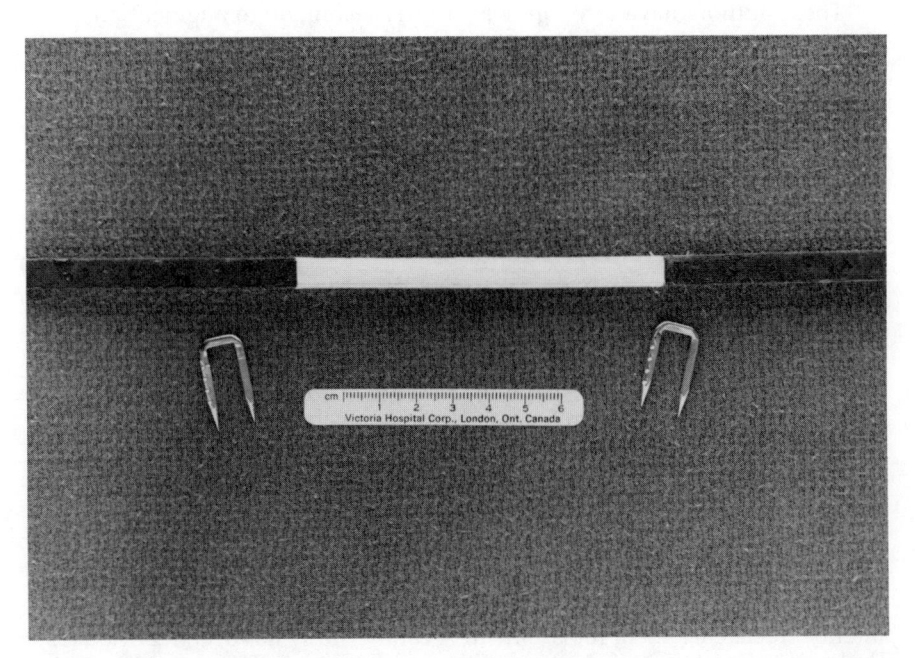

Fig. 26-2. THE PROPLAST PROSTHESIS. *This prosthesis is stabilized to the tibia and femur with staples. The coating at each end is both fibrous and porous, allowing fibrous tissue ingrowth which strengthens its fixation to bone and soft tissue attachment sites.*

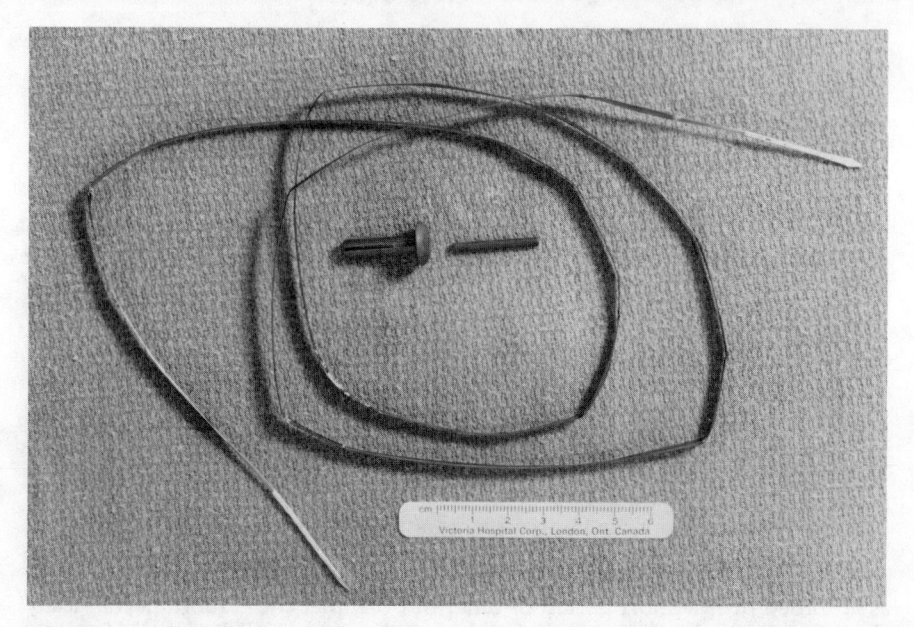

Fig. 26-3. *PLA-COATED CARBON FIBER SCAFFOLD. The strip of carbon is woven into an autograft and stabilized to bone with the use of a specially designed carbon fastener.*

These authors have developed a surgical technique to augment an autograft to reconstruct the deficient ACL. They have reported their early results (14).

Strum and Larson compared carbon fiber augmentation of autogenous ACL reconstructions with a similar group of unaugmented autogenous reconstructions and did not show any benefit with the use of carbon fibers (13).

IV—GORE-TEX PROSTHESIS

A single filament, expanded polytetrafluoroethylene (PTFE) prosthetic ligament (Fig. 26-4) has been developed to replace the anterior cruciate ligament. Following animal studies, a human clinical study has been initiated. As of December 1983, two of 130 ACL replacements at 15-month follow-up had to be removed (2). Although preliminary results are encouraging, long-term follow-up is necessary.

V—BOVINE XENOGRAFT PROSTHESIS

Glutaraldehyde cross-linked bovine xenograft is being investigated as an anterior cruciate ligament replacement. A canine study has been reported (10). The major component of the bioprosthesis is collagen. The natural intermolecular cross-link is the key to maintenance of the collagenous form and chemical stability and glutaraldehyde is an effective cross-linking agent. Glutaral-

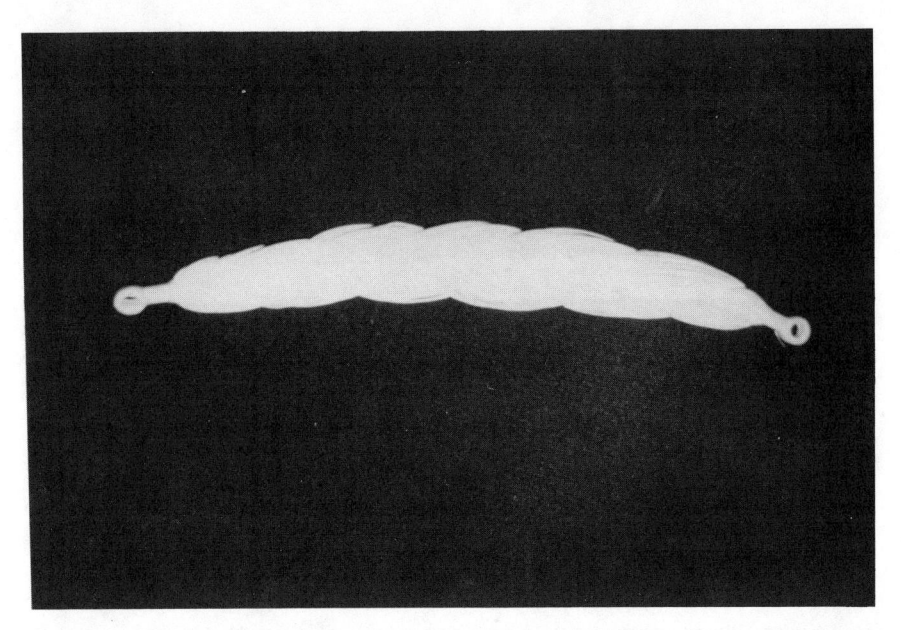

Fig. 26-4. *THE GORE-TEX PROSTHETIC LIGAMENT. The prosthesis is inserted through tibial and femoral tunnels and internally fixed to bone with screws inserted through the loops at either end.*

dehyde-stabilized collagen is resistant to mechanical, chemical, and biological degradation and becomes a histological prosthesis. Human clinical trials began in Europe in late 1980. Clinical trials were initiated in North America in 1982. Long-term follow-up results are not available.

VI—POLYPROPYLENE BRAID LIGAMENT AUGMENTATION DEVICE

A diamond weave polypropylene braid has been developed to function as a ligament augmentation device (Fig. 26-5). Extensive bench and in-vivo testing have demonstrated that the device is safe. Improved efficacy of the polypropylene braid-augmented reconstructions compared to the unaugmented reconstruction is suggested (9,11).

In June of 1979, the late Dr. J. C. Kennedy performed the first human anterior cruciate ligament reconstruction using the polypropylene braid to synthetically augment an autograft composed of a portion of the quadriceps tendon, prepatellar periosteum, and patellar tendon. The key technical points are that the polypropylene braid be sutured to the autograft with multiple sutures and that there be biological fixation only at one end.

Prior to his untimely death, Dr. Kennedy performed 144 polypropylene-augmented procedures. One hundred-and-thirty-four of these have been reviewed. Results have been very satisfactory. The polypropylene braid is safe in humans when used as an augmentation device. Improved efficacy in augmented patients compared to unaugmented patients has been demonstrated.

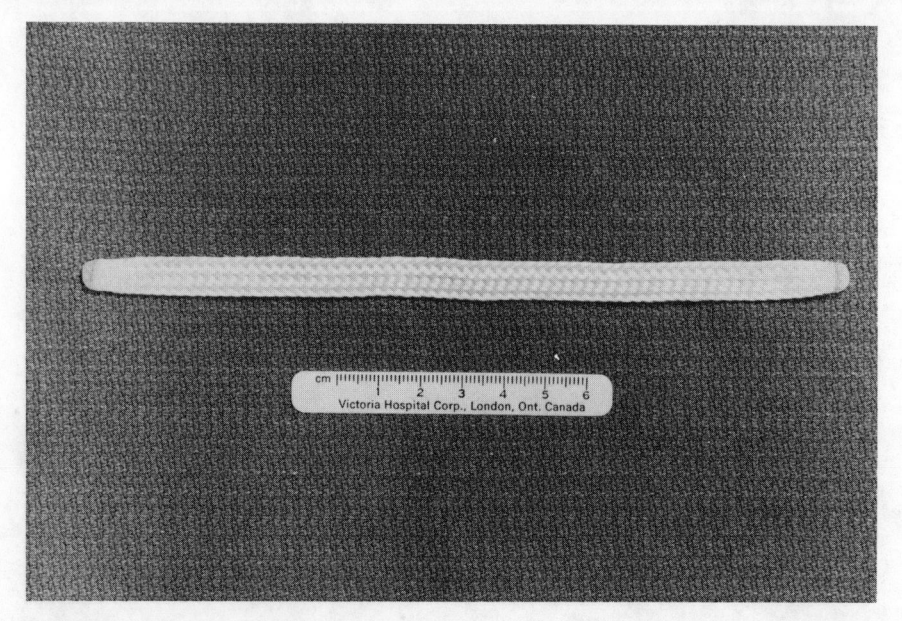

Fig. 26-5. THE POLYPROPYLENE BRAID LIGAMENT AUGMENTATION DEVICE. *The device is sutured to an autograft. Fixation of the composite graft created is by internal fixation at one end, and biological fixation only at the other end to prevent total stress shielding of the autograft by the device.*

We continue to use the polypropylene braid-augmented intra-articular anterior cruciate ligament reconstruction technique at our center. We feel that the polypropylene braid offers what we desire. It is safe and protects the autograft from elongation or breakage and allows early knee motion post-reconstruction, preventing the morbidity related to prolonged cast immobilization.

This technique allows the autograft portion of the composite graft to re-collagenize, preventing the problem of fatigue associated with the prosthetic ACL replacements.

REFERENCES

1. Aragona, J., J. R. Parsons, H. Alexander, and A. B. Weiss. Soft tissue attachment of a filamentous carbon-absorbable polymer tendon and ligament replacement. *Clin. Orthop.* 160:268–278, 1981.
2. Bolton, C. W., and W. C. Bruchman. The Gore-Tex (TM) expanded polytetrafluoroethylene prosthetic ligament—an in-vitro and in-vivo evaluation. *Clin. Orthop.* 196:202–213, 1985.
3. Butler, D. L., E. S. Grood, and F. R. Noyes. On the interpretation of our anterior cruciate ligament data. *Clin. Orthop.* 196:26–34, 1985.
4. Dandy, D. J., J. P. Flanagan, and J. Steenmeyer. Arthroscopy and the management of the ruptured anterior cruciate ligament. *Clin. Orthop.* 167:43–49, 1982.
5. Friedman, M. J., O. H. Sherman, J. M. Fox, W. Del Pizzo, S. J. Snyder, and R. J. Ferkel. Autogenic anterior cruciate ligament reconstruction of the knee—a review. *Clin. Orthop.* 196:9–14, 1985.
6. Grood, E. S., and F. R. Noyes. Cruciate ligament prosthesis: Strength, creep and fatigue properties. *J. Bone Joint Surg.* 58A:1083–1088, 1976.
7. Jenkins, D. H. R., and B. McKibbon. The role of flexible carbon-fiber implants as tendon and ligament substitutes in clinical practice. *J. Bone Joint Surg.* 62B:497–499, 1980.

8. Kennedy, J. C. Application of prosthetics to anterior cruciate ligament reconstructions and repair. *Clin. Orthop.* 172:125–128, 1983.
9. Kennedy, J. C., J. H. Roth, H. V. Mendenhall, and J. B. Sanford. Intra-articular replacement in the anterior cruciate ligament-deficient knee. *Am. J. of Sports Med.* 8:1–8, 1980.
10. McMaster, W. C. A histologic assessment of canine anterior cruciate substitution with bovine xenograft. *Clin. Orthop.* 196:196–201, 1985.
11. McPherson, G. K., H. V. Mendenhall, D. F. Gibbons, H. Plenk, W. Rottmann, J. B. Sanford, J. C. Kennedy, and J. H. Roth. Experimental mechanical and histologic evaluation of the Kennedy ligament augmentation device. *Clin. Orthop.* 196:186–195, 1985.
12. Rushton, N., D. J. Dandy, and C. P. E. Naylor. The clinical, arthroscopic and histological findings after replacement of the anterior cruciate ligament with carbon fiber. *J. Bone Joint Surg.* 65B:308–309, 1983.
13. Strum, G. M., and R. L. Larson. Clinical experience and early results of carbon fiber augmentation of anterior cruciate reconstruction of the knee. *Clin. Orthop.* 196:124–138, 1985.
14. Weiss, A. B., M. D. Blazina, M. D. Goldstein, and H. Alexander. Ligament replacement with an absorbable copolymer carbon fiber scaffold—early clinical experience. *Clin. Orthop.* 196:77–85. 1985.

27
Osteoarthritis, Athletes, and Arthroscopic Management

JAMES R. ANDREWS, M.D.
RICK K. ST. PIERRE, M.D.

Hughston Orthopaedic Clinic, P.C.

ABSTRACT

Athletes under 30 years of age typically have knee injuries produced by trauma while older athletes present with knee disorders secondary to degenerative changes. For older athletes, the objectives of treatment following meniscal and ligamentous injuries are to restore function and minimize further degenerative changes. For younger athletes, who characteristically experience bucket-handle tears of the menisci, the objective of treatment should be to preserve joint function. This is best achieved by arthroscopic partial meniscectomy as opposed to open total meniscectomy.

Osteoarthritis, frequently seen by the orthopedic surgeon in older athletes, is due to repetitive stress and trauma on the knee joint from continued participation in sports. Arthroscopic treatment of the older athlete's knee includes treatment of degenerative meniscal disorders such as flap tears or horizontal cleavage tears. Chondral lesions and chondromalacia of the patella and the femoral and tibial condyles can also be debrided arthroscopically. Abrasion arthroplasty has also been a viable treatment modality in those athletes with moderate to severe degenerative changes with eburnation of bone. Thus, arthroscopic treatment of both the younger and older athlete's knee enables the orthopedic surgeon to minimize the amount of surgical trauma and maintain the function of the joint compartments of the knee.

Increased participation in sports by older individuals has caused osteoarthritis to become a common presentation in sports medicine clinics. The degenerative changes are due to continuous competitive athletics, or they may follow ligament or meniscal injury.

It is necessary to differentiate between knee disorders in the older and

---

This work was supported in part by the Hughston Sports Medicine Foundation, Inc., 6262 Hamilton Road, Columbus, Georgia 31995.

younger athlete. The younger athlete (less than 30 years of age) has knee injuries produced by trauma, while the older athlete presents with knee disorders secondary to degenerative changes. Operative arthroscopy is useful in the treatment of knee disorders in both younger and older athletes.

The objectives of treatment following meniscal and ligamentous injuries are to restore function and minimize further degenerative changes. Meniscal tears with or without ligamentous laxity and complete ligamentous disruption contribute to the development of degenerative arthritis following injury. Treatment includes: removal of obstructions blocking joint motion, smoothing of the joint surfaces, restoration of normal pathways of motion through ligamentous repair and reconstruction, decreasing joint overload by ensuring full motion, and development of maximum muscular support of the knee. Early diagnosis and treatment of the injury is essential. Arthroscopic surgery alone or in combination with open ligament repair and thorough rehabilitation is the best prophylaxis against consequent degenerative arthritis (1).

The knee joint is a highly complex structure. Full coordination of all its components is essential to normal static and kinetic function. Experimental evidence suggests that joints wear out by repetitive impulsive loading. Changes in the bone or soft tissue which render them less effective as shock absorbers have deleterious effects on the articular cartilage. Experimental studies by Radin et al. (11) show the rapidity with which fully developed osteoarthritis manifests itself after what could be considered mild to moderate mechanical insults.

The meniscus is a primary stabilizer and weight transmitter within the knee and is, therefore, a frequent site of knee injury. Arthroscopic partial meniscectomy involves excision of the mobile fragment of the meniscus, leaving behind a stable peripheral rim anchored to both the anterior and posterior tibia. Partial meniscectomy should remove mechanical interference, relieve pain and meniscal instability, and continue weight acceptance of the meniscal rim. Theoretically, degeneration should be minimized (2, 7, 11).

Meniscal lesion in younger athletes is usually the result of trauma. In middle-aged and older athletes, it is more often a degenerative phenomenon. The most common type of lesion in the younger athlete is the bucket-handle tear. Trauma is the initiating factor in many ways. A traumatic episode may produce a bucket-handle tear that must be resected arthroscopically or a peripheral detachment amenable to arthroscopic repair (Fig. 27-1). Rotational instability resulting from ligamentous injury leads to abnormal meniscal mechanics with an altered pattern of flexion and extension. Repeated trapping of either of the menisci may take place between the articular surfaces with eventual formation of a tear. The most frequent predictable symptom complex of a significant tear is pain, swelling, and giving way. Joint line tenderness is the most reliable sign according to Fowler (2).

With a torn meniscus, the mobile fragment is the cause of the symptoms. Mechanical obstruction of the fragment causes locking. Stretching of the capsule by traction of the fragment through its remaining attachments to the capsule and synovium causes pain and swelling. Treatment consists of removing the mobile fragment. The amount of meniscal tissue removed depends on conflicting factors. The surgeon must remove the fragment and yet preserve the function of the normal meniscus by leaving as much meniscal tissue as possible. It is important to preserve the intact ring, and the remaining rim should be stable and smoothly contoured (15).

Many authors (2, 5–7, 9, 10, 12) have reported better results in those patients undergoing partial rather than total meniscectomy. Fowler (2) demonstrated that the severity of degenerative joint changes depended on the amount

A
Bucket Handle Tear

B
Peripheral Detachment

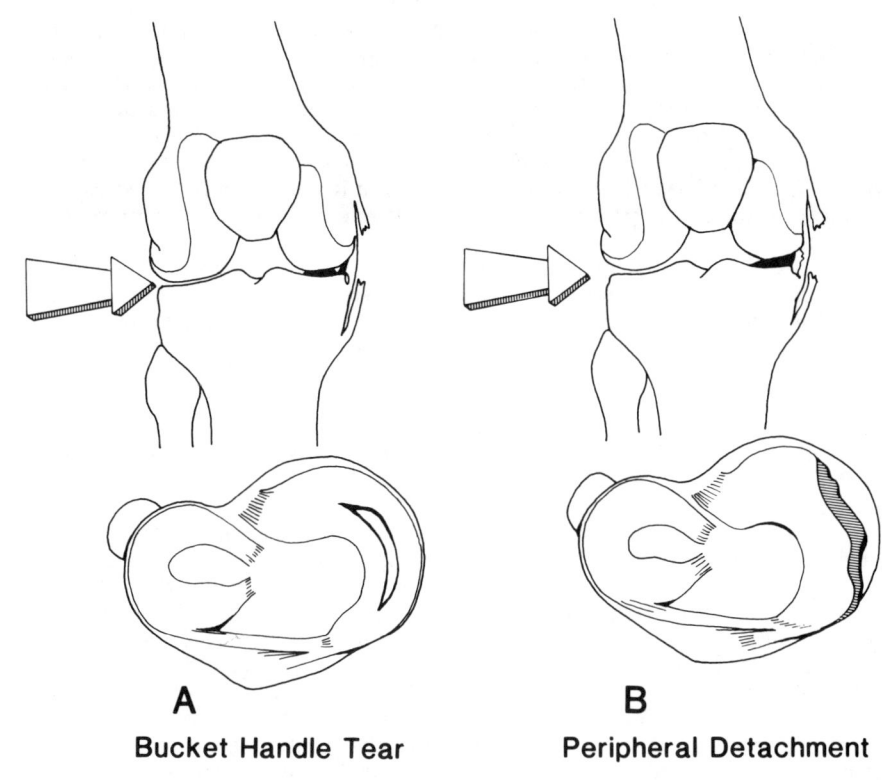

Fig. 27-1. *Common meniscal lesions in younger athletes. A: bucket-handle tear; B: peripheral detachments may be caused by pure valgus force to the knee.*

of meniscus removed. He reported that although meniscectomy eliminated load transmission of the excised area, it resulted in redistribution of the load over the remaining portion of the meniscus. Thus in the case of peripheral lesions, efforts should be made to carefully reattach the meniscus. The preservation of even a small rim of meniscus has definite merit.

In older individuals who participate in athletics, degenerative changes are due to continuous competitive athletics and are a late finding after untreated ligament and meniscal injury. Pain and stiffness after prolonged activity are common complaints. Muscle atrophy, ligament contractures, and osteophytic buildups may be present. Acute episodes of osteoarthritis of the knee are treated with rest and oral anti-inflammatory medications. In moderate to severe cases where the patient is not a candidate for a total knee replacement, arthroscopic debridement and/or abrasion arthroplasty may be performed. The morbidity is low and the patient's quality of life can be improved.

Prior to the advent of arthroscopy, the osteoarthritic knee was frequently treated by open debridement. Removal of all mechanical irritants was believed to slow the progression of the disease. This was accomplished by shaving degenerative cartilage, excising torn menisci, removing loose bodies and osteophytes, and patellar debriding or patellectomy. The advantages of arthroscopic debridement over open treatment are numerous. Prolonged immobilization is unnecessary. The hospital stay is decreased, and a long and difficult rehabilitation program is shortened and facilitated.

Jackson (4) states that arthroscopy is indicated to evaluate the state of the arthritic joint and determine the need for an extra-articular procedure such as an upper tibial osteotomy, or an intra-articular procedure such as meniscectomy, cartilage shaving, removal of loose bodies, or abrasion arthroplasty. Beneficial effects have been observed following irrigation only of the osteoarthritic knee (6). Many patients have reported relief of symptoms ranging from days to years.

Excessive compression is an important factor in the degenerative process of the meniscus (13). With the knee in a constantly flexed position, there is increased compression and significant degeneration of the posterior horn of the meniscus. Horizontal cleavage and flap meniscal tears (Fig. 27-2 and Fig. 27-3) are usually the result of degenerative changes in the meniscus. They frequently occur after the age of 30 and follow a minor trauma, such as a sudden turn or rising from a kneeling position. The rotation that takes place normally between the meniscus, tibia, and femur tends to occur more or less within the substance of the meniscus, resulting in horizontal cleavage which remains closed until trauma takes place (13).

Jackson (4) has delineated several principles for the arthroscopic treatment of the osteoarthritic knee. He believes the first and most important principle is to prevent the development of degenerative changes by the early restoration of normal function. To do this, one must make an early diagnosis and then treat the abnormality correctly. Such treatment involves careful surgery (including detection and preservation of normal menisci) followed by a thorough rehabilitation program. With knees that show moderately advanced arthritic changes at the time of treatment, one should try to retard or reverse the process of degenerative arthritis by correcting the existing abnormalities. With joints that show a far advanced state of arthritis, salvage surgery is all that remains to be done and is performed solely to improve function (4).

In addition to meniscal tears, arthroscopy in the osteoarthritic knee is effective in the treatment of proliferative synovitis, articular lesions, and for removal of osteophytes and loose bodies (14). Johnson (8) has reported good results in 76% of patients undergoing arthroscopic abrasion arthroplasty. Friedman et al. (3) have also demonstrated good results with abrasion arthroplasty to stimulate a viable new surface in the diseased joint.

In conclusion, when discussing arthroscopic treatment of athletes' knee injuries, we must divide patients into 2 age groups—those patients less than 30 years of age and those over 30 years of age. In the younger age group, trauma is usually the mechanism of the knee injury. The primary intra-articular pathology found is a bucket-handle or peripheral tear of the meniscus. The importance of the meniscal cartilage and its relationship to normal joint function has been emphasized in many reports, and the high incidence of degenerative arthritis of the knee following total meniscal excision has been recognized (16). In the young athlete, an attempt should be made to preserve joint function with a partial rather than a total meniscectomy. Complications following arthroscopic meniscectomy are rare. Shahriarie (12) arthroscopically removed 205 displaced bucket-handle tears and reports no early degenerative arthritis of the tibial femoral joint.

Arthroscopy is beneficial in the treatment of meniscal damage in the older athlete's knee as well. Flap tears and horizontal cleavage tears of the menisci can be excised. Chondral lesions and chondromalacia of the patella, femoral, and tibial condyles can also be debrided arthroscopically. Similarly, osteophytes and loose bodies may be removed. In those athletes with moderate to

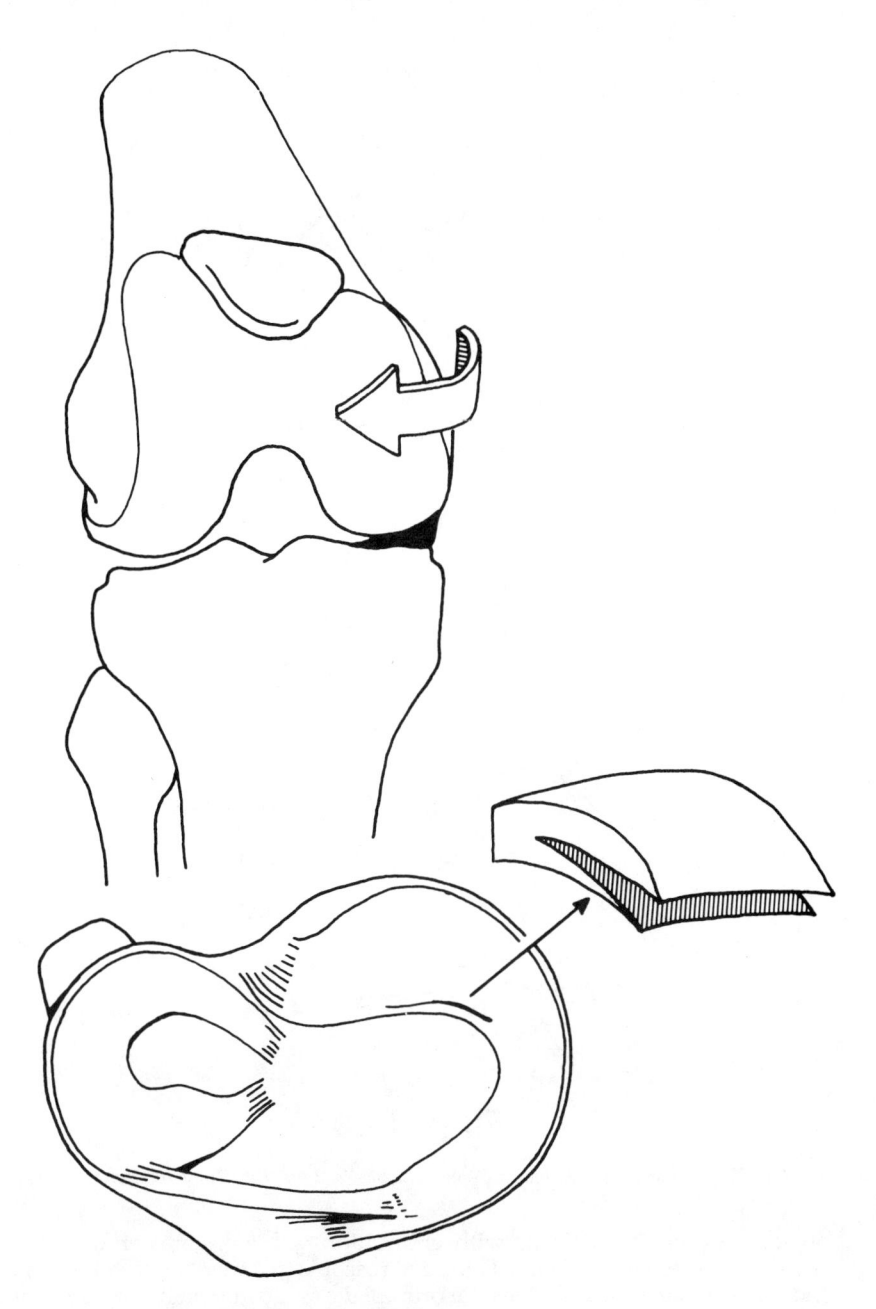

Degenerative Horizontal Cleavage Tear

Fig. 27-2. *Horizontal cleavage tears, common in the older athlete, are frequently due to rotation of the knee with the foot fixed to the ground.*

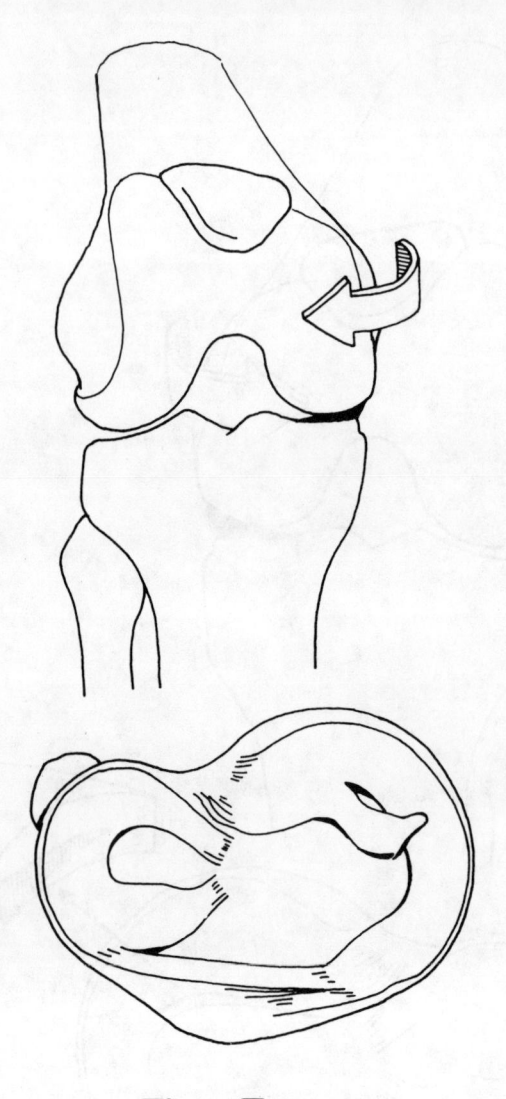

Flap Tear

Fig. 27-3. *Flap tears, common in older athletes, are often due to a rotational injury.*

severe degenerative arthritis with eburnation of bone, abrasion arthroplasty is a viable treatment modality. Thus, arthroscopic treatment of both the younger and older athlete's knee enables the orthopedic surgeon to minimize the amount of surgical trauma and maintain the function of the knee joint.

REFERENCES

1. Early Degenerative Arthritis of the Knee. Symposium Report. *J. Bone Joint Surg.* 51A:1026–1028, 1969.

2. Fowler, P. J. Meniscal lesions in the adolescent. The role of arthroscopy in the management of adolescent knee problems. In: *The Injured Adolescent Knee.* 42–75. J. C. Kennedy (ed.) Baltimore: Williams and Wilkins, 1979.
3. Friedman, M. J., C. C. Berasi, J. M. Fox, W. Del Pizzo, S. J. Snyder, and R. D. Ferkel. Preliminary results with abrasion arthroplasty in the osteoarthritic knee. *Clin. Orthop.* 182:200–205, 1984.
4. Jackson, R. W. The role of arthroscopy in the management of the arthritic knee. *Clin. Orthop.* 101:28–35, 1974.
5. Jackson, R. W., and I. Abe. The role of arthroscopy in the management of disorders of the knee. *J. Bone Joint Surg.* 54B:310–322, 1972.
6. Jackson, R. W., and K. E. Dehaven. Arthroscopy of the knee. *Clin. Orthop.* 107:87–92, 1975.
7. Jackson, R. W., and D. W. Rouse. The results of partial arthroscopic meniscectomy in patients over 40 years of age. *J. Bone Joint Surg.* 64B:481–486, 1982.
8. Johnson, L. L. Abrasion arthroplasty (videocassette) *Arthroscopy Video Journal* (3):1982.
9. Johnson, R. J., D. B. Kettelkamp, W. Clark, and P. Leaverton. Factors affecting late results after meniscectomy. *J. Bone Joint Surg.* 56A:719–729, 1974.
10. Orbon, R. J., and G. G. Poehling. Arthroscopic meniscectomy. *South Med. J.* 74:1238–1242, 1981.
11. Radin, E. L., I. L. Paul, and R. M. Rose. Role of mechanical factors in pathogenesis of primary osteoarthritis. *Lancet* 1:519–522, 1972.
12. Shahriarie, H. Six years follow-up on arthroscopic excision of bucket handle tears. *Arthroscopic surgery of the knee seminar.* March 26–28, 1981. The Alamos Resort, Scottsdale, Arizona.
13. Smillie, I. S. *Injuries of the Knee Joint,* 5th ed. Edinburgh: Churchill Livingstone, 1978.
14. Sprague, N. F. Arthroscopic debridement for degenerative knee joint disease. *Clin. Orthop.* 160:118–123, 1981.
15. Sprague, N. F. Arthroscopic meniscectomy. Patterns of meniscal tears and general approaches. *Arthroscopic Surgery of the Knee Seminar,* March 26–28, 1981. The Alamos Resort, Scottsdale, Arizona.
16. Tapper, E. M., and N. W. Hoover. Later results after meniscectomy. *J. Bone Joint Surg.* 51A:517–526, 1969.

28

Principles of Resistance Exercise in Rehabilitation Following Knee Injuries

D. G. SALE, PH.D.

McMaster University

A common feature of knee injuries is a loss of voluntary muscular strength in the muscle groups acting on the knee joint. The loss of strength may be a direct result of injury or a result of treatment such as surgery and immobilization. Rehabilitation consists in part of restoring strength to at least the pre-injury level.

Voluntary strength of a muscle group is determined by the quantity and quality of the muscle and by the extent to which the muscle mass can be activated by the central nervous system. Consequently, it is not surprising that the loss of strength following knee injuries is related to both atrophy of muscle (17) and reduced neural activation of muscle during voluntary effort (12). Similarly, increases in voluntary strength with rehabilitation exercise or training in normal conditions might be expected to be associated with muscle hypertrophy (23) and increased neural activation (16, 28).

The basic unit of neuromuscular function is the motor unit, which consists of a motoaneuron and the muscle fibers it innervates. The large muscles acting at the knee joint would consist of several hundred to a few thousand motor units. Each motor unit would consist of a few to several hundred muscle fibers. The concept of the motor unit is a suitable focus for the consideration of principles of rehabilitation exercise; thus, the successful rehabilitation program is one which enables the patient to fully activate all the motor units of the appropriate muscle groups, and which stimulates hypertrophy of the muscle fibers of the motor units.

In the following sections, the principles of rehabilitative exercise will be discussed in relation to achieving 2 objectives: 1) attaining complete motor unit activation; 2) stimulating adaptation in muscle fibers. The relative merits of common types of exercise equipment will also be discussed. Finally, some aspects of program design and evaluation will be considered.

PRINCIPLES OF RESISTANCE EXERCISE

Achieving Complete Motor Unit Activation

OVERLOAD: Motor units in human muscles are of 2 main types. Slow-twitch motor units are relatively small and therefore, according to the size principle (18), are recruited easily with mild voluntary effort. These motor units are resistant to fatigue and are thus suitable for maintaining posture and maintaining low intensity activity for prolonged periods. Fast-twitch motor units are larger and therefore more difficult to recruit. The largest and highest threshold fast-twitch motor units are recruited only during maximal or near-maximal efforts. Application of the overload principle consists of imposing an exercise task which requires a high degree of voluntary effort to complete, thereby ensuring that all motor units have been activated. The overload condition may be imposed in 2 ways. First, the patient may be required to perform a series of brief maximal contractions, as might be done on an isokinetic dynamometer. Second, the patient may be required to perform a series of submaximal contractions until failure (i.e., until fatigue prevents further contractions) as might be done on weight lifting apparatus. The relative merits of the 2 methods of overload will be discussed below in relation to adaptation in muscle fibers and in relation to exercise equipment.

LIMITATIONS TO ACHIEVING THE OVERLOAD CONDITION: Several factors may affect the patient's ability to achieve complete motor unit activation during rehabilitation exercise.

Motivation: An obvious factor is motivation. Patients who are unwilling to make maximal efforts will fail to activate the highest threshold motor units.

Pain: Pain may limit voluntary effort and prevent full motor unit activation. Even if the patient disregards the pain, pain-induced reflex inhibition may still limit complete motor unit activation (10).

Reflex Inhibition: Even in the absence of pain, surgical intervention may result in reflex inhibition of motor units (32).

Immobilization: If the treatment of the knee injury has included a period of immobilization, the immobilization itself may cause impairment of the patient's ability to fully activate motor units (12, 29).

Specificity of Movement Pattern: A change in joint position (22) or in the movement performed by a muscle group (34) can affect the motor unit activation achieved by a patient during maximal effort. Based on these observations, there would be merit in selecting a variety of exercises involving different movements and ranges of movement in the rehabilitation program. This would ensure acquisition of complete motor unit activation of a muscle group in a variety of conditions.

Specificity of Velocity: Increases in strength following training are to some extent specific to the velocity of contraction at which the training is performed (5, 9, 20). The specificity may be the result of specific changes in the muscle (9), but also the result of specific changes in motor unit activation (5). In the specific case of knee extension, voluntary contractions at the low velocity, high force portion of the concentric contraction force-velocity relationship may cause reflex inhibition of motor units (3, 4). Within the constraints of safety and suitable equipment, it may be valuable to perform exercises at a variety of velocities.

Potentiation by Precontraction of Antagonists: Motor unit activation of a muscle group can be enhanced if its activation is immediately preceded by a contraction of the antagonists (3, 4). The potentiation is most pronounced when the ensuing contraction is performed at low velocity (3). Therefore, there would be an advantage to an arrangement whereby reciprocal contractions of antagonistic muscle groups could be performed.

Unilateral vs. Bilateral Contractions: There is impairment of motor unit activation when the same movement must be performed simultaneously with both limbs (26, 31, 35). Consequently, it would be easier for a patient if one limb was exercised at a time. On the other hand, the impairment isn't present if the two limbs are performing opposite movements (e.g., extension of one knee simultaneous with flexion of the other knee) (26).

Inducing Adaptation in Muscle Fibers

Once the patient can regularly activate a motor unit during rehabilitation exercise, the muscle fibers will begin to adapt. The nature of the adaptation will depend on which method of overload is used.

STRENGTH VS ENDURANCE: If the exercise consists of high resistance, low repetition exercise (strength training), the muscle fibers will hypertrophy (23), and the hypertrophy will be due in part to increased contractile protein (24). If the exercise consists of low resistance, high repetition exercise (endurance training), the muscle fibers will undergo little or no hypertrophy; however, adaptations related to endurance will have occurred, such as increased capillary density (1) and mitochondrial volume density (19). Because immobilization and hypoactivity following knee injuries are associated with losses in both the strength and endurance components of the muscle fibers (6), the rehabilitation program should include both forms of training. While the foregoing is valid when comparing the extremes of strength and endurance training (2), many common programs contain both strength and endurance elements, even if they are considered as only a strength or endurance program. Short-term experiments comparing these so-called strength and endurance programs have demonstrated an apparent lack of specificity in the results obtained (8). In these studies, the overriding common factor of overload has prevailed over any specific elements in the two programs compared.

VELOCITY OF CONTRACTION: Performing exercises at different velocities of contraction may affect the intrinsic contractile properties of muscle. Isometric contraction training may increase shortening velocity with heavy but not light loads, whereas ballistic training with light weights will increase shortening velocity with light but not heavy loads (9). The velocities of contraction used in the patient's normal and sporting activities should be considered when designing the rehabilitation program.

EVALUATION OF EXERCISE EQUIPMENT

Several types of resistance training equipment are now available for rehabilitation. The types include weight training, hydraulic, pneumatic, and electro-mechanical machines. As might be expected, there are now computer-controlled machines which allow velocity, tension, and contraction type to be programmed and monitored. The relative merits of the various types of equipment will be evaluated against selected criteria.

Matching the Strength Curve

In maximal voluntary contractions, the torque that can be developed by a muscle group at a joint will vary as the joint position (angle) changes. The variation in torque with changing joint angle, which is referred to as a strength curve, is caused by variation in muscle length, leverage, and motor unit activation. To ensure that motor unit activation is near-maximal at all joint positions through a range of movement, it would be desirable to exercise with a device that provided a resistance curve that closely matched the strength curve.

Cam or lever systems have been incorporated into weight, pneumatic, and spring and cable machines to provide appropriate resistance curves. Various manufacturers have been more or less successful with this approach. There are limitations to cam and lever systems. First, while these systems can be successful in providing an average resistance curve, they cannot provide for normal variations in strength curves. Second, an injury may cause a marked alteration in a strength curve; cam and lever systems cannot accommodate such alterations. Third, a strength curve may alter during the performance of an exercise due to fatigue; cam and lever systems cannot adjust precisely to the effects of fatigue. Finally, cam and lever systems which are incorporated into weight machines must contend with inertia and momentum. Performing the exercise at different speeds can alter the resistance pattern.

Velocity-controlled hydraulic or electro-mechanical machines (most commonly isokinetic or quasi-isokinetic machines) by design are able to provide resistance which precisely matches any strength curve. Variations caused by fatigue or injury are automatically accommodated.

Velocity Control

Velocity-controlled hydraulic and electro-mechanical machines by design permit velocity-controlled exercise. The most common machine is isokinetic; that is, once a velocity of contraction is set, it remains constant regardless of the torque produced. A range of velocities may be selected, allowing exercise to be performed at various controlled velocities. Two problems can arise when using some isokinetic devices for high velocity exercise. One problem is that no resistance is offered by the device until the limb has accelerated up to the preset velocity. At high velocities, a significant portion of the range of movement can be traversed before resistance is encountered. Thus, the device fails to provide full range resistance. The second problem is related to the first one. When the device is finally engaged after acceleration of the limb, there is an impact event (30, 37) as the limb is suddenly decelerated by the device. This impact could be traumatic to the joint or muscle structure. Some manufacturers have dealt with these problems by providing a ramp increase in velocity up to the target velocity. These ramp increases occur over a period of a few hundred milliseconds. Resistance is met at the initiation of the movement; therefore, there is full range resistance and the impact event is avoided. Some devices can be programmed so that the entire movement is an acceleration against resistance. With computer control, innumerable velocity patterns are possible.

In the case of weight, pneumatic, and cable and spring devices, control of velocity is indirect. Setting a high resistance ensures a low velocity of movement, while a low resistance will permit accelerations to high velocities. These movements are similar to the full range accelerations of the velocity-controlled devices. A problem with weight machines is that inertia can impose excessive resistance at the beginning of the movement, while momentum can unload the resistance toward the end of the movement. The inertia of pneumatic and cable and spring systems is minimal by comparison.

Vanishing Resistance

There may be occasions during rehabilitation exercise when pain causes a sudden reduction or complete cessation of force output. A corresponding reduction or cessation of resistance would be a desirable feature of exercise equipment. The velocity-controlled devices possess this feature of vanishing resistance, for resistance exists only as a reaction to muscular force output. In contrast, the resistance (resistive force) of weight, pneumatic, and spring and cable machines does not dissipate with cessation of muscular force output. The resistance in this situation could be the source of inconvenience, added discomfort, or even injury. In the rehabilitation of injured or reconstructed knees, these machines should not be used until the healing phase is completed.

Eccentric Resistance

Muscles can develop their greatest tension when they are forcibly lengthened (eccentric contraction). Because the stimulus to protein synthesis and muscle hypertrophy is positively related to muscle tension (13), it could be argued that high force eccentric contraction training would be superior to stimulate muscle growth. There is some evidence to support this argument (21). Eccentric muscle training may also stimulate beneficial adaptations in connective tissue.

Weight lifting exercise consists of alternating concentric and eccentric contractions. To permit high force eccentric contractions to be made, adjustments are necessary. With some apparatus it is possible to raise the weight (concentric phase) with both limbs and to lower the weight (eccentric phase) with one limb. Another technique is to have assistance with the concentric phase and then perform the eccentric phase without assistance. These same modifications can be used with pneumatic and spring and cable equipment. Until recently, velocity-controlled equipment (isokinetic and quasi-isokinetic) permitted the performance of concentric and isometric exercise only. Now two manufacturers offer velocity-controlled eccentric loading. Eccentric exercise is perhaps safest with this equipment.

High force eccentric training can cause muscle damage and severe soreness (11) in its initial stages, but this problem can be minimized by gradual progression in the training.

Two-Way Resistance

As discussed earlier, it may be easier for the patient to fully activate motor units if antagonistic muscle groups can contract alternately. Most of the velocity-controlled devices permit alternate concentric contractions of antagonistic muscle groups, and two now permit alternate eccentric exercise. One-way resistance devices (weight, pneumatic, spring and cable machines) do not allow this kind of exercise to be performed.

Unilateral and Reciprocal Exercise

It had been observed that patients may have difficulty fully activating motor units if bilateral rather than unilateral exercise must be performed. Most types of resistance equipment allow unilateral exercise to be performed. Bilateral exercise is not a hindrance if it is reciprocal; that is, if extension in one limb is simultaneous with flexion in the other limb and vice versa. Reciprocal exercise is only possible with two-way resistance equipment.

Other Features

Other features of rehabilitation exercise equipment to be considered are ease and convenience of use, extent of feedback to patient while exercising, data analysis features, and adaptability to different movement patterns and to patients of varying sizes.

ADDITIONAL CONSIDERATIONS

Electrical Stimulation

In the early phase of rehabilitation when it may be difficult for the patient to fully activate motor units by voluntary effort, therapeutic electrical stimulation could, in theory, be useful for training the muscle fibers of motor units. Electrical stimulation could be phased out as the patient regained control of the motor units. To be effective, the stimulation must be tetanic so that the evoked tension is great enough to stimulate hypertrophy or prevent further atrophy. To ensure a high probability that muscle fibers of units not activated voluntarily are stimulated, the intensity of stimulation must be great enough to activate a large proportion of the muscle mass. Fulfillment of these two conditions of electrical stimulation may be associated with discomfort to the patient. A gradual increase in the intensity and frequency of stimulation will allow the patient to habituate to the discomfort. The effectiveness of programs of electrical stimulation will depend upon the degree to which the two conditions of stimulation have been satisfied and upon the measurements used to evaluate effectiveness (7, 10, 27).

Early Range of Movement Techniques

There is some evidence that early range of movement techniques following some types of knee surgery can accelerate the recovery of voluntary strength (15, 33). Early range of movement activities may allow the patient to more quickly regain full activation of motor units.

Flexor/Extensor Balance

When the treatment of a knee injury has involved a period of immobilization, the knee extensors tend to atrophy to a greater extent than the knee flexors (17, 36). It would seem reasonable, therefore, to emphasize the extensors in the rehabilitation exercise. The flexors should not be neglected, however; otherwise, an imbalance may develop in favor of the extensors.

Criteria for Recovery and Return to Activity

Setting criteria for recovery is complicated by specificity of training. Thus, an isokinetic rehabilitation program may achieve complete restoration of isokinetic voluntary strength, yet there will still be apparent atrophy of the affected muscle groups (14). Another possibility is that the rehabilitation will have restored strength completely but not endurance (6). Whenever possible, there should be among the criterion tests one or more which closely simulate the activities to which the patient will be returning.

Age

The basic principles of resistance exercise for rehabilitation can be applied similarly for all age groups. In the case of older individuals, the rate of healing and adaptation to training will be slower. Furthermore, there will be a greater susceptibility to tissue strain and injury as well as muscle soreness in this age group. A gradual progression in the exercise can prevent or minimize difficulties arising from these characteristics.

REFERENCES

1. Anderson, P., and J. Henriksson. Capillary supply of the quadriceps femoris muscle of man: Adaptive response to exercise. *J. Physiol.* (Lond.) 270:677–690, 1977.
2. Anderson, T., and J. T. Kearney. Effects of three resistance training programs on muscular strength and absolute and relative endurance. *Res. Quart. Exerc. Sport* 53:1–7, 1982.
3. Caiozzo, V. J., W. S. Barnes, C. A. Prietto, and W. C. McMaster. The effect of isometric precontractions on the slow velocity—high force region of the in-vivo force-velocity relationship. *Med. Sci. Sports Exerc.* (abs) 13:128, 1981.
4. Caiozzo, V. J., T. Laird, K. Chow, C. A. Prietto, and W. C. McMaster. The use of precontractions to enhance the in vivo force-velocity relationship. *Med. Sci. Sports Exerc.* (abs) 14:162, 1982.
5. Caiozzo, V. J., J. J. Perrine, and V. R. Edgerton. Training-induced alterations of the in vivo force-velocity relationship of human muscle. *J. Appl. Physiol: REEP* 51:750–754, 1981.
6. Costill, D. L., W. J. Fink, and A. J. Habansky. Muscle rehabilitation after knee surgery. *Phys. Sports Med.* 5:71–74, 1977.
7. Currier, D. P., J. Lehman, and P. Lightfoot. Electrical stimulation in exercise of the quadriceps femoris muscle. *Phys. Ther.* 59:1508–1512, 1979.
8. DeLateur, B. J., J. F. Lehman, and W. E. Fordyce. A test of the Delorme axiom. *Arch. Phys. Med. Rehab.* 49:245–248, 1968.
9. Duchateau, J., and K. Hainaut. Isometric or dynamic training: Differential effects on mechanical properties of a human muscle. *J. Appl. Physiol: REEP* 56:296–301, 1984.
10. Eriksson, E. Sports injuries of the knee ligaments: Their diagnosis, treatment, rehabilitation, and prevention. *Med. Sci. Sports* 8:133–144, 1976.
11. Friden, J., M. Sjöström, and B. Ekblom. A morphological study of delayed muscle soreness. *Experientia* 37:506–507, 1981.
12. Fuglsang-Frederiksen, A. and U. Scheel. Transient decrease in number of motor units after immobilisation in man. *J. Neurol. Neurosurg. Psychiat.* 41:924–929, 1978.

13. Goldberg, A. L., J. D. Etlinger, D. F. Goldspink, and C. Jablecki. Mechanism of work-induced hypertrophy of skeletal muscle. *Med. Sci. Sports Exerc.* 7:248–261, 1975.
14. Grimby, G., E. Gustafsson, L. Peterson, and P. Renstrom. Quadriceps function and training after knee ligament surgery. *Med. Sci. Sports Exerc.* 12:70–75, 1980.
15. Haggmark, T., and E. Eriksson. Cylinder or mobile cast-brace after knee ligament surgery. *Am. J. Sports Med.* 7:48–56, 1979.
16. Hakkinen, K., and P. V. Komi. Electromyographic changes during strength training and detraining. *Med. Sci. Sports Exerc.* 15:455–460, 1983.
17. Halkjner-Kristensen, J., and T. Ingemann-Hansen. Wasting and training of the human quadriceps muscle during the treatment of knee ligament injuries. *Scand. J. Rehab. Med.*, Suppl. 13, 1985.
18. Henneman, E., and C. B. Olson. Relation between structure and function in the design of skeletal muscle. *J. Neurophysiol.* 28:581–598, 1965.
19. Hoppeler, H., P. Luthi, H. Claassen, E. R. Weibel, and H. Howald. The ultrastructure of the normal human skeletal muscle. A morphometric analysis on untrained men, women and well-trained orienteers. *Pfluegers Arch.* 344:217–232, 1973.
20. Kanehisa, H., and M. Miyashita. Specificity of velocity in strength training. *Eur. J. Appl. Physiol.* 52:104–106, 1983.
21. Komi, P. V., and E. Buskirk. Effect of eccentric and concentric muscle conditioning on tension and electrical activity of human muscle. *Ergonomics* 15:417–434, 1972.
22. Lindh, M. Increase of muscle strength from isometric quadriceps exercises at different knee angles. *Scand. J. Rehab. Med.* 11:33–36, 1979.
23. MacDougall, J. D., G. C. B. Elder, D. G. Sale, J. R. Moroz, and J. R. Sutton. Effects of strength training and immobilization on human muscle fibres. *Eur. J. Appl. Physiol.* 43:25–34, 1980.
24. MacDougall, J. D., D. G. Sale, G. Elder, and J. R. Sutton. Ultrastructural properties of human skeletal muscle following heavy resistance training and immobilization. *Med. Sci. Sports* (abs) 8:72, 1976.
25. Moritani, T., and H. A. de Vries. Neural factors vs hypertrophy in the time course of muscle strength gain. *Am. J. Phys. Med. Rehab.* 58:115–130, 1979.
26. Ohtsuki, T. Decrease in human voluntary isometric arm strength induced by simultaneous bilateral exertion. *Behav. Brain Res.* 7:165–178, 1983.
27. Romero, J. A., T. L. Sanford, R. V. Schroeder, and T. D. Fahey. The effects of electrical stimulation of normal quadriceps on strength and girth. *Med. Sci. Sports Exerc.* 14:194–197, 1982.
28. Sale, D. G., J. D. MacDougall, A. R. M. Upton, and A. J. McComas. Effect of strength training upon motoneuron excitability in man. *Med. Sci. Sports Exerc.* 15:57–62, 1983.
29. Sale, D. G., A. J. McComas, J. D. MacDougall, and A. R. M. Upton. Neuromuscular adaptation in human thenar muscles following strength training and immobilization. *J. Appl. Physiol: REEP* 53:419–424, 1982.
30. Sapega, A. A., J. A. Nicholas, D. Sokolow, and A. Saraniti. The nature of torque "overshoot" in Cybex isokinetic dynamometry. *Med. Sci. Sports Exerc.* 14:360–375, 1982.
31. Secher, N. H., S. Rorsgaard, and O. Secher. Contralateral influence on recruitment of curarized muscle fibers during maximal voluntary extension of the legs. *Acta Physiol. Scand.* 103:456–462, 1978.
32. Shakespeare, D. T., M. Stokes, K. P. Sherman, and A. Young. Reflex inhibition of the quadriceps after meniscectomy: Lack of association with pain. *Clin. Physiol.* 5:137–144, 1985.
33. Sherman, W. M., D. R. Pearson, M. J. Plyley, D. L. Costill, J. A. Habansky, and D. A. Vogelgesang. Isokinetic rehabilitation after surgery. *Am. J. Sports Med.* 10:155–161, 1982.
34. Thorstensson, A., J. Karlsson, J. H. T. Viitasalo, P. Luhtanen, and P. V. Komi. Effect of strength training on EMG of human skeletal muscle. *Acta Physiol. Scand.* 98:323–336, 1976.
35. Vandervoort, A. A., D. G. Sale, and J. Moroz. Comparison of motor unit activation during unilateral and bilateral leg extension. *J. Appl. Physiol: REEP* 56:46–51, 1984.
36. Vegso, J. J., S. E. Genuario, and J. S. Torg. Maintenance of hamstring strength following knee surgery. *Med. Sci. Sports Exerc.* 17:376–379, 1985.
37. Winter, D. A., R. P. Wells, and G. W. Orr. Errors in the use of isokinetic dynamometers. *Eur. J. Appl. Physiol.* 46:397–408, 1981.

29

Factors Influencing the Throwing Arm of the Masters Athlete

FRANK W. JOBE, M.D.

Kerlan-Jobe Orthopedic Clinic

This chapter will discuss factors allowing masters athletes to continue throwing. In reviewing 1,600 shoulder patients in our office, we subdivided them by age into 5-year cohorts. There were no distinctive age-related patterns of pathology. We do see rotator cuff tears in masters athletes which are, in appearance, similar to those found in non-athletes of the same age. In other words, the athletic activity hasn't kept the tissue looking like that of a 21-year-old. It might be that a kind of natural selection is going on in that problems which arise tend to force throwing athletes out of the highly competitive arena, and since there is no separate masters' circuit in the throwing sports on which they can still compete, they simply stop throwing.

On the other hand, more and more throwing athletes are remaining in the major leagues to an older age. Sports writer Mark Heisler of the *Los Angeles Times* recently wrote a piece on the growing number of older baseball players. He noted that of the 650 players now in the majors, about 80 are 35 years old or older, 8 are 40 or older, and 6 of these 8 are pitchers. Certainly the performances of the throwing athletes at these games are further testimony to the potential for prolonged excellence in the throwing sports. Since others will discuss in detail the more common throwing injuries of the shoulder, it would be appropriate to review important concepts in shoulder stability, and look at the more important factors that allow masters athletes to continue to excel in the throwing sports.

The first factor is genetic makeup. It has been said by Ernst Jokl and others that the most important factor in becoming a world class athlete is the careful selection of one's parents. Genetic constitution sets the outer limits of one's performance capacity. Unfortunately, lack of opportunity, inadequate coaching, and absence of motivation often prevent individuals from exploring or achieving much of their potential. Another factor influenced by genetics is the individual's healing potential. The manner in which and the time frame within which an athlete is able to respond to a micro or macro injury is largely inherited and will certainly play a role in the longevity and quality of performance.

The second factor is the psychological makeup. Those who are successful in sports have mental toughness and attitudes which allow them to perform highly skilled acts while under great stress. Those who pursue excellence at the masters level must have strong motivating factors, such as a deep love for the game or a fierce competitive drive.

The third factor is individual style and technique. It is predictable that there will be a greater number of finesse pitchers than flamethrowers lasting in the major leagues. Those who do rely on speed will be able to do so only if their timing and mechanics are such that maximum efficiency is possible with minimum stress.

The fourth factor is an individually correct training and competition program. When one considers the fine line between those who are able to compete at the highest levels and those who cannot, the added decrease in flexibility, healing rate, strength, and stamina which occurs with increasing age, it becomes obvious that those who have a customized and physiologically sound training and competition program will have an edge.

It is in the areas of style, technique, training, and competition that one has the most control. The throwing motion is a complex series of events which requires proper sequencing and timing to be efficient and effective. Because of the very high stresses involved, a slight deficiency in sequencing or timing, muscle balance or stamina, and/or recovery periods will have a cumulative detrimental effect. Not only will this potentially create shoulder problems, but they will be manifested in the weakest link of the thrower's kinetic chain. It has been my experience that masters' level throwers as a group do not show any dramatic increase in the common shoulder problems of impingement, instability, or overuse. Interestingly enough, it is problems of the spine, hip, knee, and foot that seem to surface as they continue to throw.

If you review videotapes of throwing, you will be better able to appreciate the high levels of stress involved in throwing, how much of the body is actually involved in the throwing act, and the importance of proper sequencing and timing to maximize efficiency while minimizing stress. With a better appreciation of the demands, the order, and the complexity of the throwing act, let us look at some important concepts of shoulder stability.

First, stability of the shoulder depends on glenohumeral contact with labral enhancement, static stabilizers (the capsule and ligamentous thickenings), and dynamic stabilizers (primarily the rotator cuff). The scapula must anticipate humeral motion and adjust its position to maximize the ability of the static and dynamic stabilizers to work. Failure to do so results in increasing the destabilizing and impingement potential. As an example, if the scapula moves first with the humerus lagging, anterior forces are increased; if the scapula is slow with the humerus ahead, posterior forces are increased; and if the scapula is immobile, all forces are increased at some point in the range.

The second concept is that scapular positioning occurs via trunk and scapulo-thoracic motion. Obviously, the scapula must follow the trunk; what is not so obvious is the use of truncal positioning as a mechanism for scapular positioning. All planes of motion are possible. For example, the baseball pitcher has more than 180 degrees of trunk rotation. Proper mechanics and flexibility are important to allow this optimal truncal positioning. Scapulo-thoracic motion has a much smaller excursion but is faster moving, thus allowing fine tuning of this positioning.

Muscles important for scapulo-thoracic motion include: the serratus anterior, the trapezius, levator scapulae, rhomboids, and the pectoralis minor. Proper mechanics, flexibility, balanced muscles, and muscular stamina are important for proper scapulo-thoracic positioning.

In summary: 1) the throwing act requires a complex sequence of events which involve much of the trunk; 2) the stability of the shoulder requires glenohumeral contact with labral enhancement, static plus dynamic stabilizers, and scapulo-thoracic synchrony; and 3) proper individual style, mechanics, training, and competition are important to all athletes but are essential to those who pursue continued excellence at the masters level.

30

Arthroscopy of the Shoulder

JAMES R. ANDREWS, M.D.
WILLIAM G. CARSON, M.D.
JOSEPH J. CALANDRA, M.D.

Hughston Orthopedic Clinic, P.C.

ABSTRACT

We present our technique of diagnostic and operative arthroscopy of the shoulder. Constant attention to technical detail and consistent patient positioning is crucial to the success of the procedure. In using a systematic approach we can use our knowledge of the normal anatomy and its variations to diagnose and treat the pathological processes of the joint. Posterior and anterior portals are accurately located by outlining the bony landmarks of the shoulder. Using a large 4-millimeter (mm) diameter angled arthroscope, structures within the shoulder are systematically and sequentially examined. Diagnostic shoulder arthroscopy can be accurate and reproducible provided the surgeon has a thorough knowledge of normal anatomy and its normal variations. The surgeon must give attention to accurate placement of the arthroscopic portals and to the surgical technique.

INTRODUCTION

During the past decade, arthroscopy has become firmly established as a diagnostic and therapeutic modality for the knee joint. However, its more recent applications to other joints has led to the need for safe and effective techniques.

The shoulder joint is a common source of pain and in throwing athletes it is a common source of injury (4). Many physicians are familiar with the usual diagnostic modalities such as physical examination, radiography, arthrography, and various radioactive scans. More recently, arthrotomography

---

This work was supported in part by the Hughston Sports Medicine Foundation, Inc., 6262 Hamilton Road, Columbus, Georgia 31995.

and nuclear magnetic resonance scans have increased our knowledge of the shoulder (9, 21, 22, 25). These, however, cannot compare to the knowledge and understanding of the intra-articular anatomy and pathology we have acquired with the use of the arthroscope (3, 5, 17, 19).

To be effective, an arthroscopic examination of any joint must be systematic and reproducible. In this report, we present our technique for shoulder arthroscopy and describe a sequential examination of the shoulder joint.

TECHNIQUE

After general endotracheal anesthesia is administered, the patient is placed in the lateral decubitus position and supported by a bean bag or kidney rest. The forearm and wrist are placed in a prefabricated wrist gauntlet or skin traction apparatus. This traction device is connected to an overhead pulley with the arm in 15° of forward flexion and 70° of abduction (Fig. 30-1). The traction rope is then secured and suspended by a 7- to 9-kilogram (kg) weight. Ideally the pulley system is attached to the table so that when the table is raised or lowered, the entire unit (pulley, weight, and table) will move as one.

The shoulder is prepped in a sterile fashion from the elbow to, and including, the axilla (which is not shaved) and then draped. The bony landmarks are identified and outlined with a sterile marking pen. These are: the anterolateral and posterolateral borders of the acromion, the distal clavicle, the coracoid process, and the posterior aspect of the glenohumeral joint.

The posterior portal is the preferred portal for diagnostic arthroscopy. It

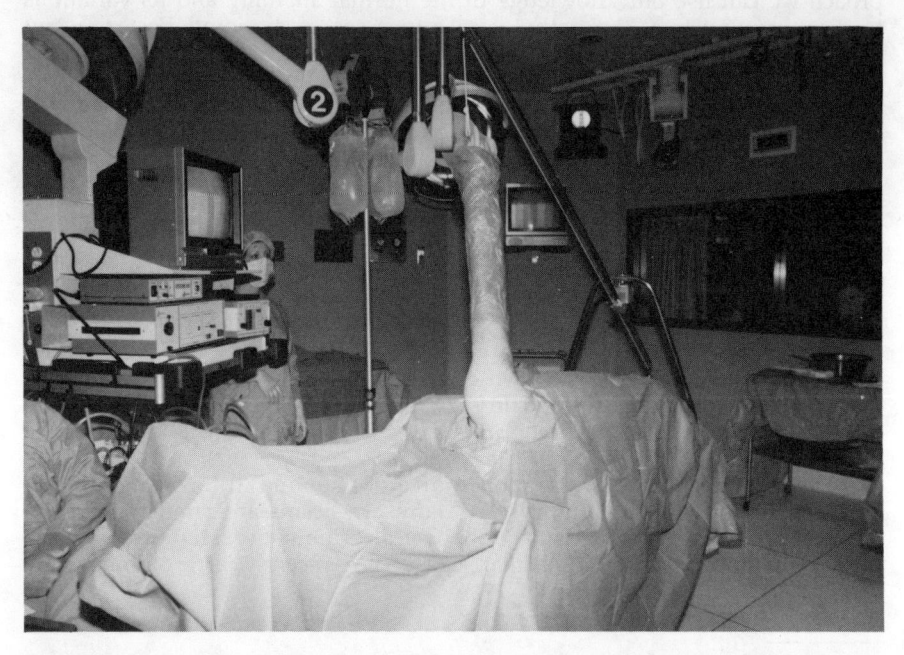

Fig. 30-1. *The patient is placed in the lateral decubitus position with the arm in 70° of abduction and 15° of forward flexion.*

is located 3 centimeters (cm) inferior and slightly medial to the posterolateral tip of the acromion. This corresponds to the soft spot on the posterior aspect of the shoulder, which is defined by the interval between the teres minor and the infraspinatus muscles. It is identified by anteriorly palpating the coracoid process with the index finger and feeling for the soft spot posteriorly with the thumb. As the arm is internally and externally rotated, the humeral head can be palpated beneath the thumb to confirm the location of the glenohumeral joint.

An 18 gauge spinal needle is inserted into the soft spot and aimed anteriorly at the coracoid process, which is being palpated by the surgeon's index finger (Fig. 30-2). Approximately 50 cubic centimeters (cc) of normal saline is injected into the joint to distend it. The presence of free backflow will confirm the correct placement of the needle within the joint. After removing the spinal needle, a small skin incision is made. The arthroscope sleeve and sharp trocar are then inserted in the same anterior direction (toward the coracoid). When the capsule is reached, a dull trocar is substituted. The joint is then entered and the scope is inserted. The capsule of the shoulder joint is considerably more difficult to penetrate than that of the knee joint.

Adequate distension is essential and is maintained throughout the procedure by a continuous inflow cannula. We use normal saline suspended in 3-liter bags on intravenous poles as our medium.

An anterior portal may be required for improved inflow or for additional instruments. This portal is located half-way between the coracoid process and the anterolateral edge of the acromion. Once again, an 18 gauge needle is

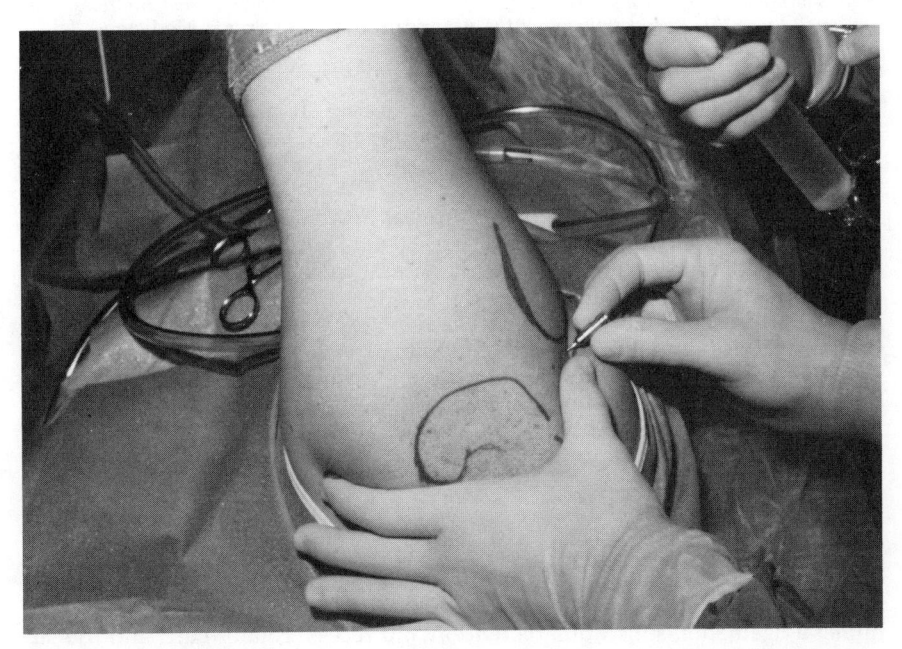

Fig. 30-2. *The spinal needle is inserted through the posterior portal and directed anteriorly toward the coracoid process, which is palpated by the surgeon's index finger. (Reproduced from Andrews, Carson, and Ortega (5), with permission of the* American Journal of Sports Medicine.*)*

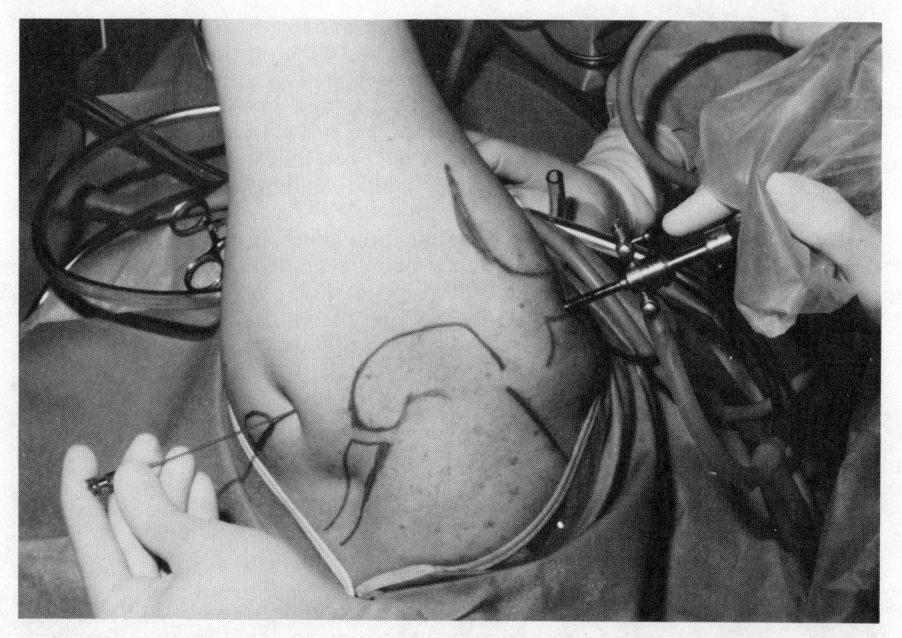

Fig. 30-3. *The anterior portal is established by inserting the spinal needle one-half of the distance between the anterolateral border of the acromion and the coracoid process. Intra-articular placement is facilitated by direct visualization with the arthroscope. (Reproduced from Andrews, Carson, and Ortega (5), with permission of the* American Journal of Sports Medicine.*)*

used to facilitate entry into the joint. The needle should enter the joint just medial to the tendon of the long head of the biceps. Direct intra-articular visualization is preferred in order to aid its placement and avoid piercing the tendon (Fig. 30-3).

A third portal is often used for surgical arthroscopy. It lies directly adjacent to the primary anterior portal (Fig. 30-4). The needle, trocar, and other instruments should enter the joint just lateral to the biceps tendon. Again, direct intra-articular visualization is the key.

The arthroscope and instruments may be exchanged between the portals to improve visibility and access to the joint. Upon completion of the procedure, 30 cc of 0.5% bupivacaine (Marcaine) is injected into the joint through the sleeve of the arthroscope. The incisions are then covered with petroleum jelly, gauze, and a sterile bulky dressing.

Arthroscopic Anatomy

A thorough knowledge of shoulder anatomy is necessary for a complete examination. The following structures should be identified and examined in sequential order: the biceps tendon, humeral head, glenoid labrum, glenohumeral ligaments, subscapularis tendon and recess, rotator cuff, and the superior recess.

BICEPS TENDON: The biceps tendon is the key to maintaining proper orientation during the arthroscopic examination (2, 5). With the patient po-

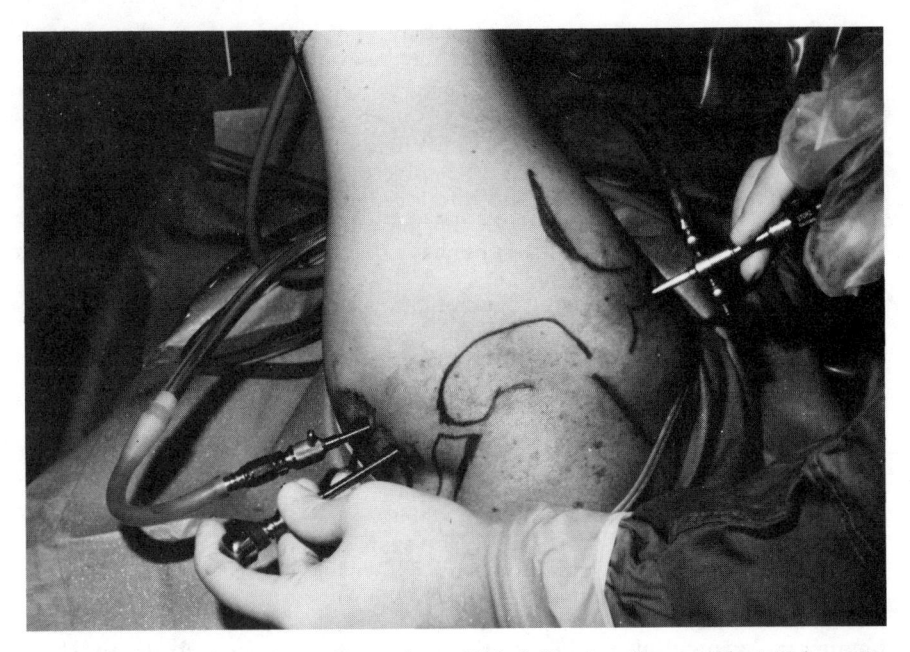

Fig. 30-4. *A second anterior portal may be established directly adjacent to the initial anterior portal. The spinal needle should enter the capsule just lateral to the biceps tendon. (Reproduced from Andrews, Carson, and Ortega (5), with permission of the* American Journal of Sports Medicine.*)*

sitioned as described, the tendon is oriented 10 to 15° away from an imaginary vertical line. It attaches to the supraglenoid tubercle at the posterosuperior aspect of the glenoid rim. It is in this region that the tendon becomes continuous with the glenoid labrum. When the patient's arm is externally rotated, the biceps tendon may be followed anteriorly into the bicipital groove. The normal tendon will glisten, appear smooth and free of adhesions, fraying, and/or tears.

HUMERAL HEAD AND GLENOID: Articular surfaces of the humeral head (superiorly) and glenoid (inferiorly) are examined next. To facilitate examination of the entire head, one must rotate the arthroscope superiorly and rotate the humerus internally and externally. The glenoid is much smaller than the humeral head and its surface is smooth.

GLENOID LABRUM: The glenoid labrum is a wedge-shaped structure which borders the entire glenoid cavity, thus adding depth to the cavity. It restricts anterior and posterior excursion of the humeral head, thereby providing inherent stability to the joint (6, 12).

Inspection begins at the biceps tendon's insertion through the superior portion of the labrum into the supraglenoid tubercle and continues anteriorly and inferiorly. The labrum should appear smooth without fraying or tearing and should not be hypermobile.

The labrum consists of hyaline cartilage, fibrocartilage, and fibrous tissue (6, 8, 14, 16, 23, 26). The glenoid surface of the labrum is continuous with the hyaline cartilage of the glenoid cavity, while the capsular surface blends with the joint capsule. The inferior rim may be visualized by further distraction of the arm, while the posterior rim may be examined by slightly retracting the scope and rotating it posteriorly.

GLENOHUMERAL LIGAMENTS: When viewed arthroscopically, the glenohumeral ligaments are anteriorly displaced due to fluid distension within the joint. The superior, middle, and inferior glenohumeral ligaments stabilize the anterior and inferior portions of the joint capsule (7, 8, 23, 27, 29). Occasionally, the glenohumeral ligaments have distinct labral origins rather than the usual capsular one.

The superior glenohumeral ligament, together with the coracohumeral ligament, stabilizes the shoulder when the arm is adducted (7, 23). The ligaments can usually be seen near the insertion of the biceps tendon into the superior aspect of the glenoid. It has two proximal attachments. One is to the superior aspect of the labrum (along with the biceps tendon), and the other to the base of the coracoid (29). The ligament takes a lateral course to insert on the anterior aspect of the anatomical neck of the humerus. Arthroscopic view of this ligament may be obscured by the biceps tendon (5).

The middle glenohumeral ligament stabilizes the glenohumeral joint when the shoulder is abducted to 45° (29). The wide attachments of this ligament are difficult to visualize arthroscopically. However, one can usually see the midportion of the ligament just posterior to the subscapularis tendon to which it sometimes fuses. The ligament extends from just beneath the superior glenohumeral ligament along the anterior border of the glenoid to the junction of the middle and inferior one-third of the glenoid rim. It blends with the capsule of the antero-inferior aspect of the shoulder joint and inserts near the lesser tuberosity over the anterior aspect of the anatomical neck of the humerus.

The inferior glenohumeral ligament provides anterior stability to the glenohumeral joint when the arm is abducted to approximately 90° (29). This triangular ligament can be seen when the arm is abducted. It arises from the antero-inferior margin of the labrum and inserts into the inferior aspect of the surgical neck of the humerus.

SUBSCAPULARIS TENDON AND RECESS: The posterosuperior edge of the subscapularis tendon may be seen when the arm is abducted. It lies in the anterior aspect of the shoulder between the superior and middle glenohumeral ligaments. However, the tendon may be obscured by or appear to blend with the middle glenohumeral ligament. The subscapularis recess is located over the anterior aspect of the shoulder near the middle glenohumeral ligament. However, there may be significant variation of normal anatomy in the relationship between the middle glenohumeral ligament and the subscapularis recess (11, 12). In one series (2), 70% of the shoulders examined had a superior subscapularis recess above and an inferior recess below the middle glenohumeral ligament, while 30% of the shoulders had a single subscapularis recess below the middle glenohumeral ligament.

ROTATOR CUFF: The biceps tendon is, again, the key to proper orientation when examining the rotator cuff. The supraspinatus tendon is located just superior to the biceps tendon. Visualization will be facilitated by rotating the arthroscope superiorly and slightly toward the humeral head. Slight posterior retraction of the arthroscope will reveal the insertion of the tendinous portion of the rotator cuff muscles into the humeral head.

By directing the arthroscope posteriorly and superiorly, one can identify the infraspinatus and the teres minor portion of the cuff.

SUPERIOR RECESS: The superior recess is in the region superior and slightly anterior to the superior aspect of the glenoid and the insertion of the biceps tendon.

DISCUSSION

The variations of the glenohumeral ligaments have been previously described (6, 13, 15, 23, 28, 30). These descriptions were based upon traditional cadaveric dissections. Turkel et al. (29) and Moseley and Overgaard (23) found the inferior glenohumeral ligament to be the most consistent of the glenohumeral ligaments. However, Depalma et al. (12, 13) found the superior glenohumeral ligament to be consistently well defined.

The variable relationship of these ligaments can result in variations in the subscapularis recess. (The recess may be found superior, inferior, or both, to the middle glenohumeral ligament.) Or, in the absence of the middle glenohumeral ligament, a single large subscapularis recess may be found (13).

As in other diagnostic and therapeutic modalities, the arthroscopic examination of the shoulder must be systematic and reproducible to be effective. The most technically demanding aspect of the procedure is entering the glenohumeral joint. In shoulder arthroscopy, the instruments must pass through thick layers of fat, muscle, and a thick capsule. Because the glenohumeral joint is located deep in these layers, proper orientation is essential to avoid entrance into the subdeltoid bursa or the axilla. We achieve this by outlining the bony landmarks with a pen and by adhering to the technique previously described.

Once the examination is completed and the pathology discerned, treatment may proceed. Operative arthroscopy of the shoulder is effective for removal of loose bodies, tears of the glenoid labrum, supraspinatus tendon, the biceps tendon, and for rheumatoid pathology. It is less effective for adhesions due to trauma. Excision of the anterior portion of the glenoid labrum increases the risk of subsequent anterior subluxation or dislocation.

The time spent in performing an arthroscopy of the shoulder must be monitored. A significant amount of fluid can extravasate through the subscapularis bursa and the bicipital groove. The resultant tissue swelling may present technical difficulties such as allowing the instruments to slip out of the capsule more easily (5).

Complications such as musculocutaneous or ulnar nerve neuropraxia can be caused by over-distraction of the glenohumeral joint, thus stretching the brachial plexus. These complications can be avoided by proper positioning of the patient's arm, using the correct pulley apparatus and limiting the weight to 7 to 9 kg.

CONCLUSION

Diagnostic arthroscopy of the shoulder can be systematic and reproducible. The surgeon must know the normal and normal variational anatomy of the shoulder and must give attention to accurate placement of the arthroscopic portals and to consistent surgical technique.

REFERENCES

1. Andren, L., and G. J. Lundberg. Treatment of rigid shoulders by joint distension during arthroscopy. *Acta Orthop. Scand.* 36:45–53, 1965.
2. Andrews, J. R., and W. G. Carson. Shoulder joint arthroscopy. *Orthopaedics* 6:1157–1162, 1983.
3. Andrews, J. R., and W. G. Carson. The arthroscopic treatment of glenoid labrum tears in the throwing athlete. *Orthrop. Trans.* 8:44, 1984.
4. Andrews, J. R., and W. G. Carson. Operative arthroscopy of the shoulder in the throwing athlete. In: *Injuries to the Throwing Arm.* 89–93. Philadelphia: W. B. Saunders Co., 1985.
5. Andrews, J. R., W. G. Carson, and K. Ortega. Arthroscopy of the shoulder. Technique and normal anatomy. *Am. J. Sports Med.* 12:1–7, 1984.
6. Bankart, A. S. B. The pathology and treatment of recurrent dislocation of the shoulder joint. *Br. J. Surg.* 26:23–29, 1938.
7. Basmajian, J. V., and F. J. Bazant. Factors preventing downward dislocation of the adducted shoulder. *J. Bone Joint Surg.* 41A:1182–1186, 1959.
8. Bost, F. C., and V. T. Inman. The pathological changes in recurrent dislocation of the shoulder. A report of Bankart's operative procedure. *J. Bone Joint Surg.* 24A:595–613, 1942.
9. Braunstein, E. M., and G. O'Connor. Double-contrast arthrotomography of the shoulder. *J. Bone Joint Surg.*, 64A:192–195, 1982.
10. Caspari, R. B. Shoulder arthroscopy: A review of the present state of the art. *Contemp. Orthop.* 4:523–534, 1982.
11. DePalma, A. F. Degenerative lesions of the shoulder joint at various age groups which are compatible with good function. In: *Instructional Course Lectures of the American Academy of Orthopaedic Surgeons,* 7:168–180, 1959.
12. DePalma, A. F. *Surgery of the Shoulder.* Philadelphia: J. B. Lippincott, 1973.
13. DePalma, A. F., G. Gallery, and G. A. Bennett. Variational anatomy and degenerative lesions of the shoulder joint. In *Instructional Course Lectures of the American Academy of Orthopaedic Surgeons,* 6:255–280, 1949.
14. DuToit, G. T., and D. Roux. Recurrent dislocation of the shoulder. A twenty-four year study of the Johannesburg stapling operation. *J. Bone Joint Surg.,* 38A:1–12, 1956.
15. Flood, V. Discovery of a new ligament of the shoulder joint. *Lancet* 672–673, 1829.
16. *Gray's Anatomy of the Human Body.* Edition 35. Warwick, R., and P. Williams (eds). Philadelphia: W. B. Saunders Co., 1973.
17. Ha'eri, G. B., and A. Maitland. Arthroscopic findings in the frozen shoulder. *J. Rheumatol.* 8:149–152, 1981.
18. Johnson, L. L. Arthroscopy of the shoulder. *Orthop. Clin. North Am.* 11:197–204, 1980.
19. Johnson, L. L. *Diagnostic and Surgical Arthroscopy.* 376–389. St. Louis: C. V. Mosby, 1981.
20. Lloyd, G. J., M. W. Older, and J. C. McIntyre. Distension arthroscopy of the shoulder joint. *Can. J. Surg.,* 19:203–207, 1976.
21. McGlynn, F. J., G. El-Khoury, and J. W. Albright. Arthrotomography of the glenoid labrum in shoulder instability. *J. Bone Joint Surg.,* 64A:507–517, 1982.
22. Mink, J. H., A. Richardson, and T. T. Grant. Evaluation of glenoid labrum by double-contrast shoulder arthrography. *Am. J. Roent.,* 133:883–887, 1979.
23. Mosely, J. F., and B. Overgaard. The anterior capsular mechanism in recurrent anterior dislocation of the shoulder. *J. Bone Joint Surg.,* 44B:913–927, 1962.
24. Pappas, A. M., T. P. Goss, and P. K. Kleinman. Symptomatic shoulder instability due to lesions of the glenoid labrum. *Am. J. Sports Med.,* 11:279–288, 1983.
25. Rokous, J. R., and J. R. Feagin, and J. Y. Abbott. Modified axillary roentgenogram. A useful adjunct in the diagnosis of recurrent instability of the shoulder. *Clin. Orthop.* 82:82–86, 1972.
26. Rowe, C. R., D. Patel, and W. W. Southmayd. The Bankart procedure. A long-term end-result study. *J. Bone Joint Surg.,* 60A:1–16, 1978.
27. Rowe, C. R., and B. Zarins. Recurrent transient subluxation of the shoulder. *J. Bone Joint Surg.* 63A:863–872, 1981.
28. Schlemm, F. Ueber die verstarkungsbander am schultergelenk. *Arch. Anat.,* 45–48, 1853.
29. Turkel, S. J., M. W. Panio, J. L. Marshall, and F. G. Girgis. Stabilizing mechanisms preventing anterior dislocation of the glenohumeral joint. *J. Bone Joint Surg.* 63A:1208–1217, 1981.
30. Weitbrecht, J. *Syndesmology, or, A Description of the Ligaments of the Human Body.* Translation by E. B. Kaplan. Philadelphia: W. B. Saunders, 1969.
31. Wiley, A. M., and M. W. J. Older. Shoulder arthroscopy. Investigation with a fibro-optic instrument. *Am. J. Sports Med.,* 8:31–38, 1980.

Section VII
Heart and Lung

31
The Heart of The Masters Athlete

PAUL D. THOMPSON, M.D.
DEANNA L. DORSEY

The Miriam Hospital, Brown University

CARDIAC FUNCTION OF THE MASTERS ATHLETE

Endurance athletic performance decreases with advancing age, as does maximal oxygen uptake ($\dot{V}O_2$ max). The rate of decline in both performance and $\dot{V}O_2$ max is approximately 1% per year. At least some of the decrease in $\dot{V}O_2$ max results from the age-related decrease in maximal heart rate. Decreases in the maximal cardiac stroke volume (SV) and the maximal arterial-venous oxygen (A-$\bar{V}$ O_2) difference also contribute to the reduction in $\dot{V}O_2$ max in untrained subjects. Firm conclusions on the rate of decline in $\dot{V}O_2$ max in masters athletes and on the role of reductions in SV and the A-$\bar{V}$ O_2 difference are prevented by the failure of most studies to differentiate the effects of aging from reductions in exercise training.

Masters athletes demonstrate patterns of ventricular enlargement on electrocardiographic and echocardiographic study similar to those seen in younger athletic subjects. The relative frequency of such abnormalities in different age groups is not known.

The risk of cardiovascular complications is increased for middle-aged athletes during exercise, and intense competition for subjects with known coronary heart disease should be avoided. Nevertheless, the absolute incidence of sudden death during exercise is extremely small, and compelling evidence suggests that the overall cardiovascular benefits of exercise training outweigh the acute risks of exercise.

INTRODUCTION

Endurance exercise performance decreases with increasing age in both the general population and in competitive athletes. Since endurance performance

---

From the Miriam Hospital Divisions of Cardiology and Nutrition and Metabolism and the Brown University Program in Medicine, Providence, Rhode Island. Supported in part by NIH Grant #HL01003.

is largely dependent on the body's ability to supply oxygen to exercising muscle, the physiological reflection of the decreased exercise capacity with age is a reduction in maximal oxygen uptake ($\dot{V}O_2$ max) (21). The Fick equation for calculating cardiac output ($\dot{Q}$) indicates that $\dot{Q}$ equals oxygen uptake ($\dot{V}O_2$) divided by the arterial-venous oxygen (A-$\bar{V}$ O_2) difference. Rearranging the Fick equation demonstrates the $\dot{V}O_2 = \dot{Q} \times$ (A-$\bar{V}$ O_2) difference and that endurance capacity is a reflection of maximal values for both $\dot{Q}$ and the A-$\bar{V}$ O_2 difference. Cardiac output is the product of heart rate (HR) and cardiac stroke volume (SV). The A-$\bar{V}$ O_2 difference refers to the systemic A-$\bar{V}$ O_2 difference. During exercise it depends on an adequate hemoglobin content, hemoglobin saturation in the pulmonary circulation, shunting of saturated blood away from nonexercising tissue to exercising muscle, and extraction of oxygen in exercising muscle. Decreases in HR, SV, or any factor affecting the A-$\bar{V}$ O_2 difference could contribute to the decrease in endurance performance with age.

This chapter will examine changes in cardiovascular performance with age in order to understand the decrease in exercise performance among masters athletes. We define masters athletes as individuals over age 40 who engage in competitive sports. We will also discuss clinical cardiac findings in masters athletes and the risk of cardiovascular complications during exercise. Because dynamic exercise exerts the greatest effects and demands on the cardiovascular system, this review is limited to the cardiac effects of dynamic exercise.

There are relatively few studies of the masters athlete, so many concepts are based on data obtained from healthy untrained individuals. Unfortunately this approach is not able to differentiate the effects of age per se from the progressive deconditioning which is common in the sedentary population. A similar problem plagues longitudinal studies of competitive athletes since few athletes maintain a high level of training throughout their competitive lifespans.

There are other problems with studies on aging which affect the present review (40). First, the effects of occult disease can be confused with the effects of age. This is especially true in studies of cardiac performance because coronary artery disease (CAD) increases with age, affects cardiac function, and may be symptomatically silent in the elderly population (30). Furthermore, CAD is notoriously difficult to detect with certainty without invasive techniques.

Second, few studies have examined exercise performance in individuals over age 60. Many studies purporting to examine exercise and aging have actually studied middle-aged subjects. Extrapolating results from these studies to persons over 60 years of age assumes that aging is a linear process. This assumption may not be true for exercise performance. The fall in $\dot{V}O_2$ max, for example, appears to accelerate after age 60 (20). Similarly, the frequency of a decrease in left ventricular ejection fraction (LVEF) from rest to exercise increases in presumably healthy individuals over age 60 (27).

Third, cross-sectional studies comparing exercise tolerance in athletes of different ages may be biased by the fact that the older subjects have been selected for their health as well as both actual and athletic survivorship. There are no guarantees that the younger athletes will be as fortunate. Also, in studies of exercise tolerance among sedentary persons, there is a bias toward subjects who are willing to be tested (4). Among older persons, this bias may select a more active or healthier group (35).

Fourth, our conclusions are based on average values. Individual variations in exercise performance are generally greater than those produced by age alone (5).

THE RATE OF DECLINE IN EXERCISE PERFORMANCE

The age-group marathon record for men 30 to 70 years of age increases linearly at the rate of approximately 1% per yr (5) (Fig. 31-1). This observation was made in 1980 before Carlos Lopes at age 38 demonstrated the power of individual variation and established a new marathon record. Despite this accomplishment, the marathon record still increases by only 1% per year between ages 40 and 70.

Alterations in mechanical efficiency are unlikely to contribute much to the increase in marathon times. There are few studies of mechanical efficiency in older runners, but oxygen uptake at identical workloads during cycle ergometry varies little in the same subjects tested over two decades (1) or among subjects of different ages tested in cross-sectional studies (9, 15, 35). Few very old subjects have been studied, however, and mechanical efficiency may deteriorate in persons over age 70 because of joint stiffness and poor coordination (2).

Both cross-sectional (3, 15, 20) and longitudinal (1) studies of exercise performance suggest that VO_2 max also decreases at approximately 1% per year. This rate is similar to the deterioration in marathon times and implies that alterations in oxygen transport explain the fall in endurance capacity. It is not clear whether this rate of decrease is similar for continually trained and untrained men or whether exercise training prevents some of the age effect.

McDonough and others studied exercise tolerance in 86 men of different ages to develop regression equations relating the decrease in VO_2 max to age (20). Physically active men demonstrated moderately higher VO_2 max values than did sedentary men of similar age. The absolute rate of decine was nearly identical (at 0.39 and 0.41 ml · kg^{-1} · min^{-1} per yr) for active and inactive men, however, and the relative rate of decline was approximately 1% per year for

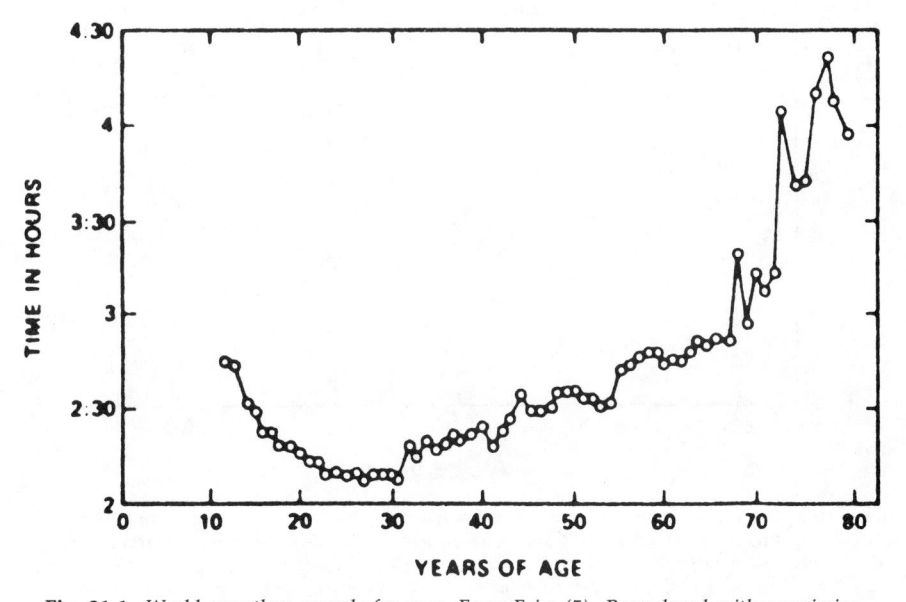

Fig. 31-1. *World marathon records for men. From Fries (5). Reproduced with permission.*

both groups. In contrast, others report that inactive men have a threefold higher rate of decline in $\dot{V}O_2$ max when compared to active men tested repeatedly over 2.3 years (4). This difference is only reduced to twofold by correcting for changes in body weight.

The rate of decline in $\dot{V}O_2$ max has recently been reviewed in detail by Heath et al. (13). These authors conclude that $\dot{V}O_2$ max decreases by approximately 9% per decade for both lean and obese untrained men (Fig. 31-2).

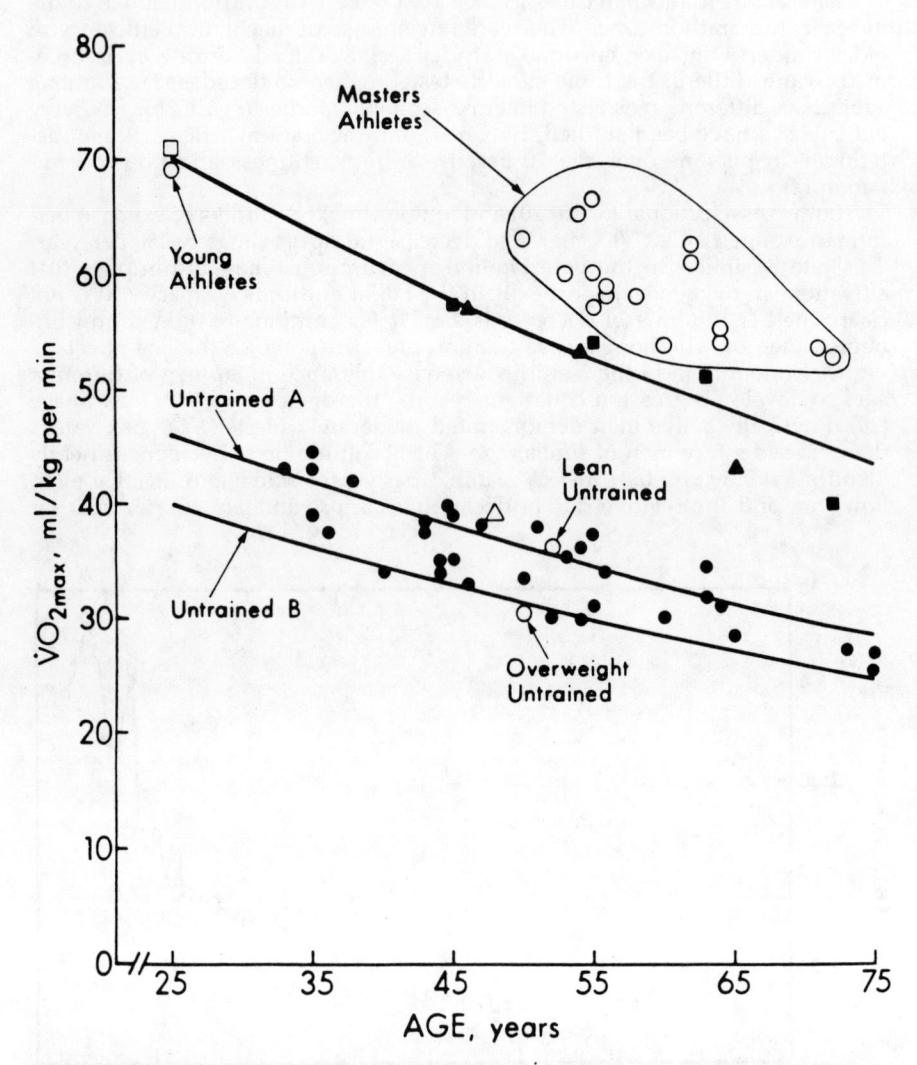

Fig. 31-2. *Decline in maximum oxygen performance ($\dot{V}O_2$ max). Open circles and labels refer to subjects studied by Heath et al. Closed circles refer to groups of untrained men, open box to active athletes, open triangle to former athletes, and closed triangle or boxes to active but aging athletes. The young athletes and masters athletes (13) were matched for current training levels and appear to show a reduced rate of decline in $\dot{V}O_2$ max in the older athletes. Reproduced with permission from Heath et al. (13).*

Cross-sectional studies of older endurance athletes reported by Grimby and Saltin (10) and by Pollock et al. (26) suggest a parallel 9% per decade decline in $\dot{V}O_2$ max for masters athletes (13). Neither of these studies of older athletes (10, 26), however, controlled for variations in training regimens. Parallel curves for the athletes and sedentary subjects might simply reflect parallel decreases in physical activity. To evaluate this possibility, 16 masters athletes, aged 59 plus or minus 6 years (mean ± SD) were matched with 16 younger athletes aged 22 plus or minus 2 years (13). Subjects were matched on the basis of training miles, training intensity, and best performance at comparable ages. $\dot{V}O_2$ max values averaged 58 ± 4.3 $ml \cdot kg^{-1} \cdot min^{-1}$ in the older athletes. If the authors assumed a 9% per decade decrement in $\dot{V}O_2$ max, the average value at age 25 for the masters athletes would have been 81 $ml \cdot kg^{-1} \cdot min^{-1}$. This possibility was unlikely since few of the subjects were elite athletes, and $\dot{V}O_2$ max values for the young comparison men averaged only 69 ± 2.3 $ml \cdot kg^{-1} \cdot min^{-1}$. If the older athletes at age 25 had $\dot{V}O_2$ max values of 69 $ml \cdot kg^{-1} \cdot min^{-1}$, identical to those of the younger subjects, then the rate of decline for the older athletes would have been only 5% per decade. Consequently, the 9% per decade decline in $\dot{V}O_2$ max for masters athletes suggested by earlier studies may reflect alterations in exercise training. Similar conclusions may apply to the decline in marathon performance. It should be noted, however, that the cross-sectional design of this study may have selected athletes who were different from their younger comparison subjects (13). Longitudinal studies of athletes who maintain the same level of training will be necessary to determine the rate of decline in $\dot{V}O_2$ max among masters athletes.

Physiological Mechanisms For The Decline In $\dot{V}O_2$ MAX

Decreases in maximal cardiac output ($\dot{Q}$ and A-$\bar{V}$ O_2 difference are the mediators of the decrease in $\dot{V}O_2$ max with age in untrained subjects. Maximal heart rate (HR) decreases at a rate of 0.4 to 0.95 $beats \cdot min^{-1}$ per yr (17, 29) and accounts for approximately 30 to 50% of the observed decrease in $\dot{V}O_2$ max (1, 3, 15). We estimate from published data that decreases in maximum SV and the A-$\bar{V}$ O_2 difference each account for an additional 25 to 30% of the decrease (3, 15). Maximal HR in trained subjects decreases at the same rate as in untrained individuals (17) and accounts for some of the decrease in $\dot{V}O_2$ max. The influence of decreases in SV and the A-$\bar{V}$ O_2 difference in masters athletes is not well defined.

Both of these variables are affected by exercise training, and variations in training have not been considered in most studies of aging athletes. Grimby et al. measured $\dot{Q}$ during exercise in masters athletes and compared the results with published values for younger subjects (9). The authors concluded that the lower $\dot{V}O_2$ max values of the older athletes were secondary to a lower A-$\bar{V}$ O_2 difference. Differences in training between age groups were not addressed. When competitive masters athletes are compared with younger athletes following similar training regimens, however, oxygen pulse (the product of SV and the A-$\bar{V}$ O_2 difference) is identical in the two groups, and HR alone accounts for all of the decrease in $\dot{V}O_2$ max with age (13). Consequently, when training is controlled for, HR may be the only independent effect of age on exercise tolerance.

Whether exercise training can increase $\dot{V}O_2$ max, SV, and the A-$\bar{V}$ O_2 difference in older subjects is also not settled. Benestad demonstrated no increase in $\dot{V}O_2$ max in 70-to-81-year-old men after 5 to 6 weeks of exercise training (2). The subjects were physically active before the study, however, and the training stimulus might not have been sufficient to affect performance. Hartley et al. reported a 14% increase in VO_2 max in men aged 38 to 53 years (12). Since maximal HR declined and the A-$\bar{V}$ O_2 difference did not change, all of the increase was due to a 16% increase in SV. In contrast, Seals et al. studied 60-to-69-year-old subjects and attributed most of the 25% increase in VO_2 max to a 14% increase in the A-$\bar{V}$ O_2 difference (32); SV increased only 6% in this study. Despite the differences in possible mechanisms, oxygen pulse and VO_2 max can be increased with exercise training in 35-to-69-year-old subjects (12, 16, 32). Consequently, in both active and sedentary men, much of the age-related decrease in VO_2 max produced by decreases in SV and the A-$\bar{V}$ O_2 difference may reflect decreases in physical activity with age. Additional studies are needed to determine the effect of training in very old subjects.

A reduction in exercise SV with age, if not caused by deconditioning, could be due to reduced myocardial contractility, increased afterload, reduced preload and left ventricular filling, or occult coronary artery disease (40). Systolic blood pressure and peripheral vascular resistance are increased during exercise in older subjects (3, 15, 35). Other sources of outflow resistance such as the characteristic impedance of the aorta (40) might also limit left ventricular function. Characteristic impedance is determined by aortic size, stiffness, and reflected pressure waves and is distinct from peripheral vascular resistance. Aortic root diameter, for example, increases with age, and this requires the heart to initiate ejection against a greater blood volume (6). Left ventricular filling pressures during exercise increase with age (35), but reduced ventricular compliance could limit ventricular filling despite higher pressures. Wall thickness increases in older subjects (6), and decreased velocity of the mitral valve filling wave implies reduced compliance of either the left ventricle or the mitral leaflets (22).

Recent radionuclide studies implicate either reduced contractility or increased afterload as the mechanism for the decreased exercise SV. Left ventricular ejection fraction (LVEF) decreases with age (27, 29, 31). Systolic blood pressure has not increased in some studies (27), but this does not exclude increased characteristic impedance, as mentioned above (40). Left ventricular compliance is probably not a limiting factor since left ventricular end-diastolic volumes increase during upright exercise in some (29, 31), but not all (27), older subjects. The Frank-Starling mechanism may actually be used in older subjects to compensate for lower peak HRs and to prevent the usual decrease in exercise stroke volume (29). Initial studies reported a fall in LVEF from rest to exercise in 73% of subjects above age 60 (27). This finding raises the possibility of occult CAD in these subjects. Average exercise LVEF still falls with age, however, even when individuals showing decreases in this parameter from rest to exercise are excluded (29). Consequently, occult CAD alone does not explain the decreased left ventricular function and either reduced contractility or increased afterload must be operative.

It should be noted that we know of no radionucleide studies of left ventricular function during exercise in masters athletes. Conclusions as to the role of left ventricular compliance, therefore, are premature in this group. Left ventricular wall thickness increases with age in professional cyclists compared to younger cyclists and to sedentary individuals (24). This increase might restrict diastolic filling in the older athletes. Also the effect of exercise training on the decrease in LVEF with age is not clear. Three months of exercise training failed to improve LVEF in subjects over age 65, but the training stimulus of only 1.5 hours per week is not comparable to that practiced by masters athletes (31).

There are also several possible causes for the lower maximal systemic A-$\bar{V}$ O_2 differences noted in older subjects. Ventilation and lung function could limit hemoglobin saturation in older subjects (7). Increased vascular stiffness could prevent vasoconstriction to nonexercising tissue and ultimately affect performance by reducing the peak exercise A-$\bar{V}$ O_2 difference. Both possibilities have been suggested (7, 12), but not fully evaluated. The capacity of the aging muscle to utilize oxygen also requires evaluation.

Clinical Abnormalities In Masters Athletes

Altered autonomic nervous control of the heart, including enhanced vagal tone and reduced sympathetic activity, is responsible for many of the electrocardiographic (EKG) abnormalities noted in young endurance athletes (14, 38). These abnormalities included sinus bradycardia, first degree arterioventricular (A-V) block, second degree A-V block of the Wenckebach type, and possible escape rhythms such as wandering arterial pacemaker and junctional rhythm. Other EKG changes, including the ST segment elevation of early repolarization and precordial T-wave changes, may also be related to increased vagal tone since both usually resolve with atropine or exercise. (38)

Identical rhythm and EKG variations are noted in masters endurance athletes (10, 11), although only rarely have studies compared their relative frequency (24). The degree of bradycardia and the incidence of ST elevation are similar in competitive cyclists aged 20 to 49 (24). The oldest athletes, however, showed more frequent ST segment depression and left precordial T-wave inversions at rest. The authors noted that such changes may be associated with depressed left ventricular function and questioned whether prolonged training may ultimately affect cardiac performance (24).

Young well-trained endurance athletes often have EKG, chest x-ray, and echocardiographic evidence of cardiac enlargement (14, 38). Although many young athletes demonstrate voltage criteria for left ventricular hypertrophy (LVH), few also demonstrate ST segment depression. EKG evidence of right ventricular hypertrophy (RVH) or incomplete right bundle branch block is also common in young endurance athletes. Increased right and left ventricular internal diameters, left ventricular wall thickness, and left atrial size have been confirmed by echocardiography.

Echocardiographic measurements in the athletes cluster at the upper limits of normal, but only a rare athlete will exceed published norms for any parameter, and estimates of ventricular function are normal. The pattern of cardiac enlargement varies with the training activity.

Endurance athletes have enlarged chamber dimensions and may have mild left ventricular wall thickening. Strength-trained men, in contrast, generally demonstrate ventricular wall thickening. Left ventricular mass is increased in both endurance and strength-trained athletes, but when left ventricular mass is normalized for body size, mass is greatest in the endurance athletes (18).

Few studies to our knowledge have compared echocardiographic dimensions in competitive men of different ages (24). Competitive cyclists aged 40 to 49 years who had trained continuously for 20 to 30 years had similar left ventricular internal dimensions but increased left ventricular wall thickness and mass compared to their younger colleagues. Sixty-five percent of the older cyclists had a cardiothoracic x-ray ratio of greater than 0.50, but this finding was present in only 29% of men aged 20 to 29 and in 35% of men aged 30 to 39 years. Although left ventricular mass and the cardiothoracic ratio increased in the older men, EKG evidence of RVH and LVH decreased from 29 to 21%

and from 100% to 65% in the youngest and oldest groups respectively. This discrepancy may relate to changes in lung volumes which might affect EKG voltage.

Exercise stress testing has been recommended by some authorities as a screening test for athletic competition among both young and master-age subjects. Abnormal EKG ST segment shifts, presumed to be falsely positive, are common in both groups of athletes. Five of 20 elite American distance runners had marked ST segment depression immediately after exercise (8). Similarly, 25% of athletes age 42 to 68 years had ST segment depression during exercise testing (11). The most marked ST segment shifts occurred in a subject with the largest heart volume by x-ray. Strandell also noted marked ST segment depressions during exercise in older subjects with the largest heart volumes (35). In contrast, only 9% of strength-trained athletes show ST segment depression during exercise, a rate not different from control subjects (34). The differences between various groups of athletes may be related to the larger left ventricular mass relative to body surface area in the runners.

These observations suggest that the high rate of ST segment depression during exercise in trained individuals represents repolarization alterations from left ventricular enlargement rather than from cardiac ischemia. Direct comparison will be required to determine the relative frequency of such changes in young and old athletes. False-positive changes may be more frequent in older athletes, however, because of the increase in left ventricular mass in these subjects (24).

THE RISK VERSUS BENEFIT RATIO OF EXERCISE

Powerful epidemiological evidence supports the hypothesis that regular exercise reduces the incidence of CHD (23, 25, 33). The factor or factors mediating the decrease are not defined, nor do we know the amount and type of exercise necessary to reduce CHD risk (36). Despite its purported beneficial effects, vigorous exercise does acutely and transiently increase the risk of sudden death. The pathological substrate for sudden death during exertion in adults is usually CAD (39), whereas other lesions such as hypertrophic cardiomyopathy, anomalous origin of a coronary artery, or aortic rupture are among the causes of exercise deaths in children and young adults (19, 28). The absolute incidence of sudden death during exertion is low. In Rhode Island, we found only 1 death per year for every 7,620 joggers aged 30 to 65 (37). Furthermore, if only deaths among healthy men are considered, the death rate is as low as 1 for every 15,200 middle-aged joggers. A similar rate of only 1 death during vigorous exercise for every 18,000 healthy men has recently been reported from Seattle (33). In both studies, however, the rate during exercise exceeded the rate during other times. Still, the total death rate for men who habitually engaged in vigorous exercise, was reduced despite the excess of deaths during activity (33). It is reassuring for the masters athlete that the greatest excess of exercise deaths occurred in men who exercised infrequently (33).

The rarity of sudden death during exertion limits the utility of routine screening tests in its prevention. Consequently, we do not recommend routine exercise testing of healthy adults prior to or during exercise training, but we do recommend such testing to evaluate possible symptoms or when occult CAD is likely. Also since exercise sudden death victims seem to ignore early signs of cardiac ischemia (39), we strongly recommend that active men know the nature of prodromal symptoms and their need for prompt medical attention.

DIRECTIONS FOR FUTURE RESEARCH ON THE MASTERS ATHLETE

Additional studies are needed of the decrease in exercise performance among masters athletes to determine the relative contributions of age per se as opposed to alterations in physical training. Such research should address the physiological mediators of the decline in performance and the possible role of alterations in mechanical efficiency during various events. These studies will require accurate measurements of cardiac output so that oxygen pulse can be divided into its component parts, stroke volume and the A-V O_2 difference. The possible limiting roles of the pulmonary system and systemic shunting should also be addressed.

Future clinical studies should compare the frequency of abnormalities on noninvasive cardiac testing in masters athletes and in middle-aged comparison subjects. The growing number of masters athletes will require that clinicians know the frequency of normal variants in this group. The frequency of non-fatal events during exercise needs to be defined since present studies on the risk of exercise have focused on sudden death and thereby underestimate the total exercise risk. Studies are also needed to identify subjects at risk for cardiovascular complications during exercise so that these complications can be prevented.

REFERENCES

1. Astrand, I., P.-O. Astrand, I. Hallback, and A. Kilbom. Reduction in maximal oxygen uptake with age. *J. Appl. Physiol.* 35:649–654, 1973.
2. Benestad, A. M. Trainability of old men. *Acta Med. Scand.* 178:321–327, 1965.
3. Conway, J., R. Wheeler, and R. Sannerstedt. Sympathetic nervous activity during exercise in relation to age. *Cardiovasc. Res.* 5:577–581, 1971.
4. Dehn, M. M., and R. A. Bruce. Longitudinal variations in maximal oxygen intake with age and activity. *J. Appl. Physiol.* 33:805–807, 1972.
5. Fries, J. P. Aging, natural death, and the compression of morbidity. *N. Engl. J. Med.* 303:130–135, 1980.
6. Gerstenblith, G., J. Frederiksen, F. C. P. Yin, N. J. Fortuin, E. G. Lakatta, and M. L. Weisfeldt. Echocardiographic assessment of a normal adult aging population. *Circulation* 56:273–278, 1977.
7. Gerstenblith, G., E. G. Lakatta, and M. L. Weisfeldt. Age changes in myocardial function and exercise response. *Prog. Cardiovasc. Dis.* 19:1–21, 1976.
8. Gibbons, L. W., K. H. Cooper, R. P. Martin, and M. L. Pollock. Medical examination and electrocardiograhic analysis of elite distance runners. *Ann. N. Y. Acad. Sci.* 301:283–296, 1977.
9. Grimby, G., N. J. Nilsson, and B. Saltin. Cardiac output during submaximal and maximal exercise in active middle-aged athletes. *J. Appl. Physiol.* 21:1150–1156, 1966.
10. Grimby, G., and B. Saltin. Daily running causing Wenckebach heart block. *Lancet* 2:962–963, 1964.
11. Grimby, G., and B. Saltin. Physiological analysis of physically well-trained middle-aged and old athletes. *Acta Med. Scand.* 179:513–526, 1966.
12. Hartley, L. H., G. Grimby, A. Kilbom, N. J. Nilsson, I. Astrand, J. Bjure, B. Ekblom, and B. Saltin. Physical training in sedentary middle-aged and older men. *Scand. J. Clin. Lab. Invest.* 24:335–344, 1969.
13. Heath, G. W., J. M. Hagberg, A. A. Ehsani, and J. O. Holloszy. A physiological comparison of young and older endurance athletes. *J. Appl. Physiol.* 51:634–640, 1981.
14. Huston, T. P., J. C. Puffer, and W. M. Rodney. The athletic heart syndrome. *N. Engl. J. Med.* 313:24–31, 1985.
15. Julius, S., A. Amery, L. S. Whitlock, and J. Conway. Influence of age on the hemodynamic response to exercise. *Circulation.* 36:222–230, 1967.

16. Kasch, F. W., W. H. Phillips, J. E. L. Carter, and J. L. Boyer. Cardiovascular changes in middle-aged men during two years of training. *J. Appl. Physiol.* 34:53–57, 1973.
17. Lester, M., L. T. Sheffield, P. Trammell, and T. J. Reeves. The effect of age and athletic training on the maximal heart rate during muscular exercise. *Am. Heart J.* 76:370–376, 1968.
18. Longhurst, J. C., A. R. Kelley, W. J. Gonyea, and J. H. Mitchell. Echocardiographic left ventricular masses in distance runners and weight lifters. *J. Appl. Physiol.* 48:154–162, 1980.
19. Maron, B. J., W. C. Roberts, H. A. McAllister, D. R. Rosing, and S. E. Epstein. Sudden death in young athletes. *Circulation.* 62:218–229, 1980.
20. McDonough, J. R., F. Kusumi, and R. A. Bruce. Variations in maximal oxygen intake with physical activity in middle-aged men. *Circulation.* 41:743–751, 1970.
21. Mitchell, J. H., and G. Blomqvist. Maximal oxygen uptake. *N. Engl. J. Med.* 284:1018–1022, 1971.
22. Miyatake, K., M. Okamoto, N. Kinoshita, M. Owa, I. Nakasone, H. Sakakibara, and Y. Nimura. Augmentation of atrial contribution to left ventricular inflow with aging as assessed by intracardiac Doppler flowmetry. *Am. J. Cardiol.* 53:586–589, 1984.
23. Morris, J. N., R. Pollard, M. G. Everitt, and S. P. W. Chave. Vigorous exercise in leisure-time: Protection against coronary heart disease. *Lancet* 2:1207–1210, 1980.
24. Nishimura, T., Y. Yamada, and C. Kawai. Echocardiograhic evaluation of long-term effects of exercise on left ventricular hypertrophy and function in professional bicyclists. *Circulation* 61:832–840, 1980.
25. Paffenbarger, R. S., and W. E. Hale. Work activity and coronary heart mortality. *N. Engl. J. Med.* 292:545–550, 1975.
26. Pollock, M. L., H. S. Miller, and J. Wilmore. Physiological characteristics of champion American track athletes 40 to 75 years of age. *J. Gerontol.* 29:645–649, 1974.
27. Port, S., F. R. Cobb, R. E. Coleman, and R. H. Jones. Effect of age on the response of the left ventricular ejection fraction to exercise. *N. Engl. J. Med.* 303:1133–1138, 1980.
28. Ragosta, M., J. Crabtree, W. Q. Sturner, and P. D. Thompson. Death during recreational exercise in the state of Rhode Island. *Med. Sci. Sports Exerc.* 16:339–342, 1984.
29. Rodeheffer, R. J., G. Gerstenblith, L. C. Becker, J. L. Fleg, M. L. Weisfeldt, and E. G. Lakatta. Exercise cardiac output is maintained with advancing age in healthy human subjects: Cardiac dilatation and increased stroke volume compensate for a diminished heart rate. *Circulation* 69:203–213, 1984.
30. Rowe, J. W. Clinical research on aging: Strategies and directions. *N. Engl. J. Med.* 297:1332–1336, 1977.
31. Schocken, D. D., J. A. Blumenthal, S. Port, P. Hindle, and R. E. Coleman. Physical conditioning and left ventricular performance in the elderly: Assessment by radionuclide angiocardiography. *Am. J. Cardiol.* 52:359–364, 1983.
32. Seals, D. R., J. M. Hagberg, B. F. Hurley, A. A. Ehsani, and J. O. Holloszy. Endurance training in older men and women. I. Cardiovascular responses to exercise. *J. Appl. Physiol.* 57:1024–1029, 1984.
233. Siscovick, D. S., N. S. Weiss, R. H. Fletcher, and T. Lasky. The incidence of primary cardiac arrest during vigorous exercise. *N. Engl. J. Med.* 311:874–877, 1984.
34. Spirito, P., B. J. Maron, R. O. Bonow, and S. E. Epstein. Prevalence and significance of an abnormal S-T segment response to exercise in a young athletic population. *Am. J. Cardiol.* 51:1663–1666, 1983.
35. Strandell, T. Circulatory studies on healthy old men. *Acta Med. Scand.* (Suppl. 414):2–44, 1964.
36. Thompson, P. D. Exercise and sudden cardiac death. *N. Engl. J. Med.* 312:183–184, 1985.
37. Thompson, P. D., E. J. Funk, R. A. Carleton, and W. Q. Sturner. The incidence of death during jogging in Rhode Island joggers from 1975 through 1980. *JAMA.* 247:2535–2538, 1982.
38. Thompson, P. D., and J. R. McGhee. The cardiac evaluation of the competitive athlete. In: *Medicine in Sports and Exercise: Non-traumatic Aspects*, R. H. Strauss (ed.). 3–12. Philadelphia: W. B. Saunders, 1984.
39. Thompson, P. D., M. P. Stern, P. Williams, K. Duncan, W. L. Haskell, and P. D. Wood. Death during jogging or running: A study of 18 cases. *JAMA.* 242:1265–1267, 1979.
40. Weisfeldt, M. L. Aging of the cardiovascular system. *N. Engl. J. Med.* 303:1172–1173, 1980.

32

The Lung of The Masters Athlete

N. L. JONES

McMaster University Health Sciences Centre

The changes that occur with age in the structure-function relationships of the respiratory system form a basis to understand what happens to breathing in exercise as you get older. It is often said that breathing never becomes a limiting factor to exercise, but one wonders if those who utter such statements have ever exercised themselves. In very heavy exercise we all become breathless, and this sensation may become severe enough to make us stop exercising. Many of the effects of aging on the respiratory system express themselves through an increase in the sense of effort in breathing during exercise. Thus the masters athlete may experience greater breathlessness during a given exercise activity than at a younger age. A number of factors contribute to breathlessness during exercise; aging may influence each of these factors to a varying degree. Several may be modified by exercise training and in doing so, training may serve to lessen breathlessness during exercise.

A number of papers have dealt with the effects of age on breathing in exercise. To supplement the information obtained from them, I have also drawn upon our own data of exercise in sedentary young and old subjects and the effects of training that form the basis of the chapter by Lydia Makrides (16).

The main structural basis for the effects of aging on the respiratory system is a gradual loss of the normal structure within the lung that supports alveoli, small airways, and the small blood vessels. The elastin and collagen fibers that form this support appear to degenerate, leading to increases in the size of alveoli and later to breakdown of alveolar walls. In its most marked form, this change is often termed senile emphysema, and of course it is often difficult to separate the effects of aging on the normal lung from the appearance of emphysema and chronic bronchitis. These have a relatively high incidence in the general population and particularly in the smoking population. The loss of these structural elements leads to increasing size of the air spaces, especially the alveolar ducts (Fig. 32-1), together with a reduction in the surface area and the alveolar-capillary bed (21), and the lack of support of small airways and blood vessels leads to secondary changes in the flow characteristics of air and blood in the lungs. Added to these effects are changes in the chest cage. The loss of elastic recoil in the lung which normally opposes the outward recoil of the chest wall is lessened and thus the chest wall tends to

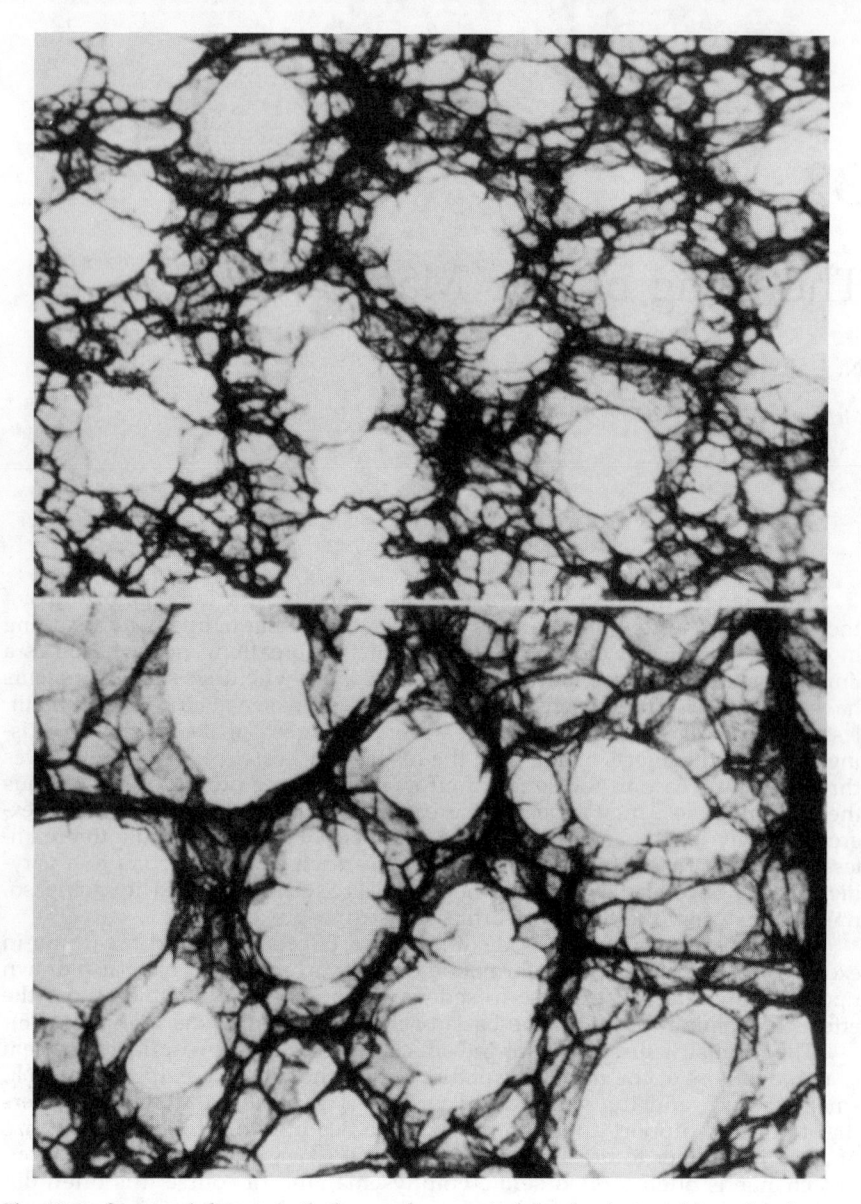

Fig. 32-1. *Structural changes in the lung; enlargement of alveolar ducts and loss of surface area in the lung of an 80-year-old man (lower) compared with that of a 26-year-old man (upper). Reprinted from Ref. 21 with permission.*

occupy a higher volume. Opposing this effect are aging changes in the joints of the ribs to the vertebral column and in the cartilage joining the ribs to the sternum. Finally, there are the effects of aging on the muscles of the respiratory system with a gradual loss in strength and aerobic metabolic capacities.

Although these structural changes are difficult to quantify, their functional effects have been well documented in a number of cross-sectional population studies. In order to present an overall picture of the changes, the predicted values at age 20 and 60 years in a male 170 centimeters (cm) tall will be used.

Pressure-Volume Characteristics

The loss of elastic recoil leads to a shift to the left in the pressure-volume characteristics of the lung (14); thus in the aging lung, less transpulmonary pressure is needed to achieve a given change in lung volume. The static lung compliance increases from 0.24 to 0.34 1/cm H_2O between 20 and 60 years (2) (Fig. 32-2). The less opposed action of the outward recoil characteristic of the chest wall acts to increase total lung capacity; however, this is accompanied by a relative stiffening of the chest wall, and the slope of the pressure-volume characteristic of the thoracic cage is flattened. There are 2 net effects of these changes. First, total lung capacity tends to fall with age to a small extent (see below). Secondly, a higher tension has to be developed by the inspiratory muscles to expand the total respiratory system with increasing age. As an increase in the thoracic cage volume is always associated with a shortening of the inspiratory muscles, it takes a greater effort of contraction to expand the lungs; this sense of effort is expressed in a feeling of breathlessness (13).

Flow-Volume Characteristics

Minor changes in the flow-volume curve occur with increasing age. In inspiration, the major factor influencing flow is the effectiveness of the inspiratory muscles. Because of the increase in lung volume and shortening of the respiratory muscles, there is a small reduction in inspiratory flow, but maximum flow is also reduced due to a reduction in respiratory muscle strength. During expiration, on the other hand, the major factors limiting flow are the lung elastic recoil and the airway resistance. Because elastic recoil is reduced and airway resistance is increased at low lung volumes because of a lack of support in the small airways, expiratory flow is reduced, particularly at low lung volumes (Fig. 32-3), when the airways tend to close. The maximum inspiratory flow at 50% of vital capacity (FIF50) falls from 5.8 liters per second (1/s) to 4.7 1/s between the ages of 20 and 60, a 17% fall occurring at a rate of 26 ml/s/yr (1). The forced expiratory volume in 1/s (FEV_1) falls to a greater relative extent, from 4.25 to 2.9 l, a 30% fall at a rate of 32 ml/yr (8, 17).

Lung Volumes

The changes in pressure-volume characteristic and the occurrence of airway closure at low lung volumes lead to a reduction in total lung capacity, an increase in residual volume, and a reduction in vital capacity with increasing age. Total lung capacity falls from 6.8 to 6.3 l, a 7% fall, between 20 and 60 years (10). Residual volume increases from 1.6 to 2.2 l (37% change) (10). Vital capacity falls from 5.2 to 4.2 l, a 19% reduction, at a rate of 25 ml/yr (8, 17). As already pointed out, small airways begin to close during an expiration at a higher lung volume with increasing age; the closing volume (CV), expressed as a percentage of the total lung capacity (CV/TLC%), doubles between 20 and 60 years, from 24.8 to 49.3% (6).

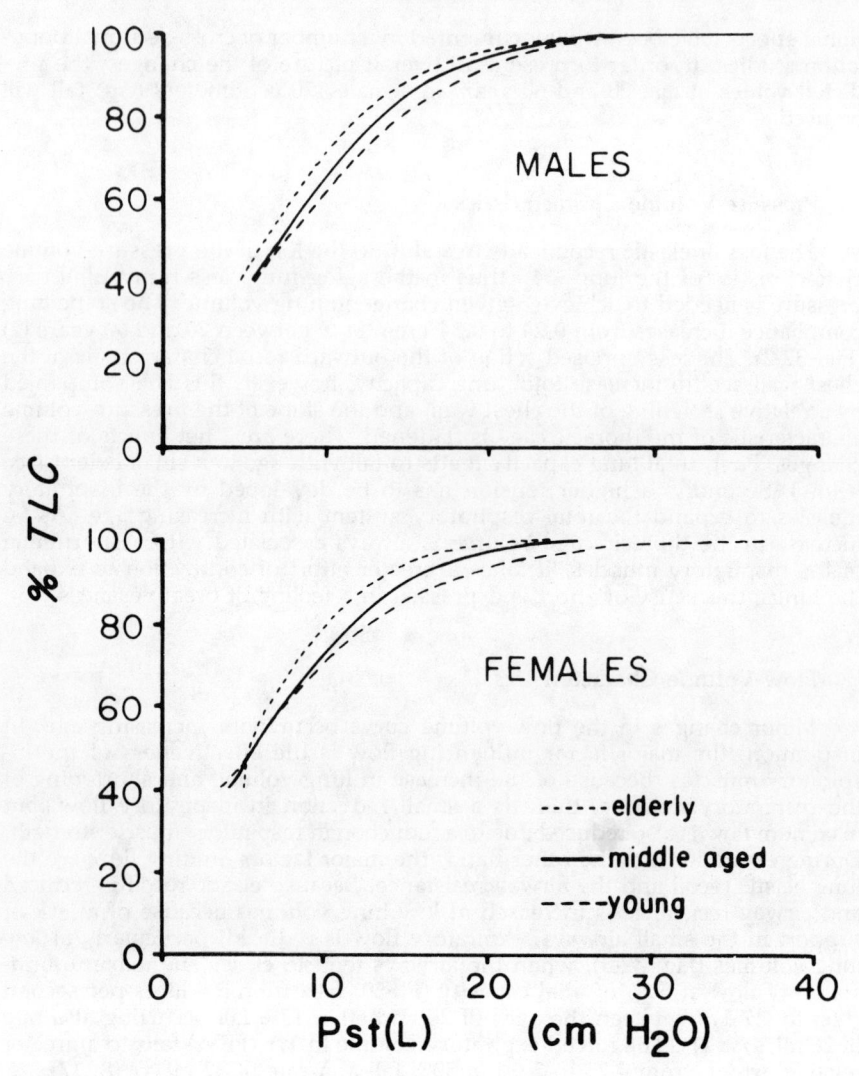

Fig. 32-2. Static pressure-volume curves obtained in males and females at different ages. Reprinted from Ref. 14 with permission.

Respiratory Muscles

As with all skeletal muscles, there is a gradual loss of strength in the respiratory muscles. In other muscles this has been shown to be related to a loss of the Type II fast-twitch fibers and also a reduction in the functioning motor units. Inspiratory muscle strength is assessed by measuring maximal inspiratory pressures; these show a gradual fall with increasing age from 132 to 110 cm H_2O between 20 and 60 years (3). The maximum expiratory pressures are less affected, due partly to the fact that many muscles in addition to the respiratory muscles contribute to this pressure.

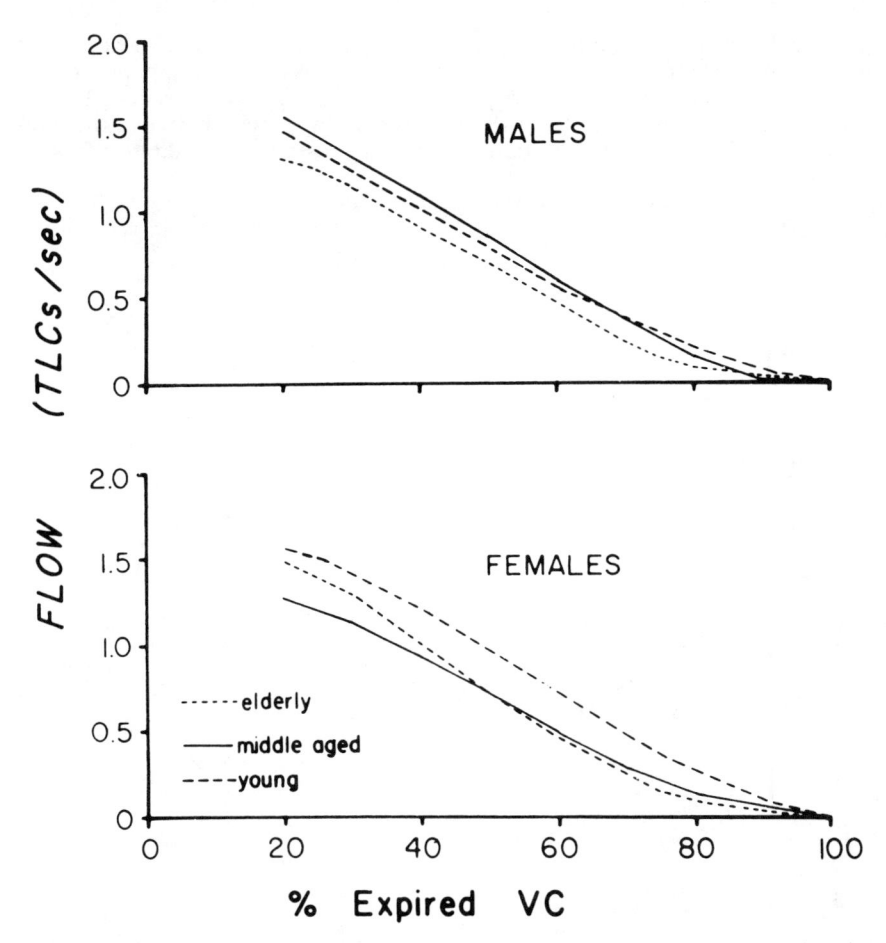

Fig. 32-3. *Expired flow-volume relationships in subjects of different ages. Reprinted from Ref. 14 with permission.*

Breathing Capacity

The changes in the pressure-volume and flow-volume characteristics of the total respiratory system, together with a reduction in respiratory muscle strength, account for a gradual fall in maximal voluntary ventilation or breathing capacity from 182 to 125 l/min, a 31% fall, between 20 and 60 years (8, 10). One may easily appreciate that this fall in breathing capacity will contribute to dyspnea during exercise and perhaps also to a ventilatory limitation to continued maximal exercise.

Pulmonary Blood Flow

With increasing age there is a gradual loss of the small vessels in the lung and the resistance to flow through small vessels increases. These changes influence the distribution of blood flow in the lung and also lead to the requirement for a greater perfusion pressure at a given rate of flow, for example during exercise. Inevitably, this leads to greater pressures being generated in the right ventricle. Systolic mean pulmonary artery pressure increases from 12 to 15 mmHg at rest, and from 18 to 30 mmHg in exercise between the ages of 20 and 60 (7), implying a doubling of arterial resistance from 0.6 to 1.2 units (Fig. 32-4).

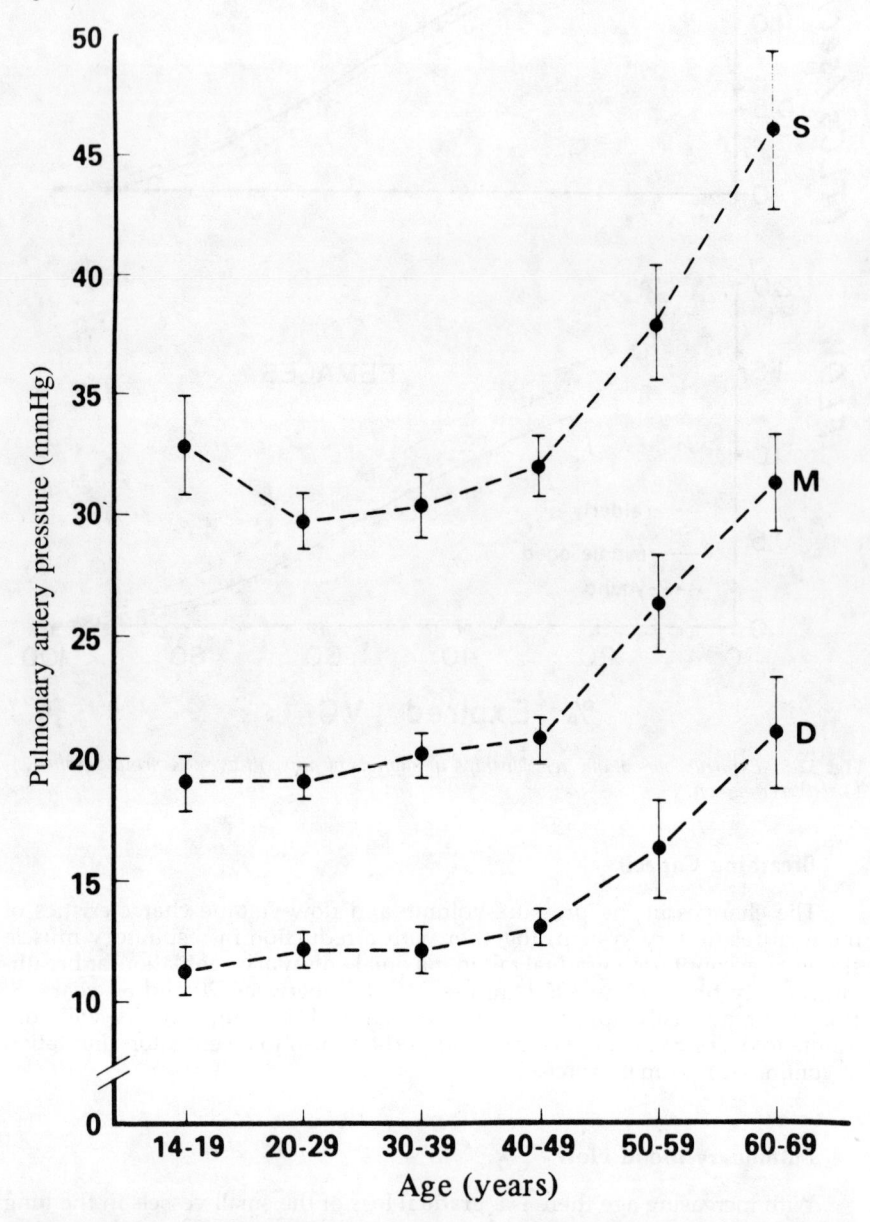

Fig. 32-4. *Pulmonary artery pressures in subjects free of heart disease, during exercise. Reprinted from Ref. 7 with permission.*

Pulmonary Gas Exchange

The transport of oxygen from alveolar gas into blood depends upon diffusion of oxygen across the alveolar capillary membrane and an efficient balance between the ventilation and perfusion of lung units. Because of the reduction in surface area available for gas transfer and the increased resistance to pulmonary blood flow (7), the capacity for diffusion gradually falls. As measured by the carbon monoxide technique, diffusing capacity falls from 35 to 21 ml/min/mmHg, a 40% reduction between 20 and 60 years (9, 22). Also, the changes in the alveoli and blood vessels lead to a poor matching between ventilation and blood flow in different units, leading to areas that are poorly ventilated in relation to their blood flow (leading to venous admixture). This is particularly seen at the bases of the lung, where some alveoli may not be ventilated at all with normal resting tidal volumes because the end-inspiratory volume remains below closing volume. There is also the opposite effect, mainly in the lung apices, where blood flow is poor and the ventilation-perfusion ratio is high. This is measured as an increase in the dead space/tidal volume ratio (4, 19).

Arterial Blood Gases

The pulmonary gas exchange disturbances described above lead to a gradual fall in arterial oxygen pressure with age, amounting to about 4 mmHg for each decade (Fig. 32-5) (19, 20). Because ventilation-perfusion matching is influenced by gravity, this effect is seen mainly in the supine position. At age 60 the lowest limit of normal is 70 mmHg, compared with 85 mmHg at age 20.

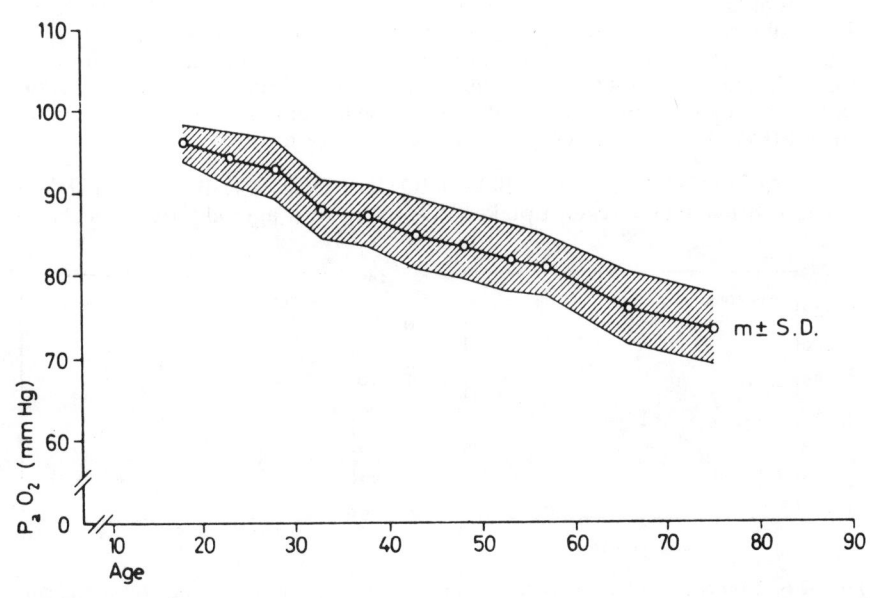

Fig. 32-5. *Arterial oxygen pressure at rest supine in healthy subjects of different ages. Reprinted from Ref. 20 with permission.*

Although at first sight this appears to be a dramatic finding which might imply a reduction in oxygen delivery to the exercising muscles, it should be noted that these changes take place on the upper flat portion of the oxygen dissociation curve. Thus, in terms of oxygen saturation of arterial blood, the effect accounts for only a 1 to 2% fall in saturation, and arterial oxygen saturation remains at about 95%, even at age 60. The fall in arterial PO_2 is associated with a widening in the alveolar to arterial PO_2 difference that is seen both at rest and during exercise (11, 19). However, the venous admixture ratio falls with exercise in both young and old, and it appears that pulmonary gas exchange function improves with exercise in the elderly (11). Arterial PCO_2 shows little change with age, a small reduction usually being seen, particularly on exercise (5).

Control of Breathing

There is some evidence that the gain in respiratory control systems falls with increasing age, but it seems likely that this effect is quite small. Studies have shown that the ventilatory response to inhaled CO_2 and hypoxic gas mixtures is lower than in younger subjects (5, 18). To some extent this effect may be accounted for by smaller lung volumes and weaker respiratory muscles. However, one study demonstrated a reduction in the pressure generated over the first 0.1 s of an occluded breath (PO.1); this has been taken as a reliable index of central respiratory drive (18). Although there is a fall in the respiratory responses to these 2 stimuli, impaired respiratory control does not appear to contribute to differences in the ventilatory responses to exercise (5).

Ventilation during Exercise

There is an increase in the ventilatory response to exercise in healthy elderly subjects (5, 15). Our own studies (12) show that this effect is really quite small, and when subjects of comparable fitness are compared, the differences are insignificant at low and moderate workloads. However, at the higher workloads, elderly subjects exhibit an increase in ventilation for a given power output (Fig. 32-6). A number of factors contribute to this:

1) AN INCREASE IN CARBON DIOXIDE OUTPUT: Because of the reduction in maximal oxygen uptake ($\dot{V}O_2$ max) with age, elderly subjects are

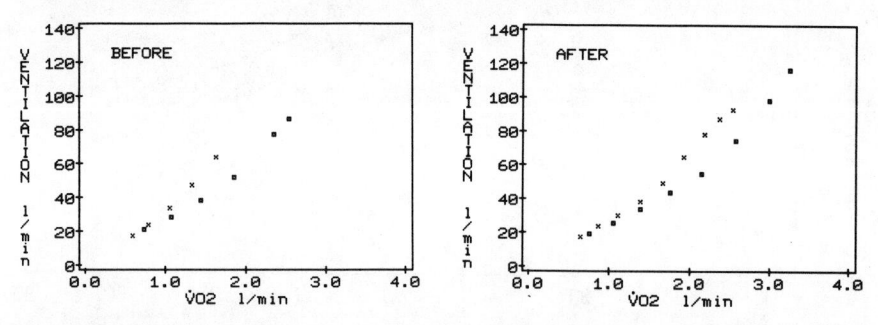

Fig. 32-6. *Ventilation during exercise in young (□) and old subjects (x) studied before and after a 12-week exercise training program (16). Both groups showed a fall in ventilation after training, but ventilation was slightly higher in older subjects at both times.*

exercising at a higher proportion of $\dot{V}O_2$ max for any given power output than are younger subjects. Related to this is a higher lactate production. An increase in the lactate concentration in blood is associated with falls in bicarbonate concentration and the evolution of CO_2 in expired ventilation. Thus when young and old are compared in terms of the ventilatory response to $\dot{V}CO_2$, the differences are less than when considered in relation to oxygen intake.

2) INCREASES IN VD/VT RATIO: The VD/VT ratio is higher in elderly subjects than younger subjects (4, 19). This is due in part to ventilation perfusion imbalance and in part to the fact that at any given power output, the tidal volume tends to be lower in elderly subjects than younger subjects due to differences in the mechanical characteristics of the lung.

3) AN INCREASE IN ALVEOLAR VENTILATION: Alveolar ventilation is reflected in the arterial PCO_2 which is lower in elderly subjects than younger subjects; this is due at least in part to a response to the metabolic acidosis (see 1 above).

Breathlessness during Exercise

Breathlessness may be defined as the consciousness of increased respiratory effort. At any given power output, elderly subjects may be expected to appreciate a greater respiratory effort because of the increase in ventilation during exercise, the increase in the mechanical work of breathing due to the changes in respiratory system mechanical characteristics, and the reduction in respiratory muscle strength. Thus, in any given individual a number of factors contribute to breathlessness, and it is to be expected that the older athlete will experience a greater degree of breathlessness during any athletic event than a younger athlete. However, training, even in the elderly, may lead to appreciable improvements in the sense of breathlessness for a number of reasons. For instance, training leads to a reduction in lactate production and thus in CO_2 output during exercise (Fig. 32-6) (16). Our study did not show any changes in the pattern of breathing with exercise, but increases in respiratory muscle strength have been shown to follow training. The combination of a reduction in ventilatory demand and an increase in respiratory muscle strength will tend to lessen the sensation of breathlessness.

We can't do anything about the structural changes in the respiratory system which occur as we get older except try to avoid exposure to cigarette smoke and environmental pollutants; but by maintaining a high level of fitness, we can maintain the efficiency of our lungs and reduce the effort required to breathe.

REFERENCES

1. Bass, H. The flow volume loop: Normal standards and abnormalities in chronic obstructive pulmonary disease. *Chest* 63:171–176, 1973.
2. Begin, R., A. D. Renzetti, Jr., A. H. Bigler, and S. Watanabe. Flow and age dependence of airway closure and dynamic compliance. *J. Appl. Physiol.* 38:199–207, 1975.
3. Black, L. F., and R. E. Hyatt. Maximal respiratory pressures: Normal values and relationship to age and sex. *Am. Rev. Resp. Dis.* 99:696–702, 1969.
4. Bradley, C. A., E. A. Harris, E. R. Seelye, and R. M. L. Whitlock. Gas exchange during exercise in healthy people. *Clin. Sci.* 51:323–333, 1976.

5. Brischetto, M. J., R. P. Millman, D. D. Peterson, D. A. Silage, and A. I. Pack. Effect of aging on ventilatory response to exercise and CO_2. *J. Appl. Physiol.: REEP* 56:1143–1150, 1984.
6. Buist, A. S., H. Ghezzo, N. R. Anthonisen, R. M. Cherniack, S. Ducic, P. T. Macklem, J. Manfreda, R. R. Martin, D. McCarthy, and B. B. Ross. Relationship between the single-breath N_2 test and age, sex, and smoking habits in three North American Cities. *Am. Rev. Resp. Dis.* 120:305–318, 1979.
7. Ehrsam, R. E., A. Perruchoud, M. Oberholzer, F. Burkart, and H. Herzog. Influence of age on pulmonary haemodynamics at rest and during supine exercise. *Clin. Sci.* 65:653–660, 1983.
8. Ericsson, P., and L. Irnell. Physical work capacity and static lung volumes in elderly people. *Acta Med. Scand.* 185:185–191, 1969.
9. Gelb, A. F., W. M. Gold, R. R. Wright, H. R. Bruch, and J. A. Nadel. Physiologic diagnosis of subclinical emphysema. *Am. Rev. Resp. Dis.* 107:50–63, 1973.
10. Grimby, G., and B. Soderholm. Spirometric studies in normal subjects: III. Static lung volumes and maximum voluntary ventilation in adults with a note on physical fitness. *Acta Med. Scand.* 173:199–206, 1963.
11. Harris, E. A., E. R. Seelye, and R. M. L. Whitlock. Gas exchange during exercise in healthy people. II. Venous admixture. *Clin. Sci.* 51:335–344, 1976.
12. Jones, N. L., L. Makrides, C. Hitchcock, T. Chypchar, and N. McCartney. Normal standards for an incremental progressive cycle ergometer test. *Am. Rev. Resp. Dis.* 131:700–708, 1985.
13. Killian, K. J., and N. L. Jones. The use of exercise testing and other methods in the investigation of dyspnea. *Clinics Chest Med.* 5:99–108, 1984.
14. Knudson, R. J., D. F. Clark, T. C. Kennedy, and D. E. Knudson. Effect of aging alone on mechanical properties of the normal adult human lung. *J. Appl. Physiol.: REEP* 43:1054–1062, 1977.
15. Mahler, D. A. Pulmonary Aspects of Aging. In: *Contemporary Geriatric Medicine*, Vol I, S. R. Gambert, (Ed.). New York: N. Y. Plenum Publishing Corporation, 45–84, 1983.
16. Makrides, L., G. J. F. Heigenhauser, N. McCartney, and N. L. Jones. Physical training in young and older healthy subjects. In: *Sports Medicine for the Mature Athlete*. J. Sutton and R. Brock, eds. Indianapolis: Benchmark. 1986.
17. Morris, J. F., A. Koski, and L. C. Johnson. Spirometric standards for healthy nonsmoking adults. *Am. Rev. Resp. Dis.* 103:57–67, 1971.
18. Peterson, D. D., A. I. Pack, D. A. Silage, and A. P. Fishman. Effects of aging on ventilatory and occlusion pressure responses to hypoxia and hypercapnia. *Am. Rev. Resp. Dis.* 124:387–391, 1981.
19. Raine, J. M., and J. M. Bishop. A-a difference in O_2 tension and physiological dead space in normal man. *J. Appl. Physiol.* 18:284–288, 1963.
20. Sorbini, C. A., V. Grassi, E. Solinas, and G. Muiesan. Arterial oxygen tension in relation to age in healthy subjects. *Respiration* 25:3–13, 1968.
21. Thurlbeck, W. M. Chronic airflow obstruction in lung disease. Philadelphia: W. B. Saunders, 190–197, 1976.
22. Van Kessel, A. L. Pulmonary diffusing capacity for carbon monoxide. In: *Pulmonary Function Testing Guidelines and Controversies*, J. L. Clausen, (Ed.). N. Y.: Academic Press, 1982.

Section VIII
Bone

33

Nuclear Medicine Techniques To Detect Exercise–Induced Changes in the Skeleton

GEOFFREY COATES, MB.B.S., F.R.C.P.(C)
COLIN WEBBER, PH.D.

McMaster University Medical Centre

During the past 10 years there have been major technical developments in the fields of radiology and nuclear medicine. Many of these techniques have been applied to the problems of sports-related injuries and to the skeletal changes that develop with age. In this chapter we will review the technical aspects of radionuclide bone imaging, measurement of bone density and bone mass, and their application to exercise-related changes in the skeleton.

BONE IMAGING WITH RADIOISOTOPES

In the absence of a suitable radioactive isotope of calcium, the first agents to be used routinely to image bones were strontium-85 and fluorine-18 (51). These were replaced in the early 1970s by phosphates labeled with technetium-99m (^{99m}Tc-P). This man-made isotope is readily available, cheap to produce, and emits a single gamma ray of 140 Kev which is ideally suited to modern imaging equipment. An image of the distribution of isotope in the skeleton is obtained with a gamma camera. Tomographic three-dimensional images of the skeleton can also be obtained with a rotating gamma camera interfaced to a digital computer. Lesions in bone such as fractures, metastases, or infection cause the bone around the lesion to accumulate more isotope than the surrounding normal bone (Fig. 33-1).

Mechanism of Increased Bone Uptake

If ^{99m}Tc-pyrophosphate is poured onto a column containing either dried powdered bone or hydroxy apatite, none of the isotope can be detected in

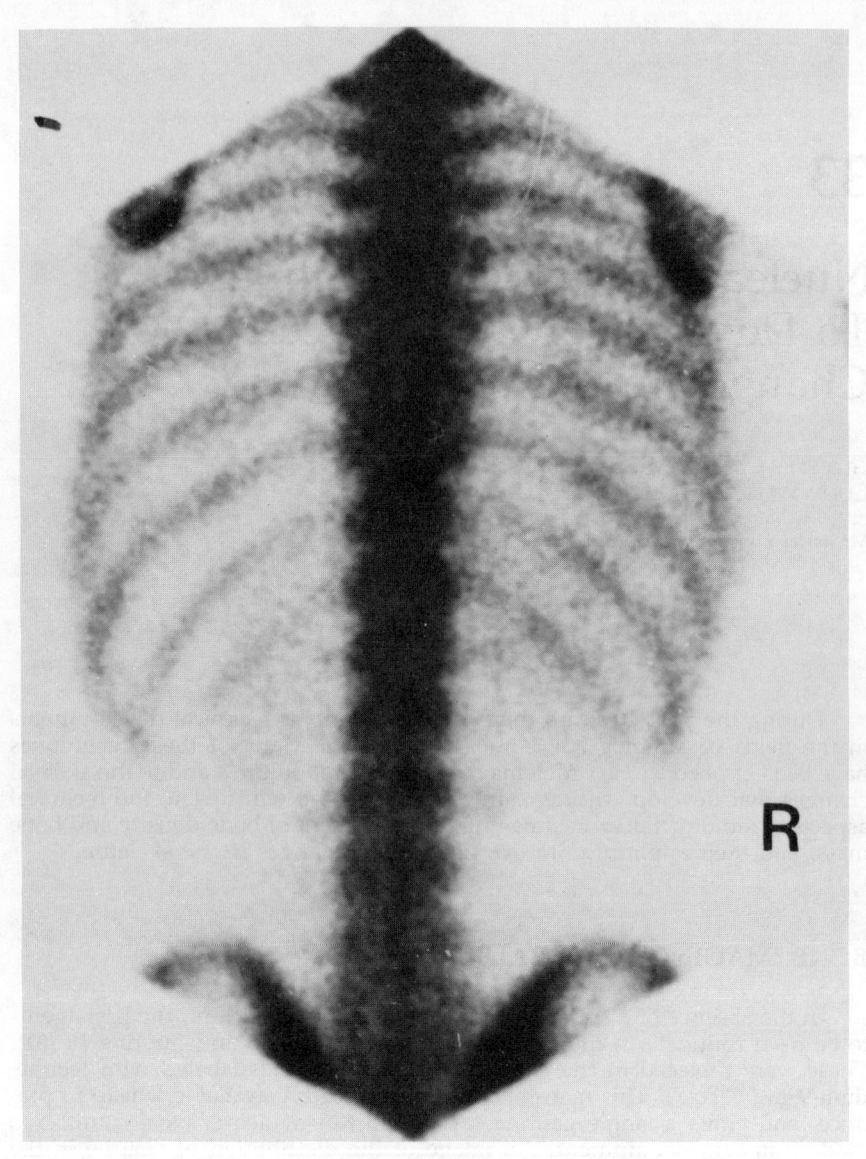

Fig. 33-1a, 1b. *Normal bone scan obtained with ^{99m}Tc-imidodiphosphate (^{99m}Tc-IDP). Accumulation of ^{99m}Tc-IDP in a patient with multiple rib fractures following auto accident.*

the effluent; i.e., the bone absorbs 100% of the isotope presented to it. So clearly, an increase in bone uptake cannot be secondary to changes in the hydroxy apatite lattice itself. Garnett et al. (25) measured the extraction efficiency of ^{99m}Tc-pyrophosphate from blood to living bone. Normal bone extracts only 60% of the isotope presented to it by the blood. On the other hand, abnormal bone (recent fracture) not only extracts isotope more efficiently but also receives an increased blood flow. Thus, an abnormal accumulation of

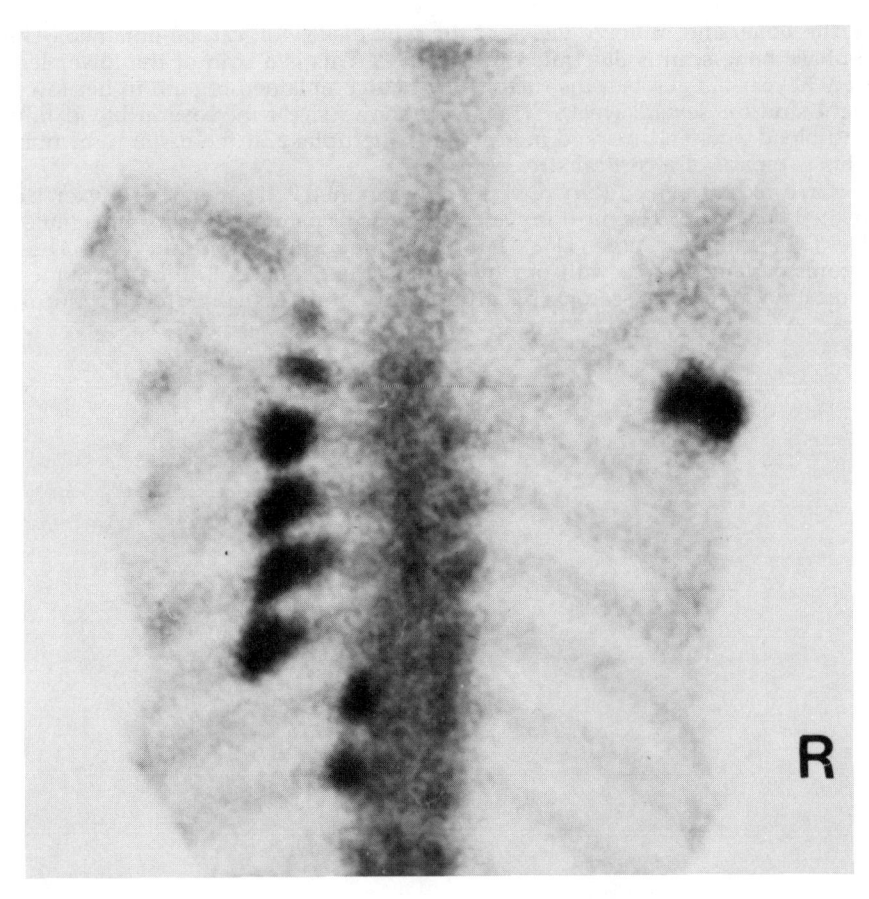

Fig. 33-1b.

^{99m}Tc-P on a bone scan results from the combined effects of a more efficient extraction, secondary to increased bone capillary permeability, and increased bone blood flow.

Radioisotope Bone Scans in Sports Injuries

Within 12 hours of a bone injury there is an easily detectable increase in uptake of ^{99m}Tc-P. In contrast to this, a radiograph of injured bone may not become abnormal for 10 days, particularly in the small bones of the hands and feet. Thus the nuclear bone scan can be used as a sensitive indicator of early bone damage such as that which occurs during intense physical activity. The bone scan is performed in three phases. Technetium-99m-P is injected intravenously and images of the region of interest are taken every 2 seconds for 30 seconds. This is the first phase of the scan, and the amount of radioactivity in any given area represents blood flow. This is similar to an angiogram. After 1 minute a second image is obtained. This represents the distribution of blood volume in the region. The third image is obtained 2 hours later, when much of the isotope has left blood and soft tissue. What is left is in the bone, and multiple views of the whole skeleton can be obtained. The 3-phase bone scan is illustrated in Fig. 33-2. This is a scan of the lower legs of a 30-year-old aerobics instructor. She had complained of pain in her lower right shin for several weeks. The study shows slight increase in blood flow and blood pool and marked increase in bone uptake in the distal right tibia. This is typical of a cortical stress fracture.

In a recent review, Rupani et al. (66) examined 238 patients with exercise-related bone pain. The most prevalent regions of pain were tibia/fibula (40%), feet (25%), lumbar spine (11%), femur (8%), and pelvis and hip (6%). These figures certainly agree with our own clinical experience. The most frequent indication for a bone scan in this group of patients was either focal or diffuse

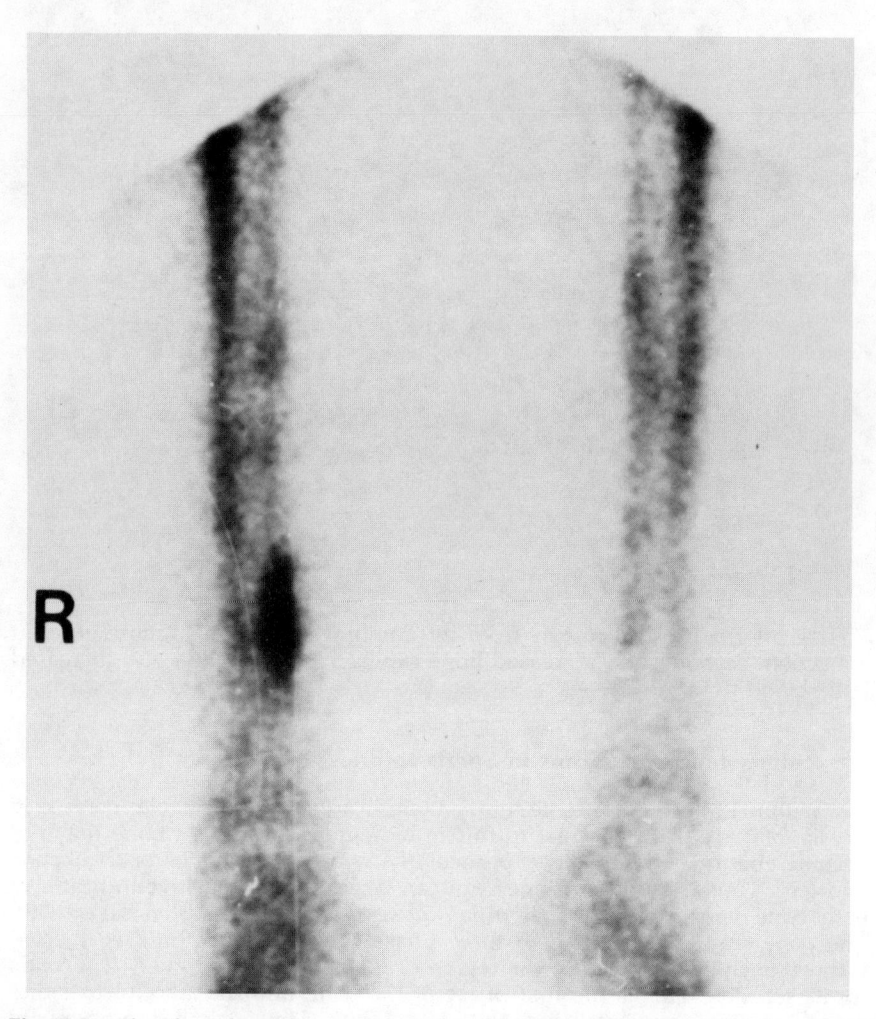

Fig. 33-2a, 2b. *Three-phase bone scan in 30-year-old aerobics instructor with pain in lower right tibia (2a). Multiple images taken 2 seconds apart of radioactivity arriving in the lower legs (blood flow). The arrow indicates a region of increased blood pool corresponding to the region of marked accumulation of ^{99m}Tc-IDP on the delayed images (2b). This is typical of a stress fracture.*

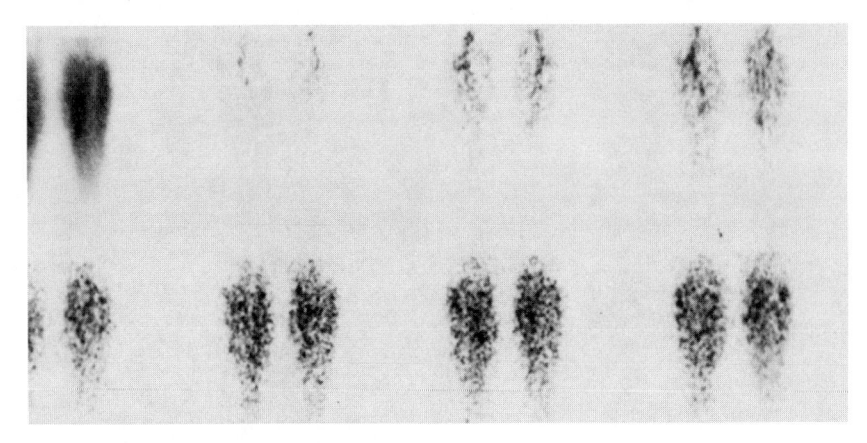

Fig. 33-2b.

pain. In Rupani's study (66), 192 patients had focal pain and 46 had diffuse pain.

The most common abnormality seen in the tibia/fibula is the stress fracture (Fig. 33-2). However, the clinical syndrome of shin splints also results in a typical bone scan appearance. Fig. 33-3 is a bone scan of a 19-year-old woman who had recently started exercise classes. She had complained of pain and tenderness in both shins for several weeks. The blood flow and blood pool phases of her scan were normal, but the delayed images demonstrate the typical finding of marked increase in isotope uptake along the middle third of the posterio-medial borders of both tibia, best seen on the antero-medial view. This has been attributed to periosteal irritation from frequent overuse of the soleus or posterior tibial muscles. It is sometimes difficult to distinguish on scan between a localized shin splint and stress fracture. In our own experience, the blood flow and blood pool phases are normal in simple shin splints but usually abnormal in stress fracture; similar findings have been reported by others (31).

Of the 238 patients in Rupani's study (66), 215 had radiographs; 149 were normal. Fractures of the carpals and tarsals are particularly difficult to see on a radiograph, and the bone scan has been the investigation of choice in these regions in both exercise-related and non-exercise-related injuries. Fig. 33-4 shows isotope uptake in the scaphoid bone and navicular in separate patients. The regions of increased uptake are readily seen, but the radiographs were initially normal.

Most reports indicate that running is by far the major cause of exercise-related bone scan abnormalities, and this is also our experience. However, the bone scan has also been found useful in a variety of injuries and activities. Fractures have been detected in the pubic arch of military recruits (52), the pars interarticularis of lumbar spine (66), the first rib (41) and the humerus (61) of tennis players and the feet of ballet dancers (28). We have seen extensive changes from shin splints in an aerobics instructor and multiple regions of increased uptake in the feet of a high jumper. Table 33-1 is taken from Rupani's study and documents the final diagnosis in patients with abnormal bone scans injured in less common sports.

The bone scan is a very sensitive indicator of bone damage, but once it is abnormal the increased uptake remains long after the normal healing phase is over. Fig. 33-5 shows an example of increased bone uptake in the tibia of

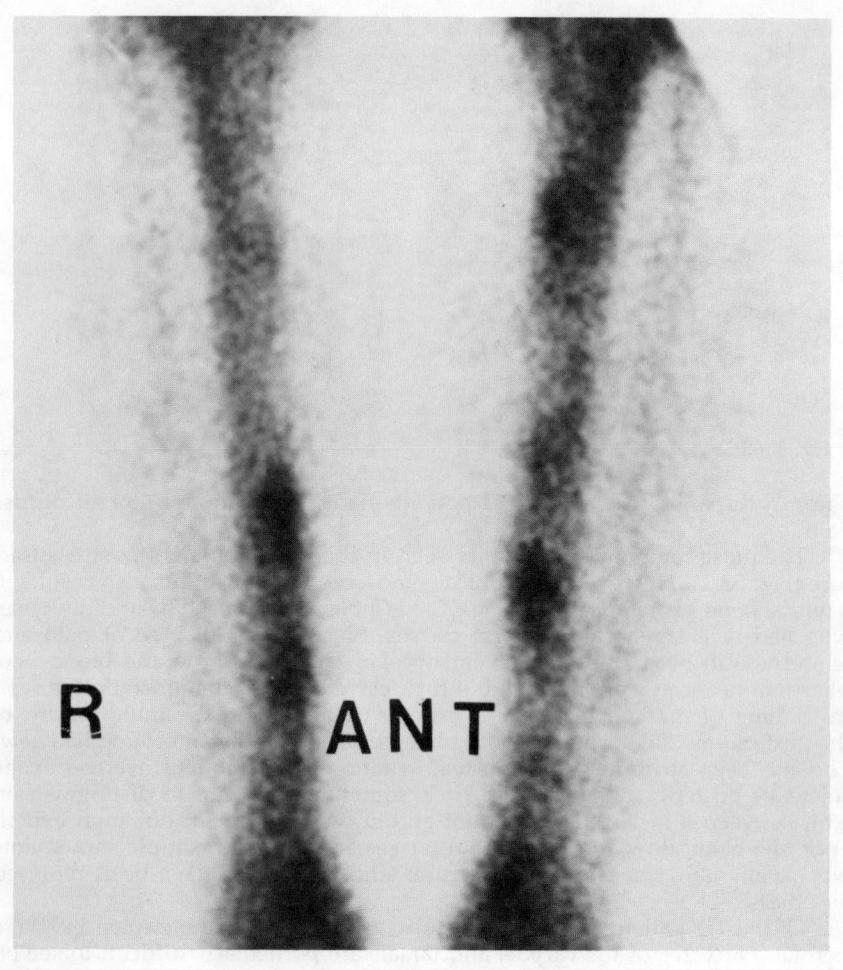

Fig. 33-3a, 3b. *This 19-year-old female recently started a fitness class and developed severe aching pain in both lower tibia. The patchy increase in isotope uptake on the anterior view (3a) is seen to be confined to the posterior cortex on the medial view (3b). This is typical of bilateral shin splints.*

a skier 8 years after the fracture. This persistence of uptake after a fracture is healed means that the scan is not a useful study to follow up the healing process. An exception to this occurs in patients with avascular necrosis when a cold rather than a hot area is an early indicator of poor bone blood flow. This has proven especially useful in evaluating the head of femur and scaphoid.

The high sensitivity of the ^{99m}Tc-P bone scan for early bone damage means that if the scan is normal, significant bone damage can be ruled out. Indeed, 22% of the patients in Raponi's study had normal bone scans, and this has major implications in terms of prognosis and treatment. In patients with alterations in gait secondary to soft tissue injury, there is frequently a generalized increase in isotope uptake by the bones in that limb (Fig. 33-6). This is

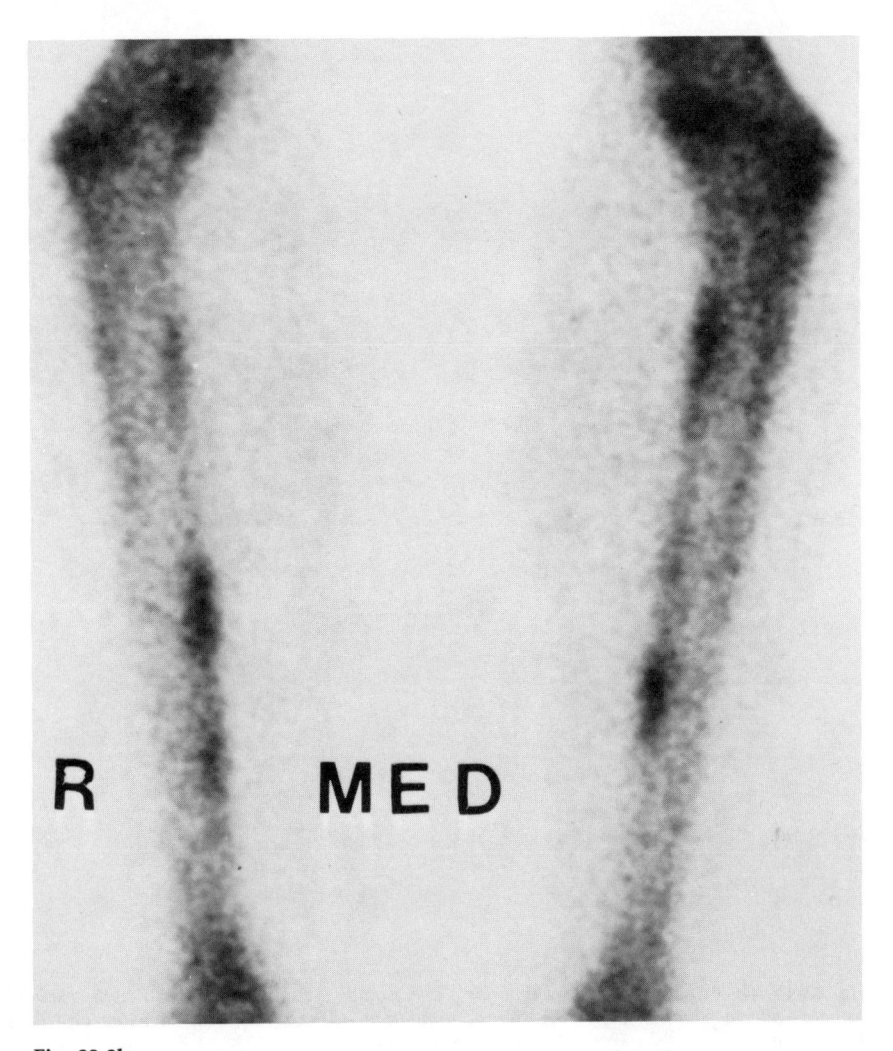

Fig. 33-3b.

secondary to disuse and can sometimes cause difficulties in interpreting the scan (29).

When the bone scan does indicate a stress fracture, this evidence can be used effectively in persuading the well-motivated athlete to take time out from his training.

Frostbite

One of the major clinical problems in patients with frostbite in their extremities is deciding when and at what level to amputate. Traditionally surgeons wait from 6 to 8 weeks until the irreversible tissue damage is well demonstrated. This long wait is trying for the patient and increases the danger of infection. There is some evidence that early imaging with ^{99m}Tc-P can accu-

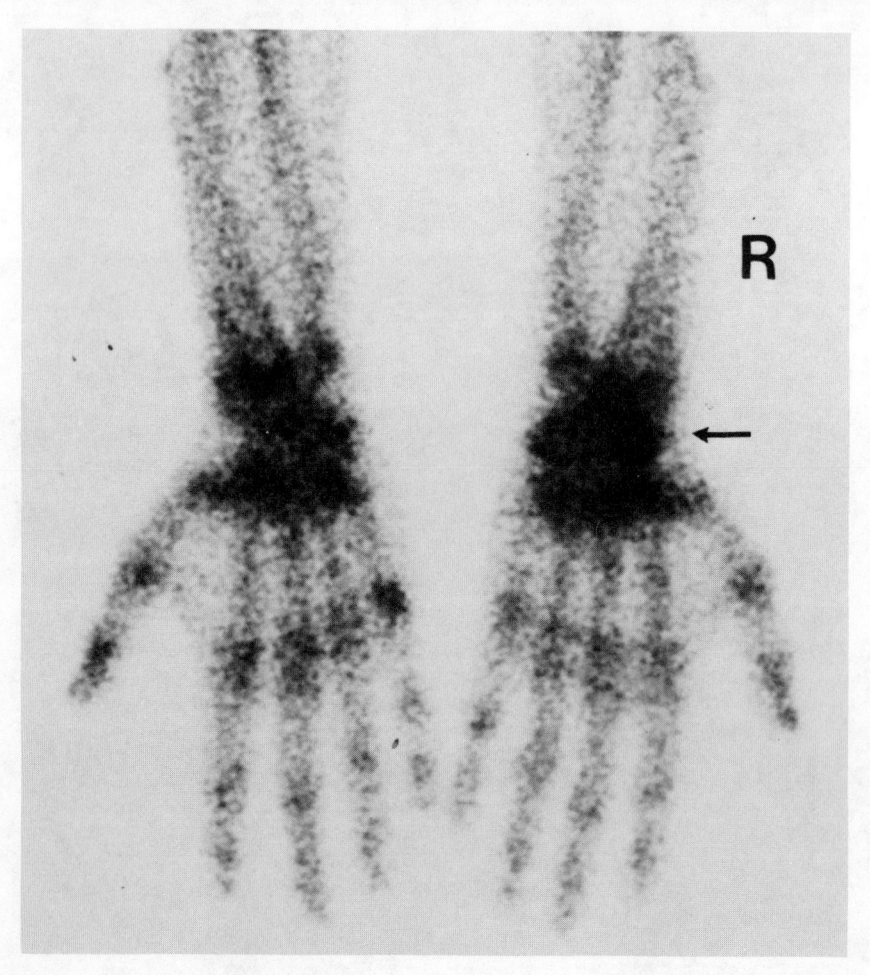

Fig. 33-4a, 4b, 4c. *Increased blood flow (4a), and isotope accumulation (4b) in right scaphoid 24 hours after a fall. Increased ^{99m}Tc-IDP accumulation in the right tarsal navicular of a long distance runner.*

rately define the eventual level of amputation (60). Fig. 33-7 illustrates a three phase bone scan on a patient with severe frostbite of the fingers 4 weeks before. The blood flow and blood pool phases indicate no flow beyond the proximal interphalangeal joints of 2nd and 5th fingers of both hands. Indeed, there is increased flow to their PIP joints probably secondary to inflammation. The lack of bone uptake beyond the PIP joints on the delayed bone scan confirms the absence of blood flow. The fingers were amputated at the PIP joints two weeks later. Although demarcation of tissue injury and mummification of the finger were well advanced in this patient when first seen 4 weeks after the injury, the scan confirmed the clinical findings and illustrated the usefulness of the technique. The high altitude studies group in Anchorage, Alaska, has experience with over 100 isotope bone scans in patients with frostbite (personal communication, W. J. Mills).

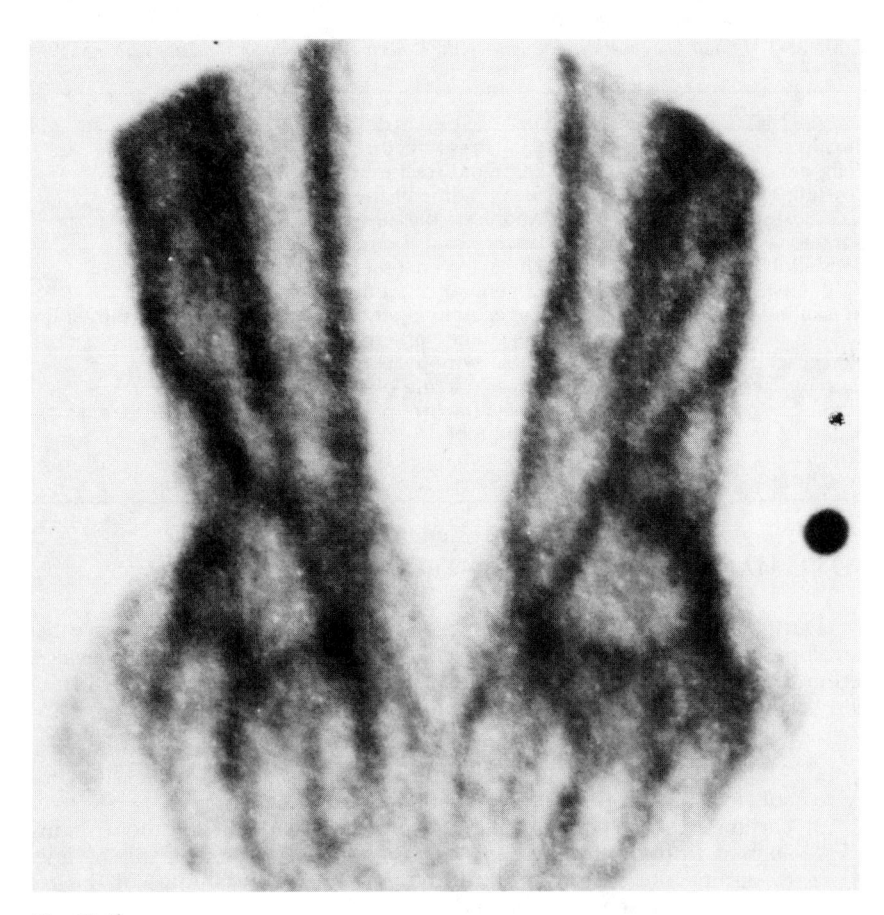

Fig. 33-4b.

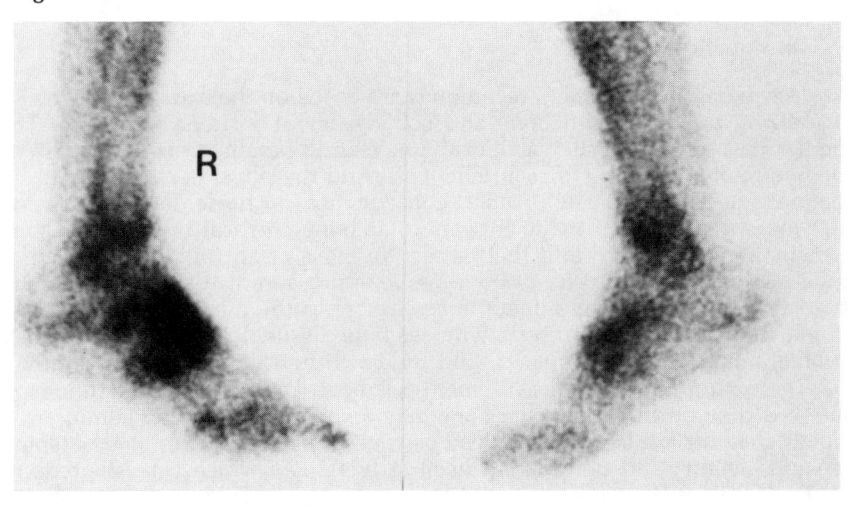

Fig. 33-4c.

NUCLEAR MEDICINE TECHNIQUES 339

Table 33-1. *Final Diagnoses in Patients with Abnormal TPB Images in Less Common Sports (66)*

Sports	Lesions
Boxing	Pars stress fracture of the lumbar spine
Belly dancing	Sesamoid fracture of the first metatarsal
Bowling	Sesamoiditis of the first metatarsal
Kick boxing	Apophyseal avulsion of the hip
Karate	Retrocalcaneal bursitis
Bobsledding	Thoracic vertebral body compression fracture
Racquetball	Degenerative joint disease of the knees
Ice skating	Degenerative joint disease of the knees, shin splints
Golf	Degenerative joint disease of the spine
Horseback riding	Pubic symphysis
Exercise bicycle riding	Stress fracture of the femoral neck
Ballet	Stress fracture of the metatarsal, stress changes of the foot
Baseball	Stress changes of the foot
Weight lifting	Pars stress fracture of the lumbar spine

BONE MASS MEASUREMENT TECHNIQUES

During the last 20 years, a number of non-invasive methods have been developed to measure bone mass *in vivo*. The stimulus for this work was the recognition of the severe consequence of osteopenic bone fractures in the elderly. It was thought that measurements of bone mass might:

1) Identify individuals with an increased risk of fracture
2) Allow quantification of the natural history of bone mass changes in subjects with and without metabolic bone disease
3) Facilitate the objective evaluation of the efficacy of treatment regimes such as fluoride, exercise, or vitamin D. The purpose of this review is to outline the various procedures and to review studies of the relationship between physical activity and bone mass.

Introduction

In general, measurement techniques are based on the extent of interaction of ionizing radiation with bone and soft tissues at a single body site. This implies that the diagnostic value of the measured parameter is dependent on the nature of bone at the measurement site and the physical characteristics of the ionizing radiation. The practical consequences of these dependencies are that measurements are made in trabecular bone, cortical bone, or in some combination of the two and that either the mass of an unknown volume of bone mineral or the density of bone tissue is measured. It should be emphasized that the term, bone mineral mass, refers to the mass of relatively high atomic number material present, whereas bone tissue density equals the mass of bone mineral, marrow, blood, and fluid within a defined tissue volume.

The optimum site of measurement has been and still is a contentious issue. It is thought that trabecular bone may respond to metabolic stimuli more rapidly than cortical bone, and indeed osteopenic fractures occur at axial (spine, proximal femur) and peripheral (distal radius) sites which consist predominantly of trabecular bone. On the other hand, appendicular cortical bone sites are readily accessible, and it is found that the variance of results in normal

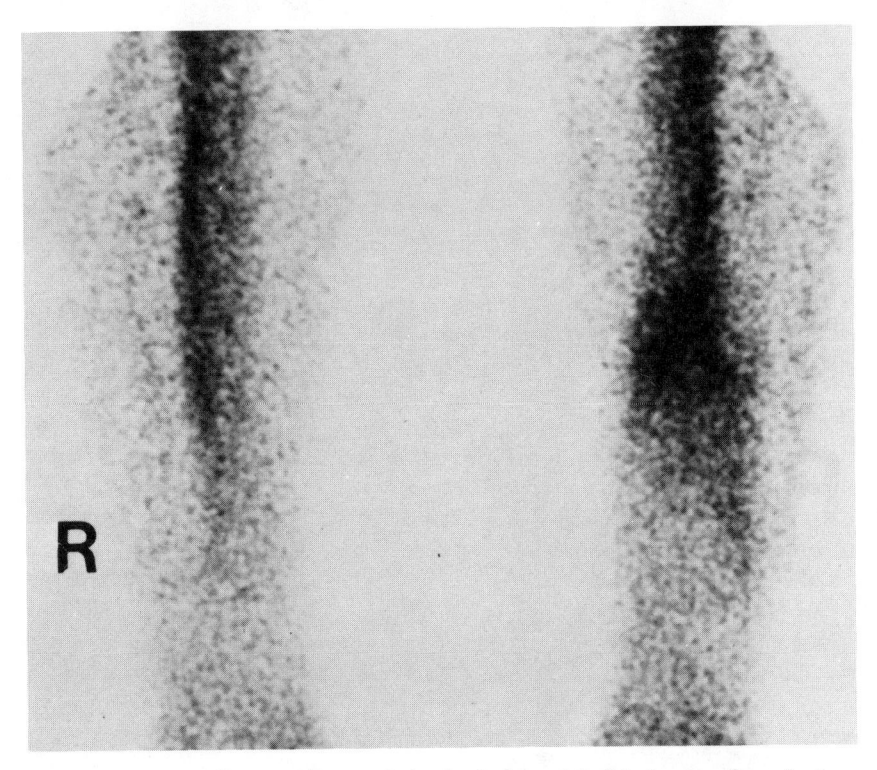

Fig. 33-5. *Increased ^{99m}Tc-IDP accumulation in the lower left tibia 8 years after a fracture.*

subject populations is generally less for cortical than for trabecular bone. This is advantageous since the discriminatory ability of a technique depends upon the ratio between the normal and abnormal population difference and the biological variance of each population. That is, it may not be appropriate to use the greater biological sensitivity of trabecular bone if measurement accuracy or population variance prevents the identification of an abnormal result.

RADIOGRAPHY: The radiographic evaluation of bone anatomy and trabecular patterns as well as subjective assessments of bone density are of little value in establishing the degree of osteopenia (3, 6, 10, 18, 22, 33, 70, 71). These factors are either not functions of bone mass or cannot be quantified objectively. In radiographic photodensitometry, objective assessments of film density are made from comparisons between the optical densities of images of bones and of a reference aluminum wedge. The technique is rarely used because of potential inaccuracies which limit its application to bones with minimal soft tissue covering (5). However, in experienced hands, useful measurements of clinical value have been obtained (16, 50).

SINGLE PHOTON ABSORPTIOMETRY: Many of the inherent sources of error in radiographic procedures are related to the polyenergetic x-ray spectrum and to the use of film as a radiation detector. The influence of such factors was eliminated by the introduction of the technique of single photon

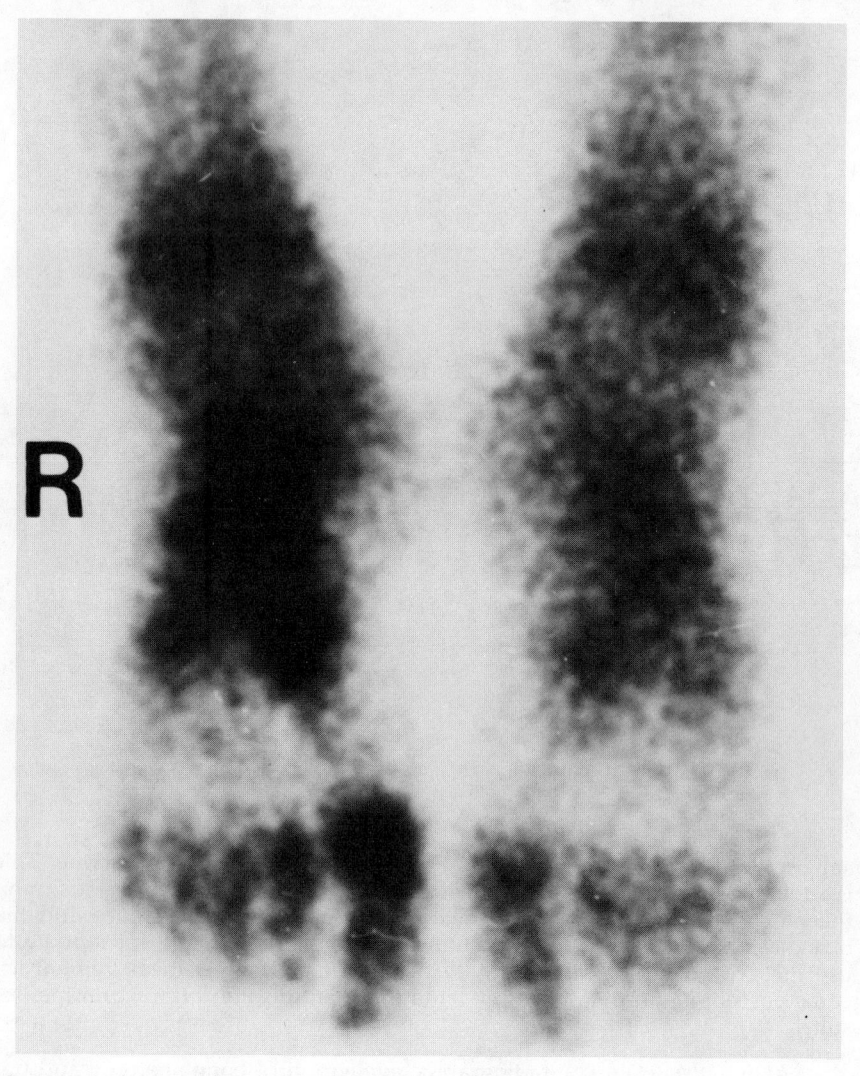

Fig. 33-6a, 6b. *Generalized increase in isotope uptake in the right ankle and foot of a runner with pain in the plantar arch. This increased uptake is frequently seen following alteration in gait (limp).*

absorptiometry (11). The transmission of a pencil beam of monoenergetic photons obtained from an ^{125}I source is measured by a scintillation detector as the beam is scanned across a limb. Changes in the transmitted intensity are proportional to the mass of bone in the beam, provided a constant thickness of soft tissue plus bone is maintained across the entire width of the scanned limb. An additional fundamental assumption is that the limb is composed only of bone material and soft tissue. Consequently, the method is restricted to peripheral bone sites such as the distal radius where constant tissue thickness can be maintained and where the fat content is acceptably small (42, 76).

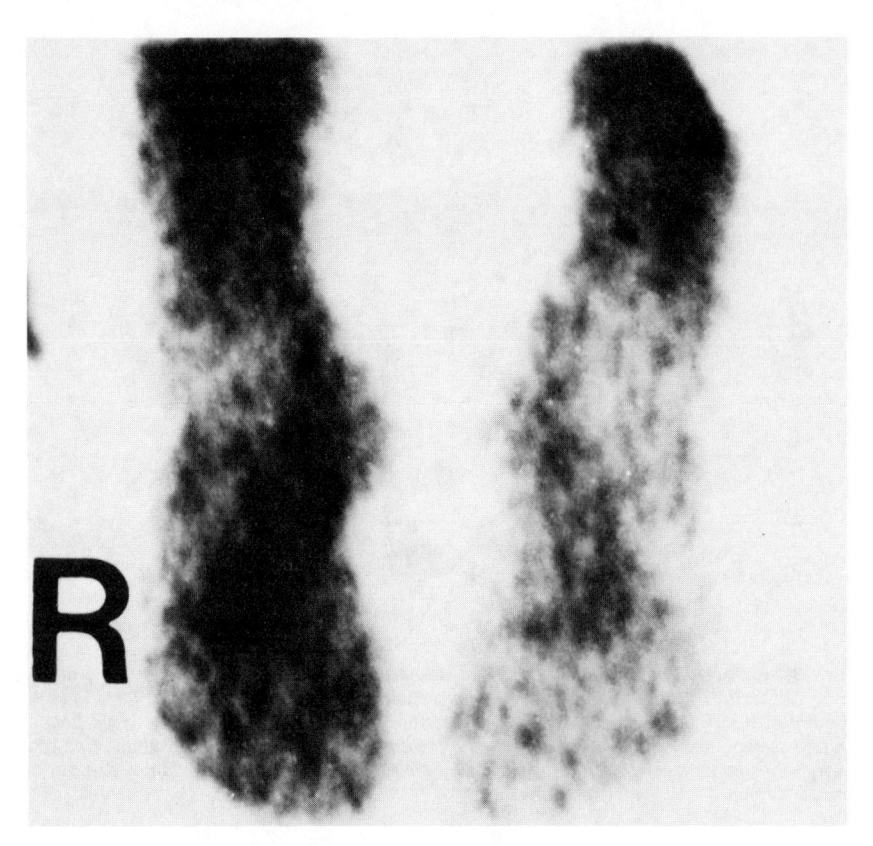

Fig. 33-6b.

The accuracy and precision of single photon transmission measurements can both be about 3% provided considerable care is taken in repositioning a limb for repeated measurements of cortical bone mass. The technique is useful for serial studies. However the mass of bone mineral measured is a function of both the degree of osteopenia and the size of the bone; consequently, the variance in normal and abnormal populations will be considerable, and the usefulness of a single measurement in an individual is limited (46, 72).

DUAL PHOTON ABSORPTIOMETRY: To eliminate the constant tissue thickness requirement of single photon absorptiometry, photons of two discrete energies are used. Bone mineral content can then be measured in otherwise inaccessible sites such as the spine and the femoral neck. It is also possible to measure the mineral content of the whole body by dual photon absorptiometry (59). The assumption still has to be made that the object consists solely of bone mineral and soft tissue; and since the ratio of fat to lean in soft tissue varies considerably from subject to subject, a correction procedure must be applied for each individual.

The precision and accuracy of dual and single photon absorptiometry are comparable. The biological variation of lumbar spine or femoral neck bone mineral measurements will be considerable since bone size and the degree of osteopenia are measured. The advantage of dual photon transmission is that

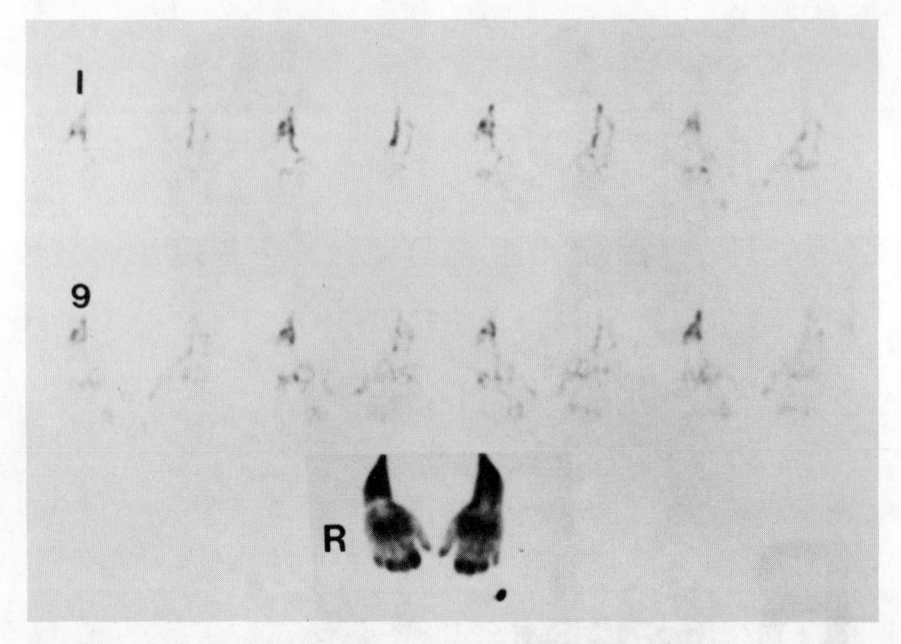

Fig. 33-7a, 7b. *Absent blood flow (7a) and delayed accumulation of isotope in the phalanges distal to the 1st IP joint in a 34-year-old climber with frostbite. He was caught for 3 days in a blizzard at the 20,000 feet level on Mt. Aconcagua in Argentina. The increased blood flow and delayed isotope uptake in the 1st PIP joint represents inflammatory reaction at the line of demarcation between viable and non-viable tissue. He subsequently had the phalanges distal to this amputated.*

fracture-prone, trabecular bone sites are measured, and thus it is to be expected that increased rates of bone mineral loss can be detected sooner than with the single photon technique.

Computed Tomography

Quantitated computerized tomography produces a cross-sectional image of the body which is a grey scale display of linear attenuation coefficients. The coefficients are derived from multiple x-ray transmission measurements through the body (8). The effective energy of the x-rays means that the coefficients predominantly reflect tissue density and it is possible to obtain the average density within a specified region from an image. If the region is restricted to a vertebral body, the result is an average of trabecular bone and marrow densities. Consequently, computed tomography yields a concentration measurement and is not a direct function of the size of a bone. The accuracy and precision of computerized tomography measurements are probably not as good as dual photon absorptiometry (27). However, it is possible to examine a vertebral body alone whereas dual photon measurements inevitably include the cortical bone of the transverse and spinous processes.

An important variation of this technique is that in which polyenergetic x-rays are replaced by a low energy radioisotope source (64). The linear attenuation coefficient will then depend on the tissue's effective atomic number rather than tissue density; the image reflects the distribution of chemical con-

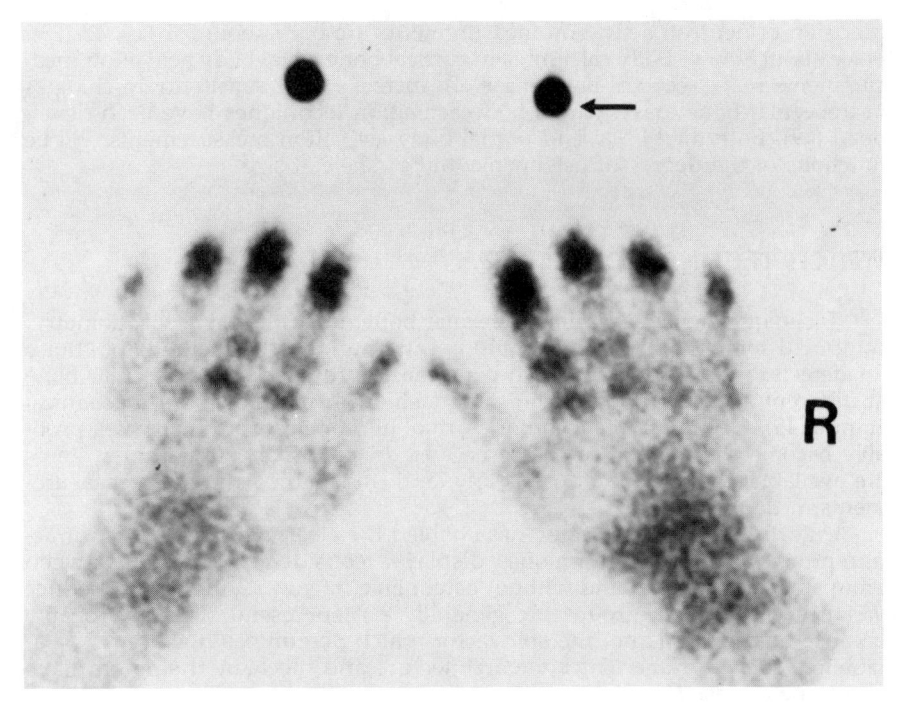

Fig. 33-7b.

stituents and the presence of fat is considerably less important. However, the lower photon energy restricts the technique to peripheral bones.

Compton Scattering

The mass of a defined volume of trabecular bone can be measured using Compton scattering of monoenergetic photons (73). This technique, together with computerized tomography, is the only method for the examination of trabecular bone without the presence of cortical bone. Scattering measurements of calcaneal trabecular bone density are simple and results are precise (63). The biological variation is smaller than transmission techniques since the measurement does not depend on the size of a bone. The disadvantage of the method, as with x-ray computerized tomography, is that the result is an average density for all substances within the scattering volume. The presence of non-bone substances reduces the sensitivity of the technique to changes in bone mineral concentration.

Neutron Activation

The calcium content of a specific region or of the whole body can be measured by neutron activation analysis. The subject is irradiated with neutrons which may interact with stable ^{48}Ca nuclei to form radioactive ^{49}Ca. Measurement of the induced ^{49}Ca activity can be related to skeletal mass since normally 99% of the total body calcium resides in the skeleton. The accuracy and precision of neutron activation measurements are both about 5% (15, 48, 75). Since about 80% of body calcium is in cortical bone, total body activation measurements reflect cortical bone mass. To increase their sensitivity to changes in trabecular bone mass, partial body activation techniques have been developed (49). Both total body and partial body activation measurements will be functions of the degree of osteopenia and of skeletal size.

WHICH TECHNIQUE TO USE?

Techniques which examine trabecular bone (dual photon absorptiometry, computed tomography, and Compton scattering) are the methods of choice for detecting temporal changes in bone mass, provided that trabecular bone at different sites responds in the same fashion to metabolic and mechanical stimuli (45). Of these three techniques, dual photon absorptrometry will probably become the method of choice because inexpensive commercial systems are available, the radiation dose is low, and this method can make measurements in the vertebrae.

Unfortunately no technique has enabled the clear identification of a fracture-prone subject. All techniques display a considerable overlap between groups of subjects with and without osteopenic fractures. Attempts to reduce variance within such groups are generally not successful. This is probably because bone mass is not the sole factor which determines fracture risk. Parameters such as trabecular bone architecture and mechanical strength have also to be assessed.

PHYSICAL ACTIVITY AND BONE MASS

Cross-Sectional Measurements in Cortical Bone

The effect of physical activity on bone mass can be studied cross-sectionally by comparing measurements in groups of individuals subjected to distinctly different levels of physical activity. Such study designs have been used to examine the influence of activity levels which were either greater or less than normal. For example, the cortical thickness of the humerus, radius, and metacarpals is consistently less on the involved side in patients suffering from hemiplegia (58). Various radiographic comparisons have been made between groups of pre- and postmenopausal women of different activity levels. In active, premenopausal women, the aluminum equivalent density of the middle phalanx of the 5th finger and the midradius bone mineral content were greater than for sedentary premenopausal women. There was no difference in the distal radius bone mineral content. Interestingly, the sedentary group were significantly heavier and their calcaneal aluminum equivalent density was greater (7). In postmenopausal women, the two most important variables which seemed to be related to the cortical thickness of the second metacarpal were the level of physical activity and the previous use of estrogen (57). Montoye et al. (1976) found in men participating in the Tecumseh Health Study that there was no relation between metacarpal morphometry and activity level. Bone hypertrophy and increased mineral mass are found in the lower extremities of professional cross-country runners (19, 56) and ballet dancers (67), and in the working arm of tennis players (35) and baseball pitchers (37).

Cross-Sectional Measurements in Trabecular Bone

Cross-sectional study designs have also been applied using those techniques in which trabecular bone is measured. Calcaneal bone density is increased in physical education students, whereas it is decreased in non-ambulant, elderly patients (63). When amenorrheic and eumenorrheic young athletes were matched for age, weight, and height as well as for type of sport, frequency, and duration of daily training sessions, it was found that the lumbar spine bone mineral content was significantly decreased in the amenorrheic group (23). This suggests that the bone loss secondary to low estrogen was not prevented by vigorous exercise. In the same subjects, there was no difference between the mineral content at either the mid- or distal radius. The only difference between the groups was that amenorrheic athletes ran a significantly greater distance per week.

Longitudinal Studies of Reduced Levels of Activity

A more appropriate study design is to search for sequential changes in bone mass in subjects whose level of physical activity has changed. Reductions in the magnitude of mechanical forces exerted on bones have been achieved with various experimental designs such as restriction of movement with a cast, confinement to bed, and space flight. When a patient or volunteer is confined to bed, trabecular bone mass decreases rapidly, at a rate of about 4% per month (43). This excessive rate slows during the next few weeks until a new steady rate is achieved (53). Upon reambulation, there appears to be complete restoration of the lost mineral (21, 32, 39).

In animals, cortical bone mass shows a rapid decrease following immobilization which is almost replaced before a second slow phase of loss eventually produces a new steady state at a bone mass of about half the original (69). The acute effects of immobilization in animals are more pronounced in trabecular bone than in cortical bone (34). During space flight, calcium losses are associated with muscle atrophy (74).

The hypercalciuria and negative calcium balance of paraplegic patients are both significantly improved by ambulation (36), although to prevent bone mass losses, it may be necessary to induce in bones the stresses and strains of normal muscle contraction (1). This is supported by experiments in rabbits in which rarefaction of the calcaneus was produced by suppression of the muscular force on the bone. The extent of bone rarefaction produced by cast immobilization was not as great when the calf muscle was stimulated (26).

Longitudinal Studies of Increased Levels of Activity

Sequential bone mass measurements have also been made in subjects whose level of physical activity has increased. Krolner et al. (40), using dual photon absorptiometry, showed that lumbar spine trabecular bone mass in postmenopausal women who had suffered a Colles fracture increased during 8 months of physical activity. The pattern of change in cortical bone mass in these women was consistent with that described by Smith et al. (68), who measured mid-radius bone mineral content in middle aged women subjected to a 3-year exercise program. During the first year mineral content fell, but rose during the subsequent two years. Neutron activation measurements showed an increased total body calcium in a group of postmenopausal women who exercised for 1 year. A matched group of non-exercising women exhibited a reduction in total body calcium (4). No significant changes were detected in the mineral content of the distal radius or in total body potassium of either group.

SUMMARY

It was inferred by Galileo in the 17th century that physical activity may influence bone structure, and it was stated by Wolff in the last century that definite changes in bone architecture follow changes in bone function (13). This means that mechanisms exist for sensing changes in the functional demands made on a bone and, as a consequence, for altering the activity of osteoclastic and osteoblastic cells within that bone. A recent conference addressed the issues concerned with such functional adaption mechanisms of bone tissue (17).

A basic bone structure and an associated bone mass are established by genetic demands. Variations in structure and increases in bone mass represent adaptations of that basic skeleton due to many factors. One of these factors is the level of physical activity. When a bone is subjected to a mechanical stress, a related strain is induced. It has been established that at least the magnitude, rate, and distribution of the induced strains are significant with respect to bone remodeling (44). These strain parameters may be sensed by a variety of mechanisms such as stress-generated electrical potentials or strain-induced release of matrix bound factors (13, 44, 74). Whatever the precise mechanism by which mechanical forces influence bone remodeling, there is little doubt that significant changes in the level of physical activity can have a profound influence on bone mass. Intuitively, increased physical activity should reduce the risk of osteoporosis and fracture in the population at risk (postmenopausal and hypo-estrogenic women), but more data are required to answer this question.

REFERENCES

1. Abramson, A. S., and E. F. Delagi. Influence of weight bearing and muscle contraction on disuse osteoporosis. *Arch. Phys. Med. Rehab.* 42:147–151, 1961.
2. Adams, P., G. T. Davies, and P. M. Sweetnam. Observer error and measurements of the metacarpal. *Br. J. Radiol.* 42:192–197, 1969.
3. Aloia, J. F., S. H. Cohn, J. A., Ostuni, R. Cane, and K. Ellis. Prevention of involutional bone loss by exercise. *Ann. Int. Med.* 89:356–358, 1978.
4. Aloia, J. F., A. Vaswani, H. Atkins, I. Zanzi, K. Ellis, and S. H. Cohn. Radiographic morphometry and osteopenia in spinal osteoporosis. *J. Nucl. Med.* 18:425–431, 1977.
5. Anderson, J. B., J. Shimmins, and D. A. Smith. A new technique for the measurement of metacarpal density. *Br. J. Radiol.* 39:443–450, 1966.
6. Ardran, G. M. Bone destruction not demonstrable by radiography. *Br. J. Radiol.* 24:107–109, 1951.
7. Bohr, H., and O. Schaadt. Bone mineral content of femoral bone and the lumbar spine measured in women with fracture of the femoral neck by dual photon absorptiometry. *Clin. Orthop. Rel. Res.* 179:240–245, 1983.
8. Brewer, V., B. M. Meyer, M. S. Keele, S. J. Upton, and R. D. Hagan. Role of exercise in prevention of involutional bone loss. *Med. Sci. Sport Exerc.* 15:445–449, 1983.
9. Brooks, R. A., and G. DiChiro. Principles of computer assisted tomography (CAT) in radiographic and radioisotope imaging. *Phys. Med. Biol.* 21:689–732, 1976.
10. Caldwell, R. A. Observations on the incidence, aetiology and pathology of senile osteoporosis. *J. Clin. Path.* 15:421–431, 1962.

11. Cameron, J. R., and J. Sorenson. Measurement of bone mineral in vivo: An improved method. *Science* 142:230–232, 1963.
12. Cann, C. E., H. K. Genant, B. Ettinger, and G. S. Gordon. Spinal mineral loss in oophorectomized women. *J.A.M.A.* 244:2056–2059, 1980.
13. Carter, D. R. Mechanical loading histories and cortical bone remodeling. *Calc. Tiss. Int.* 36:S19–S24, 1984.
14. Christensen, M. S., C. Christiansen, J. Naestoft, P. McNair, and I. Transbol. Normalization of bone mineral content to height, weight and lean body mass: Implications for clinical use. *Calc. Tiss. Int.* 33:5–8, 1981.
15. Cohn, S. H. Total body neutron activation. In: *Non-Invasive Measurements of Bone Mass and Their Clinical Application*, S. H. Cohn (ed.). Boca Raton, FL: CRC Press, 191–213, 1981.
16. Colbert, C., and R. S. Bachtell. Radiographic absorptiometry (photodensitometry). In: *Non-Invasive Measurements of Bone Mass and Their Clinical Application*, S. H. Cohn (ed.). Boca Raton, FL: CRC Press, 51–84, 1981.
17. Cowin, S. C., L. E. Lanyon, and G. Rodan. The Kroc foundation conference on functional adaptation in bone tissue. *Cal. Tiss. Int.* 36:S1–S6, 1984.
18. Dalen, N., and B. Lamke. Grading of osteoporosis by skeletal roentgenology and bone scanning. *Acta Radiol. Diag.* 15:177–186, 1974.
19. Dalen, N., and K. E. Olsson. Bone mineral and physical activity. *Acta Orthop. Scand.* 45:170–174, 1974.
20. Dequeker, J. Quantitative radiology: Radiogrammetry of cortical bone. *Br. J. Radiol.* 49:912–920, 1976.
21. Donaldson, C. L., S. B. Hulley, J. M. Vogel, R. S. Hattner, J. H. Boyers, and D. E. McMillan. Effect of prolonged bed rest on bone mineral. *Metabolism* 19:1071–1084, 1970.
22. Doyle, F. H., D. H. Gutteridge, G. F. Joplin, and R. Fraser. An assessment of radiological criteria used in the study of spinal osteoporosis. *Br. J. Radiol.* 40:241–250, 1967.
23. Drinkwater, B., K. Nilson, C. H. Chesnut, W. J. Bremner, S. Shainholtz, and M. B. Southworth. Bone mineral content of amenorrheic and eumenorrheic athletes. *N. Engl. J. Med.* 311:277–281, 1984.
24. Garn, S. M., A. K. Poznanski, and K. Larson. Metacarpal lengths, cortical diameters and areas from the 10 state nutrition survey. In: *Proceedings of First Workshop on Bone Morphometry*. 367–391. Z. F. G. Jaworski (ed.). Ottawa: Univ. Ottawa Press, 1973.
25. Garnett, E. S., B. M. Bowen, G. Coates, and C. Nahmias. An analysis of factors which influence the local accumulation of bone seeking radiopharmaceuticals. *Invest. Radiol.* 10:564–568, 1975.
26. Geiser, M., and J. Trueta. Muscle action, bone rarefaction and bone formation. *J. Bone Jt. Surg.* 40B:282–311, 1958.
27. Genant, H. K., C. E. Cann, N. I. Chafetz, and C. A. Helms. Advances in computed tomography of the musculo skeletal system. *Radiol. Clin. N. Amer.* 19:645–674, 1981.
28. Grahame, R., A. S. Saunders, and M. Maisey. The use of scintigraphy in the diagnosis and management of traumatic foot lesions in ballet dancers. *Rheumatol. Rehab.* 18:235–238, 1979.
29. Greyson, N. D., and P. S. Tepperman. Three phase bone studies in hemiplegia with reflex sympathetic dystrophy and the effect of disuse. *J. Nucl. Med.* 25:423–429, 1984.
30. Hangartner, T. N., T. R. Overton, C. H. Harley, L. van den Berg, and P. M. Crockford. Skeletal challenge: An experimental study of pharmacologically induced changes in bone density in the distal radius, using gamma-ray computed tomography. *Calc. Tiss. Int.* 37:19–24, 1985.
31. Holder, L. E., and R. H. Michael. The specific scintigraphic pattern of "shin splints in the lower leg". *J. Nucl. Med.* 25:865–869, 1984.
32. Hulley, S. B., J. M. Vogel, C. L. Donaldson, J. H. Boyers, R. J. Friedman, and S. N. Rosen. The effect of supplemental oral phosphate on the bone mineral changes during prolonged bed rest. *J. Clin. Invest.* 50:2506–2518, 1971.
33. Hurxthal, L. M., G. P. Vose, and W. E. Dotter. Densitometric and visual observations of spinal radiographs. *Geriatrics* 24:93–106, 1969.
34. Jee, W. S. S., T. J. Wronski, E. R. Morey, and D. B. Kimmel. Effects of space flight on trabecular bone in rats. *Am. J. Physiol.* 244:R310–314, 1983.
35. Jones, H. H., J. D. Priest, W. C. Hayes, C. C. Tichenor, and D. A. Nagel. Humeral hypertrophy in response to exercise. *J. Bone Joint Surg.* 59A:204–208, 1977.
36. Kaplan, P. E., B. Gandhavadi, L. Richards, and J. Goldschmidt. Calcium balance in paraplegic patients: Influence of injury duration and ambulation. *Arch. Phys. Med. Rehab.* 59:447–450, 1978.
37. King, J. W., H. J. Brelsford, and H. S. Tullos. Analysis of the pitching arm of the professional baseball pitcher. *Clin. Orth. Rel. Res.* 67:116–123, 1969.
38. Krolner, B., and P. Nielsen. Bone mineral content of the lumbar spine in normal and osteoporotic women: Cross-sectional and longitudinal studies. *Clin. Sci.* 62:329–336, 1982.
39. Krolner, B., and B. Toft. Vertebral bone loss: An unheeded side effect of therapeutic bed rest. *Clin. Sci.* 64:537–540, 1983.
40. Krolner, B., B. Toft, S. P. Nielsen, and E. Tondevold. Physical exercise as prophylaxis against involutional vertebral bone loss: A controlled trial. *Clin. Sci.* 64:541–546, 1983.

41. Lahtinen, T., A. Vaananen, and P. Karjalainen. Effect of intraosseous fat on the measurements of bone mineral of distal radius. *Calc. Tiss. Int.* 32:7–8, 1980.
42. Lancet editorial. Osteoporosis and activity. *Lancet* 1:1365–1366, 1983.
43. Lankenner, P. E., and L. J. Micheli. Stress fracture of the first rib. *J. Bone Joint Surg.* 67:159–160, 1985.
44. Lanyon, L. E. Functional strain as a determinant for bone remodeling. *Calc. Tiss. Int.* 36:S56–S61, 1984.
45. Mazess, R. B., W. W. Peppler, R. W. Chesney, T. A. Lange, U. Lindgren, and E. Smith Jr. Does bone measurement on the radius indicate skeletal status? *J. Nucl. Med.* 25:281–288, 1984.
46. Mazess, R. B. Does bone measurement on the radius indicate skeletal status? *J. Nucl. Med.* 25:1151–1152, 1984.
47. Mazess, R. B., W. W. Peppler, R. W. Chesney, T. A. Lange, U. Lindgren, and E. Smith. Total body and regional bone mineral by dual-photon absorptiometry in metabolic bone disease. *Calc. Tiss. Int.* 36:8–13, 1984.
48. McNeill, K. G. and J. E. Harrison. Partial body neutron activation—truncal. In: *Non-Invasive Measurements of Bone Mass and Their Clinical Application*, S. H. Cohn (ed.). Boca Raton, FL: CRC Press, 165–190, 1981.
49. McNeill, K. G., H. A. Kostales, and J. E. Harrison. Effects of body thickness on in vivo neutron activation analysis. *Int. J. App. Rad. Isotop.* 25:347–353, 1974.
50. Meema, H. E., M. L. Bunker, and S. Meema. Loss of compact bone due to menopause. *Obs. Gyn.* 26:333–343, 1965.
51. Merrick, M. V. Bone scanning. *Br. J. Radiol.* 48:327–351, 1975.
52. Meurman, K. O. A., and S. Elfving. Stress fracture in soldiers: A multifocal bone disorder. *Radiology* 134:483–487, 1980.
53. Minaire, P., P. Meunier, C. Edouard, J. Bernard, P. Courpron, and J. Bourret. Quantitative histological data on disuse osteoporosis. *Calc. Tiss. Res.* 17:57–73, 1974.
54. Montoye, H. J., J. F. McCabe, H. L. Metzner, and S. M. Garn. Physical activity and bone density. *Human Biol.* 48:599–610, 1976.
55. Morgan, B. Ageing and osteoporosis, in particular spinal osteoporosis. *Clin. Endocrinol. Metab.* 2:187–201, 1973.
56. Nilsson, B. E., and N. E. Westlin. Bone density in athletes. *Clin. Orthop. Rel. Res.* 77:179–182, 1971.
57. Oyster, N., M. Morton, and S. Linnell. Physical activity and osteoporosis in post-menopausal women. *Med. Sci. Sport. Exerc.* 16:44–50, 1984.
58. Panin, N., W. J. Groday, and B. J. Paul. Osteoporosis in hemiplegia. *Stroke* 2:41–47, 1971.
59. Peppler, W. W., and R. B. Mazess. Total body bone mineral and lean body mass by dual-photon absorptiometry. *Calc. Tiss. Int.* 33:353–359, 1981.
60. Purdue, G. F., S. A. Lewis, and J. L. Hunt. Pyrophosphate scanning in early frostbite injury. *Am. Surgeon* 49:619–620, 1983.
61. Rettig, A. C., and H. F. Beltz. Stress fracture in the humerus in an adolescent tennis tournament player. *Am. J. Sports Med.* 13:55–58, 1985.
62. Riggs, B. L., H. W. Wahner, E. Seeman, K. P. Offord, W. L. Dunn, R. B. Mazess, K. A. Johnson, and L. J. Melton. Changes in bone mineral density of the proximal femur and spine with aging. *J. Clin. Invest.* 70:716–723, 1982.
63. Roberts, J. G., E. Ditomasso, and C. E. Webber. Photon scattering measurements of calcaneal bone density: Results of in vivo cross-sectional studies. *Invest. Radiol.* 17:20–28, 1982.
64. Ruegsegger, P., M. A. Dambacher, E. Ruegsegger, J. A. Fischer, and M. Anliker. Bone loss in premenopausal and postmenopausal women. *J. Bone Joint Surg.* 66A:1015–1023, 1984.
65. Ruegsegger, P., U. Elsasser, M. Anliker, H. Grehm, H. Kind, and A. Prader. Quantification of bone mineralization using computed tomography. *Radiology* 121:93–97, 1976.
66. Rupani, H. D., L. E. Holder, D. A. Espinola, and S. I. Engin. Three phase radionuclide bone imaging in sports medicine. *Radiology* 156:187–196, 1985.
67. Schneider, H. J., A. Y. King, J. L. Bronson, and E. H. Miller. Stress injuries and developmental change of lower extremities in ballet dancers. *Radiology* 113:627–632, 1974.
68. Smith, E. L., P. E. Smith, C. J. Ensign, and M. M. Shea. Bone involution decrease in exercising middle-aged women. *Calc. Tiss. Int.* 36:S129–S138, 1984.
69. Uhtoff, H. K., and Z. F. G. Jaworski. Bone loss in response to long term immobilization. *J. Bone Joint Surg.* 60B:420–429, 1978.
70. Virtama, P., G. Gastrin, and A. Telkka. Bioconcavity of the vertebrae as an estimate of their bone density. *Clin. Radiol.* 13:128–131, 1962.
71. Vost, A. Osteoporosis: A necropsy study of vertebrae and iliac crests. *Am. J. Pathol.* 43:143–151, 1963.
72. Wahner, H. W., B. L. Riggs, and J. W. Beabout. Diagnosis of osteoporosis: Usefulness of photon absorptiometry at the radius. *J. Nucl. Med.* 18:432–437, 1977.
73. Webber, C. E., and T. J. Kennett. Bone density measured by photon scattering. I. A system for clinical use. *Phys. Med. Biol.* 21:760–769, 1976.

74. Whedon, G. D. Disuse osteoporosis: Physiological aspects. *Calc. Tiss. Int.* 36:S146–S150, 1984.
75. Williams, E. D., K. Boddy, I. Harvey, and J. K. Haywood. Calibration and evaluation of a system for total body in vivo activation analysis using 14 Mev neutrons. *Phys. Med. Biol.* 23:405–415, 1978.
76. Wooten, W. W., P. F. Judy, and M. A. Greenfield. Analysis of the effects of adipose tissue on the absorptiometric measurement of bone mineral mass. *Invest. Radiol.* 8:84–89, 1973.

34

Osteoporosis and the Female Masters Athlete

BARBARA L. DRINKWATER, PH.D.

Pacific Medical Center

ABSTRACT

The role of exercise in preventing osteoporosis is an intriguing area of research. While there are reports that physical activity has been successful in attenuating and even reversing bone loss in postmenopausal women, there are still many questions which must be answered before women can be assured that exercise alone or exercise plus increased calcium intake will maintain their bone density at premenopausal levels. The evidence for a beneficial effect of exercise on bone is both negative and positive. Bed rest, space flight, and immobilization of a limb all result in loss of bone mass which is regained when normal activity is resumed.

Athletes have a higher bone density than non-athletic controls, and bones in the dominant limb, such as the racquet arm in tennis, have a higher density than those in the non-dominant limb. When older sedentary women undertake a physical training program, there is a small but significant gain in bone mass, while bone density continues to decrease in the sedentary controls.

Nevertheless, it is premature to assume that exercise is the complete prophylaxis for osteoporosis. A number of questions remain unanswered regarding the mechanism of its action, its usefulness for women in the high risk group, the appropriate exercise prescription, potential detraining effects if activity is halted, and interaction with age and calcium intake. A regular program of physical activity does have a beneficial effect on health and fitness and should be encouraged. Whether exercise alone can prevent osteoporosis remains to be seen.

Osteoporosis is a major health problem for older women in many parts of the world. In the United States alone 15 to 20 million women experience one or more symptoms of the disease. Approximately 1.3 million fractures per year will occur among this group, at an annual cost of $3.8 billion (17). Fifteen to 30% of the 200,000 to 300,000 women with hip fractures will die from complications—an incidence equivalent to the death of 1 woman every 10 minutes (2, 5). Shocking as these figures are, they cannot adequately convey the pain and deterioration in the quality of life of women who suffer the crippling effects of osteoporotic fractures.

Since osteoporosis is essentially an irreversible disease, the optimal solution to the problem lies in prevention rather than treatment. The importance of instituting preventive techniques early in life is emphasized by cross-sectional studies indicating that bone mass begins to decline in women as early as the third or fourth decade (19). Since women also have a relatively low bone mass (30% less than men) and an accelerated loss following menopause (15), efforts to prevent osteoporosis must concentrate on maximizing bone mass in the early adult years and minimizing the rate of loss in later years.

The role of physical activity in augmenting and maintaining bone mass is an intriguing area of research. No one has yet isolated an aging factor to explain the decline in bone mass observed in young adults, leaving open the possibility that other factors such as a sedentary life style and/or inadequate calcium intake may play a role in the diminution of skeletal mass prior to the menopause. Since several studies (1, 12, 20) have recently reported success in halting and even reversing bone loss in older women through low-intensity exercise programs, many active women in the perimenopausal age group are wondering if their more demanding training programs will protect them from postmenopausal osteoporosis. While exercise may seem an attractive alternative to hormone replacement therapy, there is still no firm evidence that exercise alone will maintain bone density at levels which will prevent the occurrence of osteoporotic fractures.

There are many gaps in our knowledge of how exercise, calcium, estrogen, and aging interact to affect bone metabolism. While there is general agreement that bone mass declines with advancing age, it is not known what proportion of that loss can be attributed to inactivity, negative calcium balance, decreased estrogen production, or physiological changes related to aging. Before relying on exercise as a prophylaxis for osteoporosis, one would want to be assured that the positive effects of activity reported in the literature represent something other than a reversal of bone loss due to inactivity. For example, if inactivity accounts for 10% of a total decrease in vertebral density of 0.35 g/cm^2 between ages 35 and 75, an increase of 0.02 g/cm^2 in density following a physical training program may represent no more than partial recovery of the loss due to sedentary living. While even small increases in density may be important for the individual, the basic question is whether a habitual pattern of physical activity throughout adult life can also prevent that portion of the loss due to other factors.

Effect of Inactivity on Bone

The evidence for the beneficial effect of exercise on bone is both negative and positive. The results of total inactivity such as prolonged bed rest or immobilization of a limb are well known: an increased excretion of calcium in the urine, reflecting a decrease in bone density. In one 4-week study of bed rest, investigators found a 4% decrease in vertebral bone density, a rate of 1% per week (11). Bone was regained when the patients became ambulatory but at a much slower rate of 1% per month. Although it has been suggested that women might lose bone at a faster rate than men during bed rest (8), men actually have significantly higher calcium losses than women during periods of immobilization (7).

Weightlessness during space flight also results in negative calcium balance and decreased bone density, primarily in the trabecular areas (21). Because of the potentially serious consequences of this loss for astronauts, it is important to find effective methods to prevent or minimize bone loss during space flights. Prolonged bed rest is widely used to simulate weightlessness in studies addressing this problem. The selection of exercise as a technique for maintaining bone mass during bedrest has clarified some aspects of the role played by activity in protecting bone and raised more questions in other areas. Neither isotonic nor isometric exercise was successful in preventing increased urinary calcium excretion in bed rest studies (7), but both have had some success in decreasing urinary calcium loss during space flights. Attempts to mimic weightbearing by applying longitudinal pressure through the legs with a force 80% to 100% of the subject's weight for 3 to 4 hours per day was equally unsuccessful in bed rest patients (7). However, simply standing for 3 hours a day decreased urinary calcium to normal levels, an observation which emphasizes the importance of gravitational force in maintaining bone mass in the axial skeleton.

Oscillation of the bed from the horizontal to a 20-degree foot-down position and back for 8 to 21 hours each day also succeeded in slowing urinary calcium loss. Since there was minimal muscular contraction or compressional force, it was suggested that increased renal blood flow was responsible for the positive effect (7). Although the activity level of astronauts and patients with one immobilized limb is usually sufficient to maintain normal renal blood flow, they still experience some decrease in bone density. Whether bone mass can be maintained in the absence of mechanical or gravitational stress on the bone is unlikely, although it is possible that axial or appendicular sites may vary in their response to one or the other stressor. How much of this variability can be attributed to the proportion of trabecular and cortical bone in each of these areas remains to be seen.

Effect of Physical Activity on Bone

Many of the studies reporting hypertrophy of bone related to physical activity have used athletes as subjects. In one respect athletes are excellent subjects for assessing the relationship between bone density and exercise. They willingly impose on themselves training regimens that no Human Subjects Committee would approve for a random selection of subjects. On the other hand, the use of athletes raises the question of genetic selection. Are these men and women successful athletes because they are better physical specimens? Were their skeletal systems, as well as their cardiovascular, respiratory, and neuromuscular systems, superior to that of other individuals before they began training for their sport?

While biological selectivity might be a factor in total skeletal mass, it pushes credibility to the limits to suggest that the marked difference in bone mass between the dominant and non-dominant arms of tennis players is due to a genetic factor that selects for tennis! Hypertrophy of the bones of the playing arm also appears to be independent of age. Jones et al. (10) examined the cortical thickness of the right and left humerus in male and female elite tennis players, mean ages 27 and 24 respectively. Average cortical thickness of the humerus in the racquet arm was 34.9% greater for men and 28.4% greater for women than in the non-dominant arm. Jacobson et al. (9) found a smaller difference between dominant and non-dominant arms of young female tennis players at the mid (plus 15%) and distal (plus 9%) radius. Among older women, ages 45 to 64, tennis players had significantly greater bone mineral content in the radius than non-players. Even soccer players, who certainly use both legs equally during running, have a higher density in the femur of the leg used for ball control (16).

There are only a few studies comparing bone density between female athletes and non-athletes, presumably because very few women participated in sports prior to the early 1970s. However, all of the results published to date uniformly report a higher bone mineral content in active women. Brewer et al. (3) measured bone mineralization of the middle phalanx, os calcis, and the radius of 42 women who had been running for 2 to 13 years, averaging 40 miles per week, and 38 age-matched sedentary women. The runners had a higher bone mineral content and bone density at the midshaft of the radius and the finger, while the sedentary women had higher values at the os calcis. The latter finding emphasizes the importance of matching or normalizing for body weight, since the sedentary women weighed 7.5 kilograms more than the runners. Regression of bone mass against age produced interesting figures which could be misleading. An apparent increase in bone mass with age for runners is significant only for the distal radius, and while it appears as though sedentary women are losing bone with age at all 4 sites, none of the correlation coefficients are significant.

A different approach was taken by Oyster et al. (18) who recruited women aged 60 to 69, measured cortical diameter of the second metacarpal of the non-dominant hand, and correlated the results with responses to an activity questionnaire. The authors reported that activity levels and use of estrogen were the 2 variables which correlated most highly with cortical diameter. They then compared cortical diameters of the ten most active and ten least active women and found significantly larger diameters for the more active group. Among the caveats in their discussion was a reminder that the data analysis had shown a significant residual effect of estrogen supplementation early in the postmenopausal period even though none of the women had taken estrogen within 5 years of the study.

An interesting aspect of the Jacobson et al. (9) study was a comparison between swimmers and tennis players as well as between athletes and controls. While both groups of athletes had higher bone mineral content in the radius and the first metatarsal than non-athletes, only the tennis players had a higher density in the lumbar vertebrae. A similar finding was reported by Nilsson and Westlin (16) for male athletes. The density at the distal end of the femur was significantly greater for weight lifters, throwers, runners, and soccer players than for a control group, but swimmers had no evidence of increased mineralization. Apparently increased bone density in the spine and femur is a response to weight-bearing activity rather than to general systemic effects of exercise. Older female tennis players, ages 55 to 64, in the study of Jacobson et al. (9) had a 15.6% greater bone mineral content in the lumbar vertebrae and a 25.3% greater central lumbar density than their age-matched controls. Since many of these women had started playing when well into middle age, the results suggest that the positive effects of exercise on bone are not restricted to the young. A recent abstract by Lane et al. (13) is equally encouraging for masters athletes. CAT scans of the first lumbar vertabra showed that women in the Over-50 Runners Club had 40% greater bone density than expected for their age group. However, neither study reports incidence of hormone replacement therapy among either athletes or controls.

Longitudinal prospective designs eliminate some of the confounding factors associated with cross-sectional studies. Three groups of investigators (1, 12, 20), using different measurement techniques and different age groups, have reported similar improvements in the bone status of older women subsequent to a planned program of physical activity. The youngest group of women, average age 53 years, trained 1 hour 3 times a week for 1 year (1). While bone mineral content of the radius remained constant, total body calcium as measured by neutron activation analysis increased 2.6% by the end of the year. During the same period, a sedentary control group had a 2.4% decrease in total body calcium.

Dual photon absorptiometry was used to measure changes in bone mineral content of the lumbar spine in women, mean age 61 years, who participated in a walk-run-calisthenics program for one hour twice weekly over an 8-month period (12). These active women had a 3.5% increase in vertebral density by the end of the training program while sedentary controls decreased by 2.7%.

An even older group of women, averaging 81 years, was followed for 3 years by Smith et al. (20). The women exercised 30 minutes a day three times a week in a series of light exercises designed around a chair. Bone mineral content of the radius, measured by single photon absorptiometry, increased 2.29% in this group while sedentary controls decreased by 3.29%.

For the women in these three studies the beneficial effect of the exercise programs was the sum of what they gained *plus* what they would have lost had they remained inactive. The mean increase for the three groups who exercised was 2.76%; mean decrease for the sedentary controls averaged 2.80%. The overall advantage gained from activity, therefore, was 5.56%. There is no doubt that exercise can have a beneficial effect on bone; but the question still remains: can exercise offset the effect of the decrease in endogenous estrogen levels following menopause?

Recent reports (4, 6, 14) that young amenorrheic athletes with estradiol levels similar to those of postmenopausal women have significantly lower vertebral density than cyclic athletes raise questions about the effectiveness of exercise in the absence of adequate estrogen stimulation. These amenorrheic athletes are training at far greater intensities, for longer periods, and with greater frequency than the postmenopausal women. Why doesn't exercise protect them from bone loss? According to Marcus et al. (14), exercise does provide some protection since the bone density of the amenorrheic athletes is not as low as that of non-athletic hypoestrogenic women in the same age range. Both Marcus et al. (14) and Drinkwater et al. (unpublished observations) found that the cyclic athletes have vertebral densities well above those of less active young women while the amenorrheic athletes not only do not benefit from exercise-induced hypertrophy of bone, but actually lose some bone mass. In view of these data, can masters athletes approaching menopause be confident that exercise alone will preserve their bone mass?

Directions for Future Research

There are a number of other questions which need to be addressed before women can be encouraged to depend solely on physical activity as a means of maintaining bone mass. For one thing, the mechanisms underlying the response of bone to exercise must be delineated. Is the basic mechanism central, perhaps through increased circulation, local via the mechanical stress placed directly on the bone, or some combination of the two? How does exercise affect bone remodeling? Does it stimulate bone formation, reduce resorption, or both? Or might it increase resorption but increase formation even more?

Women with a familial history of osteoporosis are more at risk for the disease than other women. Is exercise equally effective with these high-risk women? There are other risk factors as well, some involving lifestyle, others related to medical or biological factors. How do these factors interact with physical activity?

Is there a threshold level at which exercise is effective in preserving bone mass? If so, does the threshold vary with age, calcium intake, and estrogen status? What is the relative importance of frequency, duration, and intensity of exercise? What are the most effective exercises? Does the activity that protects trabecular bone also preserve cortical bone?

Is the effect of exercise independent of age? How much improvement can older women expect from an exercise program? How long will it take for exercise to be effective? Does the initial status of the bone affect its response to exercise?

What happens to the bone when a training program stops? Does the skeletal system, like all other physiological systems, detrain? Must exercise be a lifelong commitment to ensure that the benefit received from activity will remain?

Eventually these questions will be answered, and women will be able to make informed decisions regarding how they wish to protect themselves against involutional bone loss. There is no doubt that a regular program of physical activity has a positive effect on health and fitness. Even small gains in bone density may be sufficient to protect some women from osteoporotic fractures. However, it is premature to assume that exercise alone can protect women from accelerated bone loss following menopause. Until the relationshp of exercise to bone homeostasis is thoroughly understood, women would be wise to assess all their options for protecting themselves from the morbidity and mortality that follow osteoporotic fractures.

REFERENCES

1. Aloia, J. F., S. H. Cohn, J. A. Ostuni, R. Cane, and K. Ellis. Prevention of involutional bone loss by exercise. *Ann. Int. Med.* 89:356–358, 1978.
2. Avioli, L. V. Postmenopausal osteoporosis: Prevention versus cure. *Fed. Proc.* 40:2418–2422, 1981.
3. Brewer, V., B. M. Meyer, M. S. Keele, S. J. Upton, and R. D. Hagan. Role of exercise in prevention of involutional bone loss. *Med. Sci. Sports Exerc.* 15:445–449, 1983.
4. Cann, C. E., M. C. Martin, H. K. Genant, and R. B. Jaffe. Decreased spinal mineral content in amenorrheic women. *JAMA* 251:626–629, 1984.
5. Christiansen, C. Postmenopausal osteoporosis—a social problem? In: *Annual Report: Novo Indrusi*, 19–27. Copenhagen, 1984.
6. Drinkwater, B. L., K. Nilson, C. H. Chesnut, III, W. Bremmer, S. Shainholtz, and M. Southworth. Bone mineral content of amenorrheic and eumenorrheic athletes. *N. Engl. J. Med.* 311:277–281, 1984.
7. Greenleaf, J. E., and S. Kozlowski. Physiological consequences of reduced physical activity during bed rest. *Exerc. Sport Sci. Rev.* 10:84–119, 1982.
8. Hansson, T. H., B. O. Roos, and A. Nachemson. Development of osteopenia in the fourth lumbar vertebra during prolonged bed rest after operation for scoliosis. *Acta. Orthop. Scand.* 46:621–630, 1975.
9. Jacobson, P., W. Beaver, D. Janeway, S. Grubb, T. Taft, and R. Talmage. Single and dual photon densitometry: Comparison of intercollegiate swimmers, tennis players, athletic adult women, and age-matched controls. In: *Proceedings, the 30th Annual Meeting of the Orthopedic Research Society*, p. 202, 1984.
10. Jones, H. H., J. D. Priest, W. C. Hayes, C. C. Tichenor, and D. A. Nagel. Humeral hypertrophy in response to exercise. *J. Bone Joint Surg.* 59A:204–208, 1977.
11. Krolner, B., and B. Toft. Vertebral bone loss: An unheeded side effect of therapeutic bed rest. *Clin. Sci.* 64:537–540, 1983.
12. Krolner, B., B. Toft, S. P. Nielsen, and E. Tondevold. Physical exercise as prophylaxis against involutional bone loss: A controlled trial. *Clin. Sci.* 64:541–546, 1983.
13. Lane, N., D. Bloch, H. Jones, P. Wood, and J. F. Fries. Running and osteoarthritis: A controlled study. (Abs) *Arthritis Rheum.* 28:S21, 1985.

14. Marcus, R., C. Cann, P. Madvig, J. Minkoff, M. Goddard, M. Bayer, M. Martin, L. Gaudiani, W. Haskell, and H. Genant. Menstrual function and bone mass in elite women distance runners. *Ann. Int. Med.* 102:158–163, 1985.
15. Mazess, R. B. On aging bone loss. *Clin. Orthop.* 165:239–252, 1982.
16. Nilsson, B. E., and N. E. Westlin. Bone density in athletes. *Clin. Orthop.* 77:179–182, 1971.
17. Osteoporosis. Conference Statement, *National Institutes of Health Consensus Development Panel*, Vol. 5, No. 3, 1985.
18. Oyster, N., M. Morton, and S. Linnell. Physical activity and osteoporosis in post-menopausal women. *Med. Sci. Sports Exerc.* 16:44–50, 1984.
19. Riggs, B. L., H. W. Wahner, W. L. Dunn, R. B. Mazess, K. P. Offord, and L. J. Melton III. Differential changes in bone mineral density of the appendicular and axial skeleton with aging. *J. Clin. Invest.* 67:328–335, 1981.
20. Smith, E. L., W. Reddan, and P. E. Smith. Physical activity and calcium modalities for bone mineral increase in aged women. *Med. Sci. Sports Exerc.* 13:60–64, 1981.
21. Wronski, T. J., and E. R. Morey. Alterations in calcium homeostasis and bone during actual and simulated space flight. *Med. Sci. Sports Exerc.* 15:410–414, 1983.

North American Life Research Award Paper

35

Physical Training In Young and Older Healthy Subjects
North American Life Research Award Paper

LYDIA MAKRIDES

Dalhousie University

George J. F. Heigenhauser
Neil McCartney
Norman L. Jones

McMaster University Health Sciences Centre

INTRODUCTION

The capacity of many physiological processes declines with age. The well established decline in maximum exercise capacity and maximum oxygen intake ($\dot{V}O_2$ max), amounting to 0.5–1.0% per year (3, 8), is accompanied by reductions in the maximum exercise heart rate and cardiac output as well as declines in breathing capacity and pulmonary gas exchange function (7). To these reductions in mechanisms influencing the delivery of oxygenated blood to the exercising muscles may be added structural and functional changes in the muscles themselves (6) and a decline in the number of functioning motor units (2). The decline in maximum muscle power with age is of a similar order of magnitude to that of $\dot{V}O_2$ max, about 0.6% per year (13).

Some of the functions which decline with age are amenable to improvement by endurance exercise training, but the extent to which each may contribute to an increase in exercise capacity is poorly understood. Furthermore, the extent to which some functions may be improved by exercise may decline with age (15).

The purpose of the present study was to examine the effects of aging on training-induced changes in the capacity to generate power in short-term exercise, and in the cardiorespiratory responses to progressive incremental exercise. The effects of a 12-week endurance exercise program were compared in a group of young subjects and a group of older subjects of comparable body

---

Supported by the Medical Research Council of Canada, Ontario Heart Foundation and Nova Scotia Heart Foundation.

size and activity level. Specific objectives included comparisons of changes in cardiac output and stroke volume, peripheral circulatory resistance, ventilation, and indices of muscle metabolism and power.

SUBJECTS AND METHODS

Twenty-four previously sedentary healthy males, 12 aged 20 to 30 years and 12 aged 60 to 70 years, entered the study (Table 35-1); 2 of the young subjects withdrew before the study ended due to their transfer to another city for business reasons. The subjects were recruited by advertising in the local community and were approximately matched for height, weight, and physical activity; occupations were similar, with most subjects being in sales, managerial, or professional occupations; 5 of the older subjects were retired and 2 of the younger subjects were students. Past or present competitive athletes were excluded, as were subjects with known history of cardiac or respiratory disease. The subjects were required to have normal spirometry, resting electrocardiogram, blood pressure below 150/90, and to be taking no medication known to influence exercise capacity. The older subjects were required to have medical examinations by their own physicians.

TABLE 35-1. *Characteristics of younger and older subjects*

		Age (yrs)	Height (cm)	Weight (kg)	Lean Thigh Volume (l)	Resting Blood Pressure Systolic (mmHg)	Resting Blood Pressure Diastolic (mmHg)
20–30 yrs	x	27.4	176.3	71.0	3.68	118.0	78.0
	SD	3.0	5.9	8.7	0.35	14.4	4.5
60–70 yrs	x	65.0	170.6	73.3	3.44	136.0	85.8
	SD	3.4	4.8	8.5	0.33	15.5	8.7

The study objectives, procedures, and possible risks were described in detail and signed informed consent was obtained. The study was approved by the university Ethics Committee. No remuneration was offered.

The subjects performed two types of exercise tests on different days, at least 2 hours after a meal. The first exercise test consisted of a multi-stage progressive incremental exercise test to maximum capacity, and the second employed an isokinetic cycle ergometer on which the subject performed 30 seconds of maximal cycling at two pedal velocities. The multi-stage progressive exercise test was performed on a calibrated cycle ergometer (Elema EM 370). The initial power setting for the younger subjects was 200 kpm/min (32.6 W) and successive increases of 200 kpm/min were made; each power setting was maintained for 4 minutes. For the older subjects the initial power setting was 150 kpm/min, with increases of 150 kpm/min after 4 minutes. The subjects exercised to a symptom-limited maximum power output; criteria were established for stopping the test (9), but no test was stopped for these reasons. Thus, the maximum power recorded was the highest power that the subject could maintain for 4 minutes, but the maximal O_2 intake, calculated as below, sometimes occurred at a higher power output, but not completed.

The electrocardiogram was monitored using lead V5, which was also used to measure heart rate; in older subjects, 12-lead electrocardiograms were also obtained at intervals during the test. Blood pressure was measured during the last minute of each power output by auscultation. Ventilation, oxygen intake ($\dot{V}O_2$), carbon dioxide output ($\dot{V}CO_2$), tidal volume, and the frequency of breathing were measured using a calibrated automated exercise metabolic system (Sensor Medics Horizon MMC). Averages were computed every 15 seconds and the mean of the highest three measurements of $\dot{V}O_2$ was taken as the maximum aerobic capacity ($\dot{V}O_2$ max).

Cardiac output ($\dot{Q}$) was measured during the last 30 seconds of each power output using the CO_2 rebreathing equilibration method (5, 10, 11). Suitable mixtures of CO_2 in O_2 were rebreathed from a small anesthesia bag to obtain equilibration of PCO_2 in the lung bag system. The mixed venous PCO_2 was derived from the equilibration PCO_2 by subtracting an alveolar-blood difference as described elsewhere (9). Arterial PCO_2 was estimated from end-tidal PCO_2 (9), and cardiac output was calculated using $\dot{V}CO_2$ and the venoarterial CO_2 content difference derived from mixed venous and arterial PCO_2.

Lean thigh volume (muscle + bone) was estimated from anthropometric and skin fold measurements (12).

The 30-second maximal cycling test was carried out on an isokinetic ergometer at pedalling frequencies of 60 and 110 revolutions per minute (rpm). The ergometer and procedure have been described in detail by McCartney et al. (14). The test allows continuous measurement of the maximum torque applied to the cranks of the ergometer; maximum power, the decline in power occurring over 30 seconds (the fatigue index), and the total work accomplished in 30 seconds are calculated. Venous blood was sampled 5 minutes after completing the exercise for measurement of plasma lactate concentration.

Following the baseline data collection, the subjects attended exercise sessions of approximately one hour's duration 3 days per week for 12 weeks. An interval training regime was used, consisting of exercise bouts of 5-minute duration on a cycle ergometer adjusted to elicit a heart rate corresponding to that obtained at 85% of $\dot{V}O_2$ max in the incremental test. The exercise bouts were initially separated by 5 minutes, pedaling at a power output corresponding to 50 to 60% of $\dot{V}O_2$ max, initially for 5 minutes, decreasing to 3 minutes as training progressed.

This procedure was repeated initially 5 times, later progressing to 7 times. Heart rate was recorded at the end of each exercise period, allowing for a gradual increase in exercise intensity over the 12-week period. Training heart rates were 165 and 140 beats/minute in the young and old groups respectively; the training power output increased from 800 and 600 kpm/min at the beginning of the 12 weeks, to 1,200 and 900 kpm/min respectively.

At the end of the 12-week training program, the testing procedures were repeated.

Results

Before training, younger subjects attained a higher maximal power output during the incremental progressive exercise test (mean 1080 kpm/min) than the older subjects (725 kpm/min; $P < 0.05$) (Table 35-2). This difference was associated with a higher $\dot{V}O_2$ max (Table 35-2, Fig. 35-1), and higher cardiac output and stroke volume measured in submaximal exercise. Ventilation, blood pressure, and total peripheral circulatory resistance were lower at a given power

TABLE 35-2. *Mean values for variables at maximum exercise before and after 12 weeks of training*

Group		Power (kpm/min)	$\dot{V}O_2$ (1/min)	$\dot{V}_E$ (1/min)	Heart Rate (beats/min)	Cardiac* output (1/min)	Systolic BP (mmHg)
20–30 y	Before	1080	2.54	86	192	19.8	190
	After	1560	3.26	116	201	23.1	170
	P	<0.05	<0.05	<0.05	ns	<0.05	ns
60–70 y	Before	725	1.60	65	161	14.5	205
	After	1125	2.21	87	173	19.6	212
	P	<0.05	<0.05	<0.05	<0.05	<0.05	ns

*Maximum cardiac output was estimated as the product of submaximal stroke volume and maximum heart rate.

output in the younger subjects, but heart rate at a given submaximal power output was similar in the two groups (Fig. 35-2).

The maximum peak power during 30 seconds of maximal cycling at 60 rpm was also higher in the younger subjects (1025 W) compared to the older subjects (743 W), and the total work in 30 seconds was also higher (16.6 kJ and 11.4 kJ respectively; $P < 0.05$) (Table 35-3). Plasma lactate concentrations at the end of this maximal test were also higher in younger subjects and the

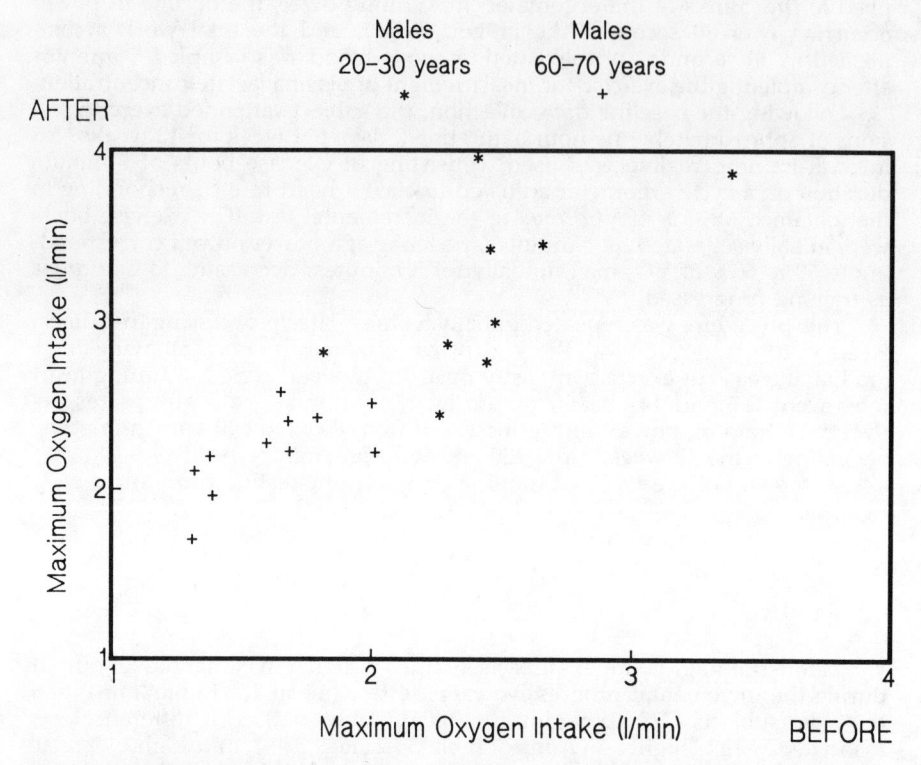

Fig. 35-1. *Individual changes in maximum oxygen intake before and after training in young (∗) and older (+) subjects.*

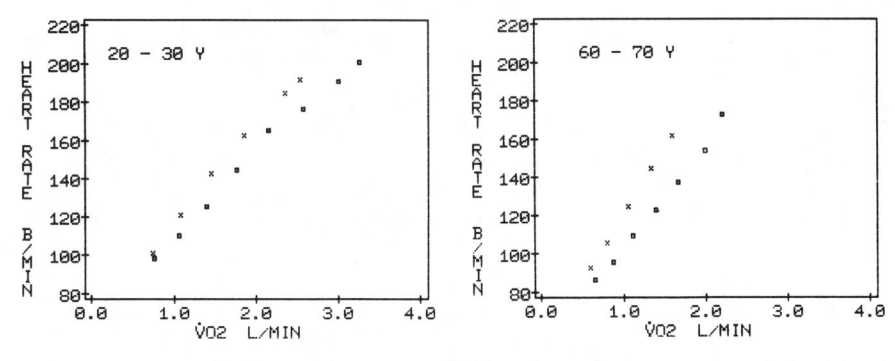

Fig. 35-2. Relationships between heart rate and VO_2 at increasing power outputs before (x) and after (□) training in the two groups. In both groups heart rate was reduced after training (P < 0.05).

fatigue index was less in this group (P < 0.05). Measurements obtained at a pedaling velocity of 110 rpm showed differences between the two groups similar to those found at 60 rpm.

After training, both groups increased the maximum power output sustained for 4 minutes during the incremental exercise test, the younger subjects increasing maximum power by 44% (Table 35-2) and the older subjects by 55%. These increases were accompanied by increases in VO_2 max (Table 35-2, Fig. 35-1) of 29% in the younger group and 38% in the older group. During submaximal exercise the older group showed an increase in cardiac output for a given VO_2 (Fig. 35-3), whereas younger subjects did not show a change in submaximal cardiac output. Both groups showed a lower heart rate (Fig. 35-2) and thus a higher stroke volume. Systolic blood pressure was reduced at a given VO_2, indicating a reduction in the peripheral circulatory resistance (Fig. 35-4) that was more marked in the older than the younger group. Ventilation at submaximal exercise was lower in both groups (Fig. 35-5). This was associated with a reduction in CO_2 output and in the respiratory exchange ratio (R) (Fig. 35-6).

In contrast to the changes in aerobic exercise capacity and submaximal exercise measurements, the changes found during the 30-second maximum exercise test were much less (Table 35-3). There were no significant differences in either age group in maximal power, but small reductions in the fatigue

TABLE 35-3. Means (±SD) of measurements during the 30-second maximal cycling test for young and older subjects before and after training

		Max Peak Power (W)		Total Work (kJ)		Fatigue Index (%)		Plasma Lactate mmol/l	
Pedal velocity		60	110	60	110	60	110	60	110
20–30 y	Before	1025	1393	16.6	15.7	29.2	62.8	12.8	14.1
	After	1004	1367	16.6	14.1	27.4	58.1	11.9	12.1
	P	ns	ns	ns	ns	ns	ns	ns	ns
60–70 y	Before	743	967	11.4	11.2	34.3	59.0	9.0	10.5
	After	746	967	11.7	12.6	30.7	54.2	7.5	7.8
	P	ns	ns	ns	<0.05	ns	ns	ns	<0.05

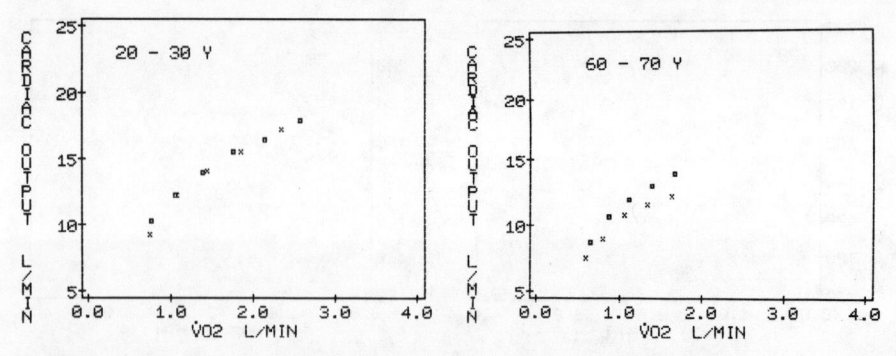

Fig. 35-3. *Cardiac output before and after training; symbols as in Fig. 35-2. Cardiac output increased in the older group post-training (P < 0.05).*

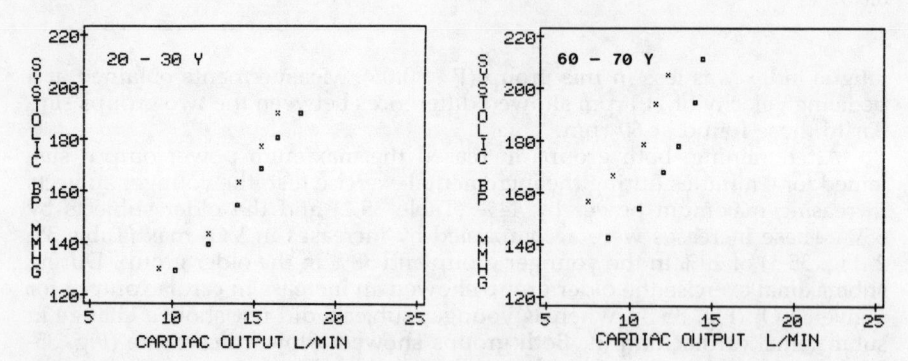

Fig. 35-4. *Systolic blood pressure measured at the same exercise level as cardiac output. The pressure was lower post-training in the older group (P < 0.05). Symbols as in Fig. 35-2.*

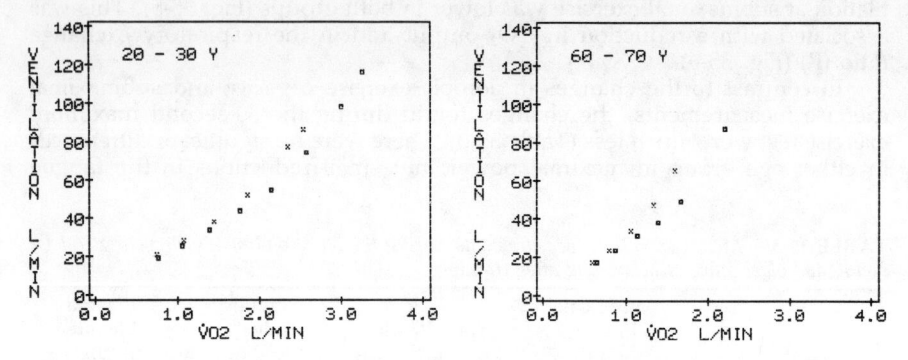

Fig. 35-5. *Ventilation was lower post-training in both groups (P < 0.05). Symbols as in Fig. 35-2.*

index occurred in both groups. This decrease was larger in the older subjects and was greatest at a pedalling velocity of 110 rpm. Although the total work accomplished during 30 seconds was unchanged at 60 rpm, an increase occurred in the older subjects when pedaling at 110 rpm (P < 0.05). In both groups the plasma lactate increase following exercise was lowered, particu-

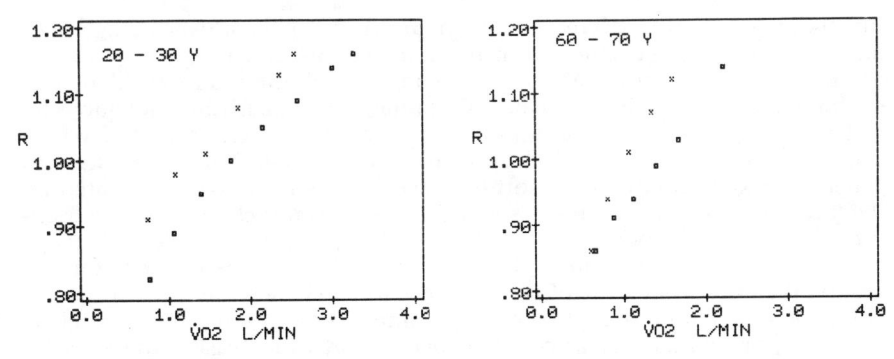

Fig. 35-6. *Respiratory exchange ratio at increasing exercise was lower post-training in both groups (P < 0.05). Symbols as in Fig. 35-2.*

larly when considered in relation to the total work accomplished during the 30 seconds, which was similar to or higher than pretraining (Table 35-3).

Discussion

The results of the present study afforded some insights into several aspects of exercise physiology—the linkage between mechanisms influencing maximum exercise performance, the aging process, and the ability of an exercise training program to improve function.

The capacity to perform maximum exercise declines with age (3, 8), and a number of factors are thought to contribute to this decline; reductions in lean body mass and in the level of physical activity are thought to be major contributing factors (16). We controlled for these factors by selecting subjects who were well matched in terms of body size and levels of everyday physical activity. The younger subjects were a little taller and lean thigh volume was 7% greater than in the older subjects (Table 35-3); in keeping with their sedentary life style, the mean $\dot{V}O_2$ max for the young subjects was 83% of predicted, and for the older subjects 87% of predicted $\dot{V}O_2$ max (8). The differences between the two groups before training were consistent with the established associations with increasing age: lower $\dot{V}O_2$ max (the older subjects' $\dot{V}O_2$ max being 63% of the younger subjects), lower maximum heart rate, and higher systolic blood pressure (Table 35-2). In addition, similar differences were found in the performance indices in the 30-second maximum exercise test; maximum power was reduced by 30% in the older compared with the younger subjects, with a similar reduction in the total work accomplished in 30 seconds (Table 35-3). Thus the age-related reduction in $\dot{V}O_2$ max was accompanied by a quantitatively similar reduction in muscle power, consistent with reductions in fast-twitch muscle fibers (6) and active motor units in aging subjects (2).

Although structural changes with increasing age occur in muscles, heart, and lungs that undoubtedly contribute to reductions in $\dot{V}O_2$ max with age, the wide variation within a given population means that an active 60-year-old may have a $\dot{V}O_2$ max to comparable an inactive 20-year-old (8). Thus there is a large potential for the maintenance of $\dot{V}O_2$ with advancing age through an increase in physical activity. Our findings confirm this with the large increase in $\dot{V}O_2$ max in both groups following training; post-training $\dot{V}O_2$ max in the older (2.2 1/min) approached the pretraining $\dot{V}O_2$ max of the younger group (2.5 1/min). Although these conclusions are at variance with the view that training responses decrease with advancing age (15), advancing age does impose a limit to the extent to which improvements may occur.

Present studies provide new information on the mechanisms that may contribute to increases in VO_2 max with training, particularly in older subjects. In both groups, large increases in aerobic exercise capacity occurred which contrasted with the relative lack of change in the ability of the muscles to generate maximum power in short-term work. This contrast is illustrated by the fact that older subjects increased VO_2 max to values close to the pretraining VO_2 max of the younger subjects (Table 35-2, Fig. 35-1), while their maximum power capacity remained at 75% of the values obtained in the younger group (Table 35-3). In view of the lack of improvement in maximum muscle power, it seems improbable that changes in muscle fiber size, fiber type characteristics, or neuromuscular coupling play a part in increasing the capacity to perform endurance exercise. However, the reduction in fatigue index and increase in the total work in 30-second pedaling at 110 rpm, together with a reduction in post-exercise plasma lactate concentration, all point to an increase in the capacity or flux rate of aerobic metabolic processes in muscle. These changes were more marked in the older group of subjects; changes in the younger group did not reach statistical significance (Table 35-3, Fig. 35-7). Another measure which indicated changes in muscle metabolism was the respiratory exchange ratio (R), which consistently fell at any given VO_2 (Fig. 35-6). Although in heavy exercise a fall in R is an indication of reduced lactate production, the reduction at all levels of exercise suggests a shift towards fat oxidation as a major fuel source. Studies of enzyme activity in muscle samples obtained by needle biopsy following training have shown increases in the activity of enzymes associated with the citric acid cycle and fat oxidation in young and old subjects (15, 16).

Increases in aerobic metabolism and in the supply of blood-borne free fatty acids are dependent on an improved blood flow to muscle. Although changes in the distribution of capillaries in muscle have been difficult to establish on histological grounds in humans (15), the reduction in systolic blood pressure at a given cardiac output (Fig. 35-4) suggests that training effects are associated with a reduction in resistance to blood flow in muscle. In older subjects this effect may be magnified by an increase in cardiac output at a given VO_2 (Fig. 35-3). Thus in older subjects, training was associated with increases in stroke volume, cardiac output, and reductions in peripheral vascular resistance which brought the state of the circulation close to that of the younger group. Maximum cardiac output remained lower in older subjects than younger subjects. Maximum cardiac output was estimated by multiplying the submaximal stroke volume by the maximum heart rate; these calculations demonstrated that maximum cardiac output increased from 20 to 23 l/min in the young subjects and from 15 to 20 l/min in the older group (Table 35-2). Although data for subjects of comparable age to our subjects are not available, these changes are similar to the 8% increase in maximum cardiac output found in 8 young subjects by Ekblom et al. (4) and the 13% increase in middle aged males studied by Hartley et al. (7).

Increases in cardiac output in the present study occurred in conjunction with reductions in heart rate at a given VO_2 (Fig. 35-2), indicating increases in cardiac stroke volume. The changes in the older group (from 90 to 113 ml, a 28% increase in stroke volume) were larger than in the younger subjects (from 103 to 115 ml, an 11% increase). These changes were accompanied by significant increases in maximum heart rate of 7% and 4% in the older and younger groups respectively (Table 35-2).

From the pulmonary point of view, it appears unlikely that important

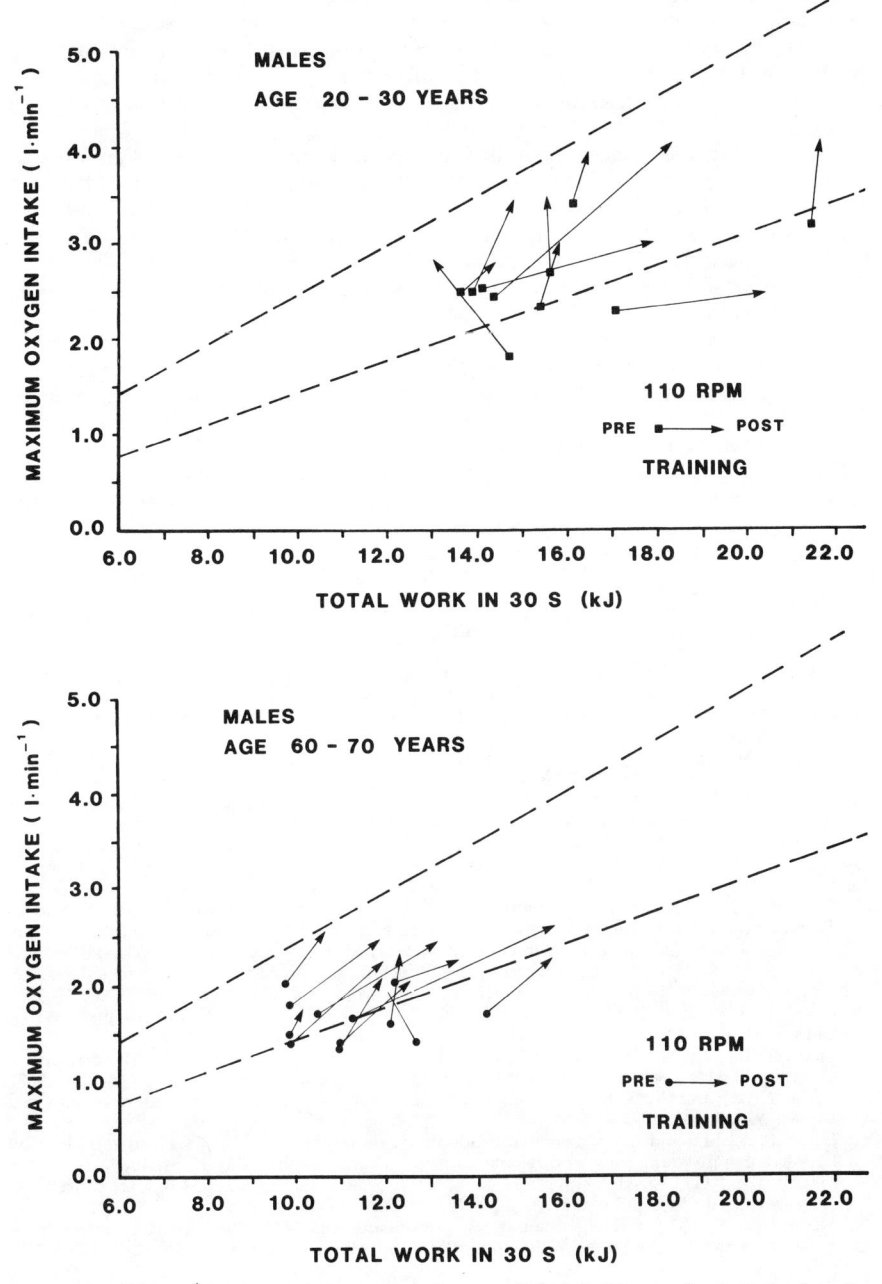

Fig. 35-7. Plot of $\dot{V}O_2$ max and the total work accomplished in 30 seconds of maximal cycling at 110 rpm, before and after training. Dashed lines are 95% confidence limits for normal subjects (Makrides et al., 1985).

changes were associated with training. Reductions in ventilation at a given $\dot{V}O_2$ (Fig. 35-5) were largely accounted for by reductions in $\dot{V}CO_2$ (reductions in R) and ventilation for a given CO_2 output were similar, suggesting unchanged pulmonary gas exchange function. Similarly, tidal volume at a given ventilation was unchanged following training, suggesting that changes in the mechanical characteristics of the lungs or respiratory muscle function did not occur.

This study confirmed the important contribution of changes in muscle metabolism and circulation in the training-related improvements in endurance exercise, particularly in elderly subjects. This influence is supported in elderly subjects by the fact that changes in $\dot{V}O_2$ max were related to changes in the total work accomplished in the 30-second maximum exercise test (Fig. 35-7). As it is impossible to separate the relative effects of peripheral muscle changes from central changes in stroke volume and heart rate, we are unable to identify whether exercise training had an independent effect on cardiac function. As the substantial improvement in $\dot{V}O_2$ max found in the younger subjects was not accompanied by convincing evidence of intrinsic muscle performance, it is probably reasonable to conclude that both central and peripheral mechanisms are involved in improvements in $\dot{V}O_2$ max. What seems clear, however, is that the effects of a training program may be at least as impressive in older subjects as in the young and that a substantial contribution in the older subjects is gained through improvements in peripheral mechanisms which are known to decline with age.

REFERENCES

1. Allen, T. H., E. C. Anderson, and W. H. Langham. Total body potassium and gross body composition in relationship to age. *J. Gerontol.* 15:348–357, 1960.
2. Campbell, M. J., A. J. McComas, and F. Petito. Physiological changes in ageing muscles. *J. Neurol. Neurosurg. Psychiat.* 36:174–182, 1983.
3. Dehn, M. M., and R. A. Bruce. Longitudinal variations in maximal oxygen intake with age and activity. *J. Appl. Physiol.* 33:805–807, 1972.
4. Ekblom, B., P. O. Åstrand, B. Saltin, J. Stenberg, and B. Wallstrom. Effect of training on circulatory response to exercise. *J. Appl. Physiol.* 24:518–528, 1968.
5. Ferguson, R. J., J. A. Faulkner, S. Julius, and J. Conway. Comparison of cardiac output determined by CO_2 rebreathing and dye dilution method. *J. Appl. Physiol.* 25:450–454, 1968.
6. Grimby, G., and B. Saltin. The ageing muscle. *Clin. Physiol.* 3:209–218, 1983.
7. Hartley, L. H., G. Grimby, A. Ekblom, N. L. Nilsson, I. Åstrand, J. Bjure, B. Ekblom, and B. Saltin. Physical training in sedentary middle-aged and older men. III. Cardiac output and gas exchange at submaximal and maximal exercise. *Scand. J. Clin. Lab. Invest.* 24:335–344, 1969.
8. Jones, N. L., L. Makrides, C. Hitchcock, T. Chypchar, and N. McCartney. Normal standards for an incremental progressive cycle ergometer test. *Am. Rev. Resp. Dis.* 131:700–708, 1985.
9. Jones, N. L., and E. J. M. Campbell. *Clinical Exercise Testing.* (2nd ed.) Philadelphia: W. B. Saunders Co., 1982.
10. Jones, N. L., E. J. M. Campbell, G. J. R. McHardy, B. E. Higgs, and M. Clode. The estimation of carbon dioxide pressure of mixed venous blood during exercise. *Clin. Sci.* 32:311–327, 1967.
11. Jones, N. L., and A. S. Rebuck. Rebreathing equilibration of CO_2 during exercise. *J. Appl. Physiol.* 35:538–541, 1973.
12. Jones, P. R. M., and J. Pearson. Anthropometric determination of leg fat and muscle plus bone volume in young male and female adults. *J. Physiol.* (Lond.) 204:63–64, 1969.
13. Makrides, L., G. J. F. Heigenhauser, N. McCartney, and N. L. Jones. Maximal short term exercise capacity in healthy subjects aged 15–70. *Clin. Sci.* (in press).
14. McCartney, N., G. J. F. Heigenhauser, A. J. Sargeant, and N. L. Jones. A constant velocity cycle ergometer for the study of dynamic muscle function. *J. Appl. Physiol.*:REEP 55:212–217, 1983.
15. Scheuer, J., and C. M. Tipton. Cardiovascular adaptations to physical training. *Ann. Rev. Physiol.* 39:221–251, 1977.
16. Suominen, H., E. Heikkinen, H. Liesen, D. Michel, and W. Hollmann. Effects of 8 weeks' endurance training on skeletal muscle metabolism in 56–70 year-old sedentary men. *Europ. J. Appl. Physiol.* 37:173–180, 1977.

FORTHCOMING INTERNATIONAL CONFERENCES

Name	Where	When	Contact
5th International Hypoxis Symposium	Chateau Lake Louise Alberta, Canada	Feb. 10–14, 1987	John Sutton Dept. of Medicine McMaster University Hamilton, Ontario L8N 3Z5
1st World Conference Heat Stroke	Sydney, Australia	Apr. 27, 1987	Roland Richards Menzies Foundation 310/84 Pacific Hwy. N. Sydney, 2060 Australia
International Conf. on Exercise Fitness and Health	Toronto, Canada	May 29–June 3, 1988	Dr. Barry McPherson Dept. Kinesiology Univ. of Waterloo Waterloo, Ontario
International Biochemistry Exercise	London, Ontario, Canada	June 1–4, 1988	Dr. A. W. Taylor Dept. of Phys. Ed., Univ. of Western Ont., London, Ontario

FUTURE FITNESS ...

The desire of people everywhere
to be physically fit,
reflects their commitment
to get more out of life.
As well, there is a growing
awareness that financial fitness
is equally important
to enhancing one's lifestyle—
today and tomorrow.
North American Life
is currently developing
the 'future fitness' concept,
to address both the physical
and financial needs of our
increasingly active population.

North American Life
salutes all participants in
the World's Inaugural MASTERS GAMES,
and is proud to sponsor
the GAMES' International
Sports Medicine Symposium
August 8–10, at the Harbour Castle
Convention Centre.

Index

ATP hydrolysis: in muscle fiber, 18, 24, 36
ATPase staining test, 18, 74
ATP/CP energy system: evaluation of, 99
Abrasion arthroplasty of knee, 261-262; arthroscopic, 279, 281, 282
Absorptiometry. *See* Photon absorptiometry
Acclimation. *See* Heat acclimation
Acid-base disturbance: heat injury and, 128
Acromion, 300
Acta Medica Scandinavica: symposium on exercise, 4
Acute hypoxia, 215
Acute mountain sickness, 214-216, 218, 226
Adipose tissue metabolism: aging and, 82
Aerobic Power. *See* Maximal oxygen uptake
Agility, 10
Aging: altitude illness and, 218, 219, 223; blood oxygen and, 69; body composition and, 104-106; bone mass reduction and, 340, 346, 347; breathing capacity and, 319-328, 363; cardiac output and, 69, 363; coordination and, 10; in endurance athletes, 59-78; energy metabolic potential and, 21; exercise studies of, 310; exhaustion time and, 76-77; flexibility of joints and, 101; heart rate reduced with, 313, 363; heat acclimation and, 139-140; hemodynamic response and, 65-70; knee injuries and, 279-285; lung structure and function, effect on, 319, 325-326; marathon record times and, 311; maximal heart rate and, 9; maximal oxygen pulse and, 313; maximal oxygen uptake reduced with, 9, 309, 310, 311, 312, 313, 363; maximal voluntary static contraction and, 23; motor units and, 363, 369; mountain travel and, 213-214; muscle capillarization and, 21; muscle fiber and, 19-21, 32, 369; muscle tissue quality and, 71-73; one-half relaxation time and, 24; orienteering performance and, 75; osteopenia and, 340, 346; pulmonary gas function and, 363; skeletal muscles and, 17; skin blood flow and, 133; sweating response and, 133, 135-137, 140; thermal regulation and, 139; trainability and, 81-83, 363-372
Alactacid anaerobic capacity and power, 98
Altitude: acclimatization to, 216, 222-223; arterial oxygen pressure, effect on, 220; concomitant illnesses, effect on, 215, 220-222; exercise performance and, 225-230; maximal oxygen uptake and, 227; oxygen delivery and, 226-229
Altitude illness: prevention of, 216, 222-223; types and descriptions of, 214-224
Alveoli: effect of aging on, 319, 325-326
Ambient temperature: core body temperature and, 134-135; warning system for, at running events, 202, 211. *See also* Corrected effective temperature; Effective temperature; Environmental heat load
Ambulances: in running events, 155, 184, 193, 199, 207
Amenorrheic athletes: bone mineral loss and, 347, 357
American College of Sports Medicine: heat injury prevention guidelines, 208-209
American Medical Research Expedition to Everest, 1981, 225, 226
Amputation, 337-338, 344
Anaerobic power, 98-99
Anaerobic threshold, 99. *See also* Fatigue
Anemia, 11
Anesthesia: in shoulder arthroscopy, 300
Arterial oxygen pressure: aging and, 325-326; altitude and, 220
Arteriography, 120
Artery wall elasticity, 69-70
Arthritis. *See* Degenerative arthritis, Osteoarthritis
Arthrofibrosis: in autograft knee surgery, 271
Arthroplasty. *See* Abrasion arthroplasty
Arthroscopy: in degenerative arthritis treatment, 261, 262, 280; in diagnosis and research, 258; in knee treatment, 259, 266, 268, 279-282, 284; in meniscectomy, 259; post-operative benefits of, 53; in shoulder examination, 299-306
Arthrotomography, 299
Arthrotomy, 52-53
Atherosclerosis, 12
Athletic Congress: running event certification by, 194
Auckland, New Zealand running event, 173-174
Auscultation, 365
Australian running events, 151-180
Autogenous reconstruction. *See* Autograft
Autograft: knee ligament reconstruction, 271

Ballet dancing: bone mass and, 346
Barometric pressure: oxygen consumption and, 226
Baseball: eye injury in, 248, 252; masters athletes in, 295; pitching, anatomy of, 295-297; pitching, bone mass and, 346
Bayes theorem: in coronary artery disease risk assessment, 119-120
Bed patients: bone density and, 347, 353, 354-355
Bicarbonate: in metabolic acidosis treatment, 202
Bicep tendon, 302, 304
Biceps, 302
Bicycling: knee rehabilitation and, 260, 262, 266
Bilateral symmetry: in quadriceps measurements, 47, 48
Biochemistry: of muscle fiber, 18-19, 21-22, 28
Blood analysis: in heat treatment diagnosis, 202; in physiological testing, 365
Blood: oxygenation of, 69, 325-326
Blood pressure: in coronary artery disease risk assessment, 120; exercise and, 66-67; in orienteers, 66; pulmonary and right ventricle, aging and, 323-324; in physiological testing, 365, 366, 368, 369, 370
Body composition: aging and, 104, 106; measurement, 102-105; sports and, 104, 105
Body fat, 102-106
Body fuel: response to exercise, 36
Body temperature: heat injury and, 127, 129, 130-131. *See also* Core body temperature

375

Body weight: heat injury and, 202; lean, 102-106; maximal oxygen uptake and, 8
Bone: density variation, 103; fractures from osteoporosis, 353; injury detection, 331-340; mass, loss of, 340-348, 353, 354-358; mass, measurement of, 340-348; mineral content, 103, 340, 347, 348, 355, 356-357; pain, 334; scanning, 331-337, 340, 341; tissue pain, 340
Bony sclerosis: following meniscectomy, 258
Braces: in knee rehabilitation, 266
Breathing: aging and, 319-328; capacity, 323, 363; control, 326; frequency, 365
Breathlessness: during exercise, 319, 321, 327
Bronchitis, 319
Buffalo-Niagara Falls marathon, 194-198
Bundle of His, 64
Bupivacaine (Marcaine), 302

CAT scan. *See* Computer-assisted tomography
CPR. *See* Cardio-pulmonary resuscitation
Calcaneal bone density, 347
Calcium: bone mass and, 347, 353, 354, 355
Calcium ion dynamics: in nerve stimulation, 28, 29
Calibrated automated exercise metabolic system, 365
Canadian Association of Sport Sciences: testing guidelines, 109-112
Canoeing: in knee rehabilitation, 262
Capillaries: aging and, 21; endurance training and, 71-72
Carbohydrate: requirements for endurance training, 11
Carbon dioxide: output, 365, 367; pressures, 365
Cardiac diseases: at high altitudes, 215
Cardiac function: in endurance athletes, 309-318
Cardiac output. *See* Maximal cardiac output
Cardiac stroke volume. *See* Maximal cardiac stroke volume
Cardio-pulmonary resuscitation: availability at running events, 199; in heat injury treatment, 155
Cardiorespiratory endurance capacity. *See* Maximal oxygen uptake
Cardiovascular disease. *See* Coronary artery disease
Casualty cards: in running events, 186, 189-190
Cataract: due to eye injury, 249
Central nervous system: disturbance of, in heat injury, 161; endorphins and, 12
Cerebral edema, masters athletes and, 130. *See also* High altitude cerebral edema
Chest: cage, 319; pain, 120; wall, 319-321
Cholesterol levels: in coronary artery disease risk assessment, 120; exercise and, 114
Chondromalacia, 261, 262, 279, 282
Chronic mountain sickness, 215
Chronic nerve stimulation, 27-29, 32
Citric acid cycle: in muscle metabolism, 21
Clavicle, 300
Cognitive psychology: in performance improvement, 241-245
Cold packs: in heat injury treatment, 131, 155, 162-163
Communication systems: for running event medical support, 155, 171, 198, 199, 207, 210
Compton scattering technique, 345
Computer-assisted tomography: in body composition assessment, 103; in bone injury detection, 331; in bone mass measurement, 344-345; in knee fracture diagnosis, 266, 268; in muscle measurement, 45, 48, 49

Conjunctival injury, 248
Concentric contraction, 100
Coordination: aging and, 10
Coracoid process, 300, 301, 304
Core body temperature: cooling strategies for, 130-131, 209; environmental heat load and, 147; exercise intensity and, 134; measurement of, 127
Corneal injuries, 249
Coronary artery disease: asymptomatic, 118-119; athletes, risk to, 113; diagnosis, 310; examination for, 120; exercise for, 115; risk assessment, 119-121
Corrected effective temperature: definition, 152; heat injury and, 156-157. *See also* Ambient temperature; Effective temperature; Environmental heat load
Cortical bone: mass of, 346, 347, 355, 356; in nuclear bone mass studies, 340-341
Cross-country skiers, 115
Cutaneous vasodilation: in thermal regulation, 134, 137-138
Cybex II isokinetic test device, 101
Cycle ergometer. *See* Ergometer

Death: during exercise, 316-317
Debridement, 261, 267; arthroscopic, 279, 282
Defibrillator: at running events, 208
Degenerative arthritis: in knee, 261-262, 269. *See also* Osteoarthritis
Dehydration: in heat injury, 127-129; running events and, 209
Densitomery: in body composition assessment, 103-104
Dextrose: heat injury treatment and, 155, 202
Diabetes, 12
Disease prevention, 4
Disseminated intravascular coagulation, 128
Dual photon absorptiometry, 343-344, 347

EKG. *See* Electrocardiogram
EMG. *See* Electromyography
Eccentric contraction: in strength test, 99-100
Eccentric resistance: in exercise machines, 291
Echocardiography: endurance athletes and, 315
Effective temperature, 152. *See also* Ambient temperature; Corrected effective temperature; Environmental heat load
Effusions: following meniscectomy, 53-54
Electrical conductivity and impedance: in body composition assessment, 103
Electrical stimulation: in resistance exercise, 292
Electrocardiogram, 120; endurance athletes and, 315, 316; at running events, 200; in training benefits study, 365
Electrogoniometer, 101-102
Electrolytes, 129-130
Electromyography, 50-51
Electron microscopy, 38, 40, 41
Elite athletes: characteristics of, in specific sports, 95-97, 104-105; physiological tests of, 91-105; testing guidelines and protocol for, 109-112
Emergency vehicles: at running events, 199
Emphysema, 319
Endorphins, 12
Endurance athletes: cardiac functions in, 309-318; ventricle enlargement in, 309, 315-316
Endurance training. *See* Training

Environmental heat load, 145-149; measurement of, 147. *See also* Ambient temperature; Corrected effective temperature; Effective temperature

Enzymes: chronic nerve stimulation and, 28-29; endurance training and, 39, 71-73; heat injury and, 128; muscle injury and, 37; muscle metabolism and, 18-19, 21-22

Ergometer: in maximal oxygen uptake test, 92, 94, 97; in training benefit study, 364; in Wingate Anaerobic Power Test, 99

Esophageal temperature: dehydration and, 129

Essential fat: in body component assessment, 102

Estrogen: bone mass and, 346, 347, 348; osteoporosis and, 354, 358

Exercise: body fuel, response to, 36; bone mass and, 346-348, 353, 354-358; bone pain due to, 334; cardiac output and, 65, 66, 69; cholesterol levels and, 114; core body temperature and, 134; coronary artery disease risk and, 113-115, 120; deaths associated with, 116-117, 316-317; heat exchange during, 135; hemodynamic response to, 65-70; importance of, 4; lack of, 104, 106; maximal oxygen uptake and, 313-315; resistance techniques, 287-294; risk/benefit ratio in, 113, 116-118, 309, 316-317; stroke volume and, 65-66; thermal regulation during, 133-143; ventilatory response to, 326-327. *See also* Trainability; Training

Exercise-induced heat exhaustion: "classical heat stroke," distinguished from, 152, 161; symptoms and treatment, 161, 162, 208. *See also* Exercise-induced heat stroke; Heat injury

Exercise-induced heat stroke: "classical heat stroke," distinguished from, 126-128, 152, 161; symptoms and treatment, 126-128, 209. *See also* Exercise-induced heat exhaustion; Heat injury

Exhaustion time, 76-77

Eye injury, 247-254; examination for, 247-248; protection from, 250-254

Face fanning: in heat injury treatment, 130-131, 164, 193, 201, 202

Face protectors, 250-252

Fast glycolitic (FG) muscle fibers, 18, 19

Fast oxidative-glycolitic (FOG) muscle fibers, 18, 19

Fast-twitch (FT) muscle fibers, 18-21, 23; aging and, 369; chronic nerve stimulation and, 28-32; resistance exercise and, 288

Fat: in long-distance runners, 73; metabolism of, 86-87; weight, in body component assessment, 102

Fatigue index, 365-367, 370

Fatty acids: in muscle metabolism, 19; oxidation of, 36

Female athletes: bone mass reduction and, 353-354, 356-357

Femoral condyles: flattening of, 258

Fick equation, 310; in high-altitude oxygen consumption, 225

Field hospitals. *See* Running events, on-site medical facilities for

First aid stations. *See* Running events, on-site medical facilities for

Fixx, James, 113-114, 117

Flexibility, 101-102

Flexor/extensor balance, 293

Football: eye injury in, 252

Forearm blood flow: aging and, 138

Fraisage: in degenerative arthritis treatment, 262

Frostbite, 337, 338, 344

Fun runs. *See* Running events

Gamma camera, 331

Genotype, 84

Glenohumeral joint, 296-297, 300, 302, 303, 304, 305

Glucose: coronary artery disease and, 120; exercise and, 36; in muscle metabolism, 19; tolerance of, 12

Glycogen: anaerobic breakdown of, 9; muscle fatigue and, 37; in muscle metabolism, 19; training and, 36

Glycolitic energy system, 99

Goal setting, 235-236

Golf: eye injury in, 252; knee rehabilitation and, 262

Hamstrings, 260, 266

Healing potential: heredity and, 295

Heart function. *See* Cardiac function

Heart rate: aging and, 313. *See also* Maximal heart rate

Heart size: in endurance athletes, 71

Heat acclimation, 145-149; aging and, 139-140. *See also* Heat tolerance

Heat cramps, 208

Heat exhaustion. *See* Exercise-induced heat exhaustion; Exercise-induced heat stroke; Heat injury

Heat injury, 125-131; aggressive behavior and, 200; body weight loss in, 202; cooling methods for, 131, 164, 193, 201, 202; core body temperature and, 127; dehydration and, 209; delay in treatment, 157-158; diagnostic difficulties, 125-128; hyperuricemia, 128; hypoglycemia and, 155, 162; hypothermia, 125, 209; hypovolemia, 202, 209; inexperienced runners and, 153, 163; instructions to runners concerning, 154; intravenous fluid for, 193, 202; mental state and, 200, 209; northern climate and, 145-149; oxygen for, 155; prevention of, 151-166, 200-202, 208-210; rectal temperature in, 127-128, 160, 161, 163, 202, 209; rehydration for, 155, 162, 193, 202, 208; renal failure in, 128; rhabdomyalysis in, 128; severe complications, 157-158; sex and, 158-159; treatment of, 127-128, 155, 157, 158-161, 162-164, 202, 208-209; weather and, 153, 156, 157, 158, 162. *See also* Exercise-induced heat exhaustion; Exercise-induced heat stroke

Heat loss mechanisms: in thermal regulation, 134

Heat stroke. *See* Exercise-induced heat exhaustion; Exercise-induced heat stroke; Heat injury

Heat tolerance: aging and, 133-143; deaths, 134, 140; training and, 134, 138-140. *See also* Heat acclimation

Heat waves: deaths from, 34, 140

Height/weight table, 102

Helium dilution, 103

Hematological disease: altitude and, 215

Hemodynamic response: aging and, 65-70

Hemoglobin deficiency: endurance athletes and, 11

Heredity: healing potential and, 295; maximal oxygen uptake and, 94; trainability and, 81-88, 295

High altitude illness, 213-223. *See also* Altitude

High-risk runners, 200

Hip fractures: osteoporosis and, 353

Histochemical staining pattern, 18, 74

Horizontal cleavage tear, 279, 282-284

Hospitals: running events and, 186, 194. *See also* Running events, on-site medical facilities for

Humerus, 301, 302, 303

Hyperthermia. See Exertion-induced heat exhaustion; Exertion-induced heat stroke; Heat injury
Hyperuricemia, 128
Hyphema, 250
Hypoglycemia, 155, 162
Hyponatremia, 129-130
Hypothalamus: thermal regulation and, 134
Hypothermia, 125, 209
Hypovolemia, 202, 209
Hypoxia. See Acute hypoxia
Hypoxic ventilatory response, 226-227

Ice hockey: eye injury and, 250-252
Immobilization: effects of, 45-54, 288, 293, 353-354
Inactivity: body composition and, 104, 106
Insulin-carbohydrate metabolism, 12
Intensive care facilities. See Running events, on-site medical facilities for
Intravenous fluids: in heat injury treatment, 193, 202
Isokinetic dynamometer, 288

Jogging: cholesterol levels and, 114; deaths and, 113-114, 116, 117
Joint flexibility, 101. See also Knee; Knee injury
Jumping sports: knee rehabilitation and, 260

Ketone oxidation, 36
Knee: angular deformity of, 266, 269; anterior cruciate ligament of, 258, 259-260, 265, 267, 271; braces or casts for, 262, 266, 269; cartilage and aging, 265, 268; chondromalacia and, 261; immobilization of, 46-54, 288, 293; instability and, 265-269; ligaments, 265-289; misalignment of, 261; osteoarthritis and, 279, 281-283; plateau fracture of, 265, 268; prostheses for ligaments, 262, 271-277; rehabilitation of, 46, 54, 262, 266, 267, 268-269, 280, 287-293. See also Meniscus; Patella
Knee injury, 257-263, 279-284; effect on muscles, 50-54; ligamental, 265-269; treatment decisions, 260, 263, 279, 280-282
Knee surgery, 259-262; arthroscopic, 279-285; future of, 262; recovery from, 259, 260-261, 262, 287-293

Lachman's sign, 267
Lactacid anaerobic capacity: and power, 99
Lactate concentration: aging and, 24, 327; anaerobic threshold and, 99; endurance training and, 14; motivation and, 9; in training benefits study, 366, 367, 368, 370; ventilating response and, 327
Lean thigh volume, 365, 369
Lean tissue density, 103
Left ventricular ejection fraction, 310, 314
Leg blood flow, 68-70
Leighton flexometer, 101-102
Ligaments. See Knee; Knee injury
Limping, 336-337, 342
Lipoproteins: training and, 12
Local government: running events and, 198, 202
London marathon, 181-192
Lungs, 319-327; capacity, 321; elastic recoil in, 319, 321; flow volume in, 321, 323; pressure-volume change in, 321, 322; structure, 319

Makkah Body Cooling Unit, 131, 164
Malnutrition, 11

Manual labor: coronary artery disease and, 114
Marathons: age/performance chart, 6; Buffalo-Niagara Falls, 194-197; deaths and, 116-117; London, 181-192; Melbourne, 174-175; New York City, 194; record times, 311; traditional, 182; U.S. Olympic Marathon Trial, 1984, 195; Vancouver International, 205, 207. See also Running events
Margaria-Kalamen Power Test, 99
Masters athletes: abnormalities in, 315-316; in baseball, 295; cardiac function in, 309-318; cardiovascular precautions for, 113-122; cartilage condition of, 268; cerebral edema and, 130; coronary artery disease and, 119-121; definition, 310; hyponatremia and, 130; knee problems of, 259, 260, 265-269, 279, 281-283; post-injury stiffness in, 265, 268; thermal regulation problems of, 125-131. See also Runners; Endurance athletes
Maximal aerobic power. See Maximal oxygen uptake
Maximal arterial-venous oxygen difference, 309, 310, 313, 314, 315
Maximal cardiac output: aging and, 24, 63, 65, 66, 69, 363; exercise and, 65, 66; Fick equation, 310; maximal oxygen uptake and, 93; in training benefits study, 364, 365, 366, 368, 370
Maximal cardiac stroke volume, 309, 310, 313, 314
Maximal heart rate: aging and, 24, 64, 363; endurance athletes and, 63; oxygen uptake and, 309, 310, 313, 314; in training benefits study, 365, 366, 367, 369
Maximal muscle power: aging and, 363; in training benefits study, 364, 365, 366, 367, 369, 370. See also Muscle power; Muscle strength; Muscular endurance
Maximal oxygen pulse: aging and, 313; in endurance athletes, 62
Maximal oxygen uptake: aging and, 24, 81-83, 94, 309, 310, 311, 312, 363; altitude and, 227; anaerobic threshold and, 99; cardiovascular functions and, 309, 310, 313, 314, 315; core body temperature and, 134; definition, 5; exercise and, 313-314; heredity and, 84-87, 94; measurement of, 92-98; in older athletes, 6, 59-65; specific sports and, 95-97; test protocol for, 97-98; in training benefits study, 364, 365, 366, 367, 369-370, 372
Maximal voluntary activation, 50-54
Maximal voluntary static contraction, 23
Maximal voluntary ventilation. See Breathing capacity
Melbourne marathon, 174-175
Meniscectomy, 279-281, 282; muscle activity and, 252-254; older athletes and, 258, 259
Meniscus, 258, 260, 262, 265-269, 279-283; flap tear in, 282-284
Menopause: bone mass reduction following, 346, 347, 348, 353-354, 356-357
Mental preparation: for running, 241-243
Mental strategies: during competition, 244
Metabolic acidosis, 202
Metabolism. See Muscle metabolism
Microfibrosis: in endurance runners, 41-42
Monge's disease. See Chronic mountain sickness
Motivation: analysis of, 234; high-altitude performance and, 229-230; lactate concentration and, 9; performance quality and, 233; psychological techniques for, 233-239; in resistance exercise, 288
Motoneurons, 287

Motor units: aging and, 363; muscular rehabilitation and, 287-289
Mountain climbing: acclimatization period for, 216, 222-223; contraindicators for, 221-222; maximal oxygen uptake and, 227; motivation and, 229-230; by older persons, 213-214; physiology of, 225-230
Mountain sickness. *See* Acute mountain sickness; Chronic mountain sickness; Subacute mountain sickness
Multi-stage progressive incremental exercise test, 364
Muscle: activity, measurement of, 50, 51; adaptation to long-term use, 27-32; aging and, 10, 17, 19, 24, 71-73, 82; capillarization of, 21, 71-72; chronic nerve stimulation and, 27, 29, 32; computer-assisted tomography and, 48; contraction of, 24, 288-289; fatigue, 36-37; heat production by, 135; immobilization of, 45-48, 54; inhibition of, 50-52; injury and repair, 35-43; metabolism, 18, 21, 28, 29, 30; movement patterns, 288; power, 99-100; quality of tissue, 71-73; rehabilitation, 288-289; resistance exercise and, 287-294; respiratory, 320, 321-322; shoulder, 296; strength, 17, 23, 47-49, 99-110, 287, 290; throwing and, 296; ultrasound measurement of, 48, 49; velocity specificity of, 288
Muscle fibers: adaptation of, 287-289; aging and, 19-23; chronic nerve stimulation and, 28-32; classification of, 18-24
Muscle mass: aging and, 10, 17, 24, 48, 49; joint injury and, 46; lean body weight and, 102
Muscle metabolism, 18, 19, 21-22; aging and, 21, 82; anaerobic power and, 98-99; genetic factors in, 85-87; muscle damage and, 38; training and, 9, 36, 364, 370
Muscular endurance, 99-101
Myocardial infarction, 208
Myofibrillar ATPase staining pattern, 74-75
Myofibrillar injury and repair, 38

National Running Data Center, 194
Needle biopsy, 17
Neuropraxia, 305
Neutron activation analysis, 345, 347
New York City Marathon, 194
Nuclear magnetic resonance, 103, 299
Nuclear medicine: bone studies and, 346-348
Nutrition, 11

Obesity, 102-103; in coronary artery disease risk assessment, 120
One-half relaxation time, 24
On-site medical facilities: for running events. *See* Running events
Orbital eye injuries, 248, 249
Orienteers, 59-77
Os calcis, 356
Osteoarthritis in knee, 279, 281-283
Osteopenia, 340, 346
Osteophyte formation, 258
Osteoporosis, 353-359; estrogen and, 348
Osteotomy: in knee treatment, 262, 266, 269
Overhydration, 129, 130
Overweight, 102-103
Oxidative phosphorylation, 18, 36-37
Oxygen cascade, 225
Oxygen extraction, aging and, 69

Oxygen pulse. *See* Maximal oxygen pulse
Oxygen uptake. *See* Maximal oxygen uptake

Patella: arthroscopic treatment of, 279, 282; injury to, 261
Performance psychology, 241-245
Peripheral circulatory resistance, 364, 370
Peroneal nerve injury, 268
Perth, Australia running events, 175
Phenotype, 84
Photon absorptiometry, 341-344
Physical training. *See* Training
Plasma lactate accumulation. *See* Anaerobic threshold
Post-injury stiffness, 265, 268
Post-operative inhibition: of muscle, 53
Progressive exercise tests, 120
Pulmonary artery pressure: aging and, 323-324
Pulmonary disease: high altitude and, 215
Pulmonary edema. *See* High altitude pulmonary edema
Pulmonary gas exchange: aging and, 325, 363
Puna. *See* Acute mountain sickness
Pyrexia: heat injury and, 128

Quadriceps: knee stability and, 266, 269; measurement of, 47-54

Race pace, 99
Racquet sports: eye injuries in, 250
Radiation heat loss, 137
Radio communication: for running events, 155, 171, 198, 199, 207, 210
Radiographic photodensitometry, 341, 346
Radiography: in body composition assessment, 103; in bone mass measurement, 341, 346
Radioisotope bone scan. *See* Bone scan; Computer-assisted tomography
Reciprocal exercise, 292
Recollagenization, 273, 276
Rectal temperature: heat injury and, 127-128, 160-161, 163, 202
Red cell destruction, 11
Reflex inhibition, 46, 50-54, 288
Rehydration: in heat injury treatment, 155, 162, 193, 202, 208
Relaxation techniques, 241-242
Renal failure: in heat injury, 128
Resistance exercise, 287-294; equipment for, 290; principles of, 288-289
Respiratory function: in masters athletes, 319-328
Respiratory muscles, aging and, 322
Retina: injury to, 250. *See also* High-altitude retinal hemorrhage
Retinaculum, 265
Rhabdomyalysis, 128
Rib: cartilage, 320; fracture, 333
Rights: of athletes, 113
Risk/benefit ratio, 117-118; in endurance training, 309, 316-317
Road races. *See* Running events
Rotation cuff, 295, 302, 304
Runners: bone mass in legs of, 346; cardiovascular function in, 61, 70-77; cholesterol levels in, 114; coronary artery disease and, 114, 116; death and, 116-117; disqualification of, 200; enzyme activity and, 71-73; exhaustion times of, 76-77; maximal

INDEX 379

oxygen pulse of, 62; maximal oxygen uptake of, 6, 60; microfibrosis in, 41-42; motivation of, 199; muscle capillarization in, 71-73; muscle repair in, 38-42; respiratory exchange ratio in, 73. *See also* Master athletes; Orienteers

Running: bone mineral content and, 356; knee rehabilitation and, 260; mental preparation for, 241-243

Running events, 151-165, 167-179, 181-192, 193-203, 205-212; Auckland, New Zealand marathon, 173-174; Australasian events, 151-165, 167-179; Buffalo-Niagara Falls marathon, 194-198; casualty protocols for, 200, 201; certification of, 193-194, 199; climate and, 145-149; common injuries, 170-172; communications, 155, 171, 198, 199, 207, 210; disqualification, 200; entry forms for, 154; finish line facilities, 155, 172, 186, 207; heat injury precautions, 151-155, 194, 199, 200-202; high-risk runners, 200; inexperienced runners, 163, 168, 182-183, 199; instructions to runners and staff, 154, 170, 174, 177, 185, 186-187, 198-199; intervention by officials, 200; local government and, 198, 202; local hospitals and, 194; London marathon, 181-192; medical staffing for, 155, 170-173, 186, 199-200, 207, 208; medical support for, 151-165, 167, 169-173, 176-179, 184-192, 193-203, 205-212; Melbourne marathon, 174-175; New York City marathon, 194; North American events, 145-148, 193-203, 205-212; on-site medical facilities for, 155, 171-172, 174, 175, 176, 184-185, 186, 193, 199-200, 205-207, 208; organizations certifying, 194; Perth, Australia events, 175; sanctioning of, 193, 194, 199; selection of runners, 200, 201; spotters for casualties during, 172, 173, 199, 200; starting order, 154; Sydney, Australia events, 151-165, 168-173, 175-176; Toronto, Ontario event, 145-146; U.S. Olympic Marathon Trial, 1984, 195; Vancouver International marathon, 205-207; waiver of liability for, 154, 183; warning flags for heat, 211; Waterloo, Ontario event, 145, 147, 148; weather conditions and, 194-195

Sedatives: heat injury and, 156
Senile emphysema, 319
Sex: body composition and, 104, 106; heat injury and, 158-159
Shin splints, 335, 336, 340
Shoulder, 295-297, 302-305
Sickle cell trait: high altitude and, 215
Single photon absorptiometry, 341-343
Skating: knee rehabilitation and, 260, 266
Skeletal mass, 102
Skiing: eye injury in, 252; knee rehabilitation and, 266
Skin blood flow: aging and, 138; heat loss and, 134-135, 137-138, 140; training and, 139
Skinfold measurements, 104
Slow-twitch (ST) muscle fibers, 18-21, 23; chronic nerve stimulation and, 28; endurance athletes and, 74-75; resistance exercise and, 288
Smoking, 120
Soccer: bone mass and, 355-356; knee injury and, 259
Space flight: calcium and muscle loss during, 347, 353, 354, 355
Spinal cord: thermoconductors in, 134
Staining pattern: for myofibrillar ATPase, 74
Strength curve, 290

Stress fracture: bone scan detection of, 334, 335, 337, 340
Stroke volume, 65-66; maximal oxygen uptake and, 93; in training benefits study, 364, 370
Subacute mountain sickness, 215
Subcutaneous edema, 215
Subscapularis tendon and recess, 303, 304, 305
Supraglenoid tubercle, 303
Sweating: aging and, 133, 135-137, 140; evaporation and, 137; heat injury patterns of, 127-128; mechanics of, 135
Swimming: bone mineral content and, 356; in knee rehabilitation, 260, 262, 266
Sydney, Australia running events, 151-165, 168-173, 175-176
Symptom-limited maximal incremental progressive exercise test, 120

Technetium-99m, 331, 333
Temperature regulation. *See* Thermal regulation
Tennis: bone mass and, 346, 353, 355
Tests (physiological), 91-107; for coronary artery disease risk, 120; guidelines for, 109-112; rights of athletes concerning, 112; specific sports, data for, 95-97, 104-105
Thallium exercise test, 120
Thermal regulation, 135-141; in northern climates, 145-149
Thermal stress: warning systems for, 211
Thermal tolerance. *See* Heat tolerance
Thermodetectors, 134
Thoracic cage. *See* Chest cage
Throwing: analysis of, 296-297
Tidal volume, 327, 365, 372
Tomography. *See* Bone scan; Computer-assisted tomography
Tourniquet ischemia, 53
Trabecular bone, 340-341; mass of, 343, 347, 353, 354-355; osteopenic fractures in, 340
Track and field associations: running events and, 194
Traction: in shoulder arthroscopy, 300
Trainability: aging and, 81-83, 363-372; heredity and, 81, 85-88
Training: aging and, 59-79, 363-372; anemia and, 11; atherosclerosis and, 12; benefits study, 363-372; cardiovascular functions and, 9, 63, 64, 68-70, 71; endorphins and, 12; glucose tolerance and, 12; heat tolerance and, 134, 138-140; lactate concentration and, 9, 366, 367, 368, 370; lipoprotein ratios and, 12; maximal oxygen pulse and, 62, 64; maximal oxygen uptake and, 60-65, 364, 365, 366, 367, 369-370, 372; motivational aids for, 233-234, 237-238; muscle fiber adaptation and, 74; muscle mass maintenance and, 10; muscle metabolism and, 9, 36, 364, 370; nutritional requirements for, 11; resistance techniques and, 289; risk/benefit ratio, 113, 116-118, 309, 316-317; thermal regulation and, 134, 138-139; ventilation and, 9. *See also* Exercise; Trainability
Training power output, 365
Traumatic glaucoma, 249
Treadmill ergometer, 92
Trick knee, 258
Triphasic body fuel: response to exercise, 36
Twins: in trainability/heredity studies, 84-87
Two-way resistance exercise machines, 291-292
Tympanic temperature, 129-131

380 SPORTS MEDICINE FOR THE MATURE ATHLETE

Type I muscle fibers. *See* Slow-twitch (ST) muscle fibers
Type II muscle fibers. *See* Fast-twitch (FT) muscle fibers

Ultra-marathon muscle injury study, 38-42
Ultrasound-B scanning, 45, 48, 49
Underwater weighing, 103-104
Unilateral exercise: with resistance equipment, 292
U.S. Olympic Marathon Trial, 1984, 195

Vancouver International Marathon, 205, 207
Vanishing resistance exercise machine, 290
Velocity-controlled resistance exercise machine, 289, 290-291
Ventilation: training and, 9
Ventilatory equivalent: for oxygen and carbon dioxide, 99
Ventilatory response to exercise: aging and, 326-327, 364, 365, 368, 372
Ventricle enlargement: in endurance athletes, 309, 315-316
Voluntary muscle strength, 287

Waiver of liability: in running events, 154, 183
Walking: benefits of, 12
War games: eye injury and, 252
Warning flag system: for thermal stress, 211
Water intoxication, 130
Weather conditions: running events and, 153, 156, 157, 158, 162, 194-195, 209, 211
Weight lifting: resistance exercise in, 288
Wet bulb globe temperature, 162, 299
Wingate Anaerobic Power Test, 99
Women: bone mass and, 346, 348, 353-354, 355, 366-367
Work. *See* Manual labor

X-ray. *See* Computer-assisted tomography; Radiography